Churchill Livingstone

Pocket Radiography and Medical Imaging Dictionary

For Elsevier:

Commissioning Editor: Dinah Thom
Development Editor: Catherine Jackson
Project Manager: Kerrie - Anne Jarvis
Designer: Stewart Larking
Illustrators: Marion Tasker, Cactus
Illustration Manager: Merlyn Harvey

Churchill Livingstone

Pocket Radiography and Medical Imaging Dictionary

Chris Gunn MA TDCR

CGTraining, Retford, Nottinghamshire, UK

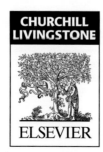

EDINBURGH LONDON NEW YORK OXFORD PHILADELPHIA ST LOUIS SYDNEY TORONTO 2008

CHURCHILL LIVINGSTONE
ELSEVIER

First published 2008

ISBN: 978 0 443 10231 8

British Library Cataloguing in Publication Data
A catalogue record for this book is available from the British Library.

Library of Congress Cataloging in Publication Data
A catalog record for this book is available from the Library of Congress.

Note
Knowledge and best practice in this field are constantly changing. As new research and experience broaden our knowledge, changes in practice, treatment and drug therapy may become necessary or appropriate. Readers are advised to check the most current information provided (i) on procedures featured or (ii) by the manufacturer of each product to be administered, to verify the recommended dose or formula, the method and duration of administration, and contraindications. It is the responsibility of the practitioner, relying on their own experience and knowledge of the patient, to make diagnoses, to determine dosages and the best treatment for each individual patient, and to take all appropriate safety precautions. To the fullest extent of the law, neither the Publisher nor the Author assumes any liability for any injury and/or damage to persons or property arising out or related to any use of the material contained in this book.

The Publisher

Working together to grow libraries in developing countries

www.elsevier.com | www.bookaid.org | www.sabre.org

ELSEVIER   BOOK AID International   Sabre Foundation

ELSEVIER your source for books, journals and multimedia in the health sciences

www.elsevierhealth.com

The Publisher's policy is to use **paper manufactured from sustainable forests**

Printed in China

Contents

. . . .

Preface

. . . .

The idea behind this dictionary was to incorporate all the terminology that may be used in an imaging department into one volume, but to keep the book small enough to be carried in a pocket and used as a quick reference guide. When I embarked on this task I had a framework to cover diagnostic and therapeutic radiography, medical ultrasound, radionuclide imaging, magnetic resonance imaging, CT, anatomy and physiology, basic nursing, medical and imaging terminology, management, and dental imaging. I also wanted to cover the many abbreviations that are becoming increasingly used in departments. In this context, I often found that for some people abbreviations were becoming so familiar that they were often being used in written publications without an explanation of what they meant.

When compiling the dictionary I made a decision not to include parts of speech (noun, adjective, etc.) after each word as is common in other dictionaries. Many of the entries include more than one word which would make the task complex and I am not convinced that current readers are familiar with or need the parts of speech identifying, for those that do I apologise.

Abbreviations are listed in the Appendix. When they do occur in the text I have included them in alphabetical order; for example, non-insulin dependent diabetes mellitus (NIDDM).

In a work of this size there are bound to be words that others feel should have been included and some which should have been left out. I have had to make decisions but have tried to keep the book as up to date as possible within the constraints of the size of the finished book and the knowledge that, at the time of writing, not all departments are fully computerised in the UK, let alone the rest of the world.

I could not have completed a work of this kind on my own and my thanks go to the following people who read, commented on and assisted with the specialist entries: Barry Carver, Director of Postgraduate Studies, University of Wales, for the CT entries; Rowan Spriggs, Superintendent Radiographer, Sherwood Forest Hospital NHS Trust, for the Radionuclide Imaging entries; Jane Payne, Senior Radiographer, Bassetlaw NHS Trust, for the Ultrasound entries; Janet Johnson, Pre-treatment Superintendent Radiographer, Sheffield Teaching Hospitals NHS Foundation Trust, and Helen Gregory, Senior Lecturer, Radiotherapy, School of Health and Emergency Professions, University of Hertfordshire, for the Radiotherapy entries.

The illustrations in the text are all taken from published works and I would like to thank Elsevier and the authors of the following books for their permission to use the following illustrations:

Waugh A and Grant A, 2001 *Anatomy and Physiology in Health and Illness* for Figure 1; Kenyon J and Kenyon K, 2004 *The Physiotherapist's Pocket Book* for Figure 2; Sutherland R (ed) 2007 *Pocket Book of Radiographic Positioning* for Figures 3, 4, 5, 9, 12, 13, 14, 15, 16, 17, 18, 19, 20 and 28, and Table 3; Gunn C,

2002 *Radiographic Imaging* for Figures 6, 24 and 29; Graham D T, 1996 *Principles of Radiological Physics* for Figures 7, 8, 10, 11, 25, 27 and 30 and Tables 5 and 6; Bushlong SC, 2004 *Radiologic Science for Technologists* for Table 1; Bomford C K and Kunkler I H, 2003 *Walter and Miller's Textbook of Radiotherapy* for Table 2 and the Box; Gunn C, 2002 *Bones and Joints: a Guide for Students* for Figures 21, 22, 23 and 26.

Retford, 2008   Chris Gunn

Contributors

. . . .

Kim Carey DCR(T)
Superintendent Therapy Radiographer
Weston Park Hospital
Sheffield

Barry Carver PgDipCT PCGE DCR(R)
Director of Postgraduate Studies
School of Radiography, University of Wales
Bangor, Wales

Margaret Jewitt DCR(T)
Superintendent Therapy Radiographer
Weston Park Hospital
Sheffield

Janet Johnson MSc BSc(Hons) DCR(T)
Superintendent Therapy Radiographer
Weston Park Hospital
Sheffield

Peter Mitchell BSc(Hons)
Superintendent Therapy Radiographer
Weston Park Hospital
Sheffield

Jane Payne DCR(R) PgDip(Medical Ultrasound)
Senior Radiographer
Doncaster and Bassetlaw Hospitals NHS Foundation Trust
Worksop

Paula Rusby DCR(T)
Superintendent Therapy Radiographer
Weston Park Hospital
Sheffield

Helen Simpson PgDip DCR(T)
Superintendent Therapy Radiographer
Weston Park Hospital
Sheffield

Sally Spence DCR(T)
Superintendent Therapy Radiographer
Weston Park Hospital
Sheffield

Rowan Spriggs
Superintendent Radiographer
Sherwood Forest Hospital NHS Trust
Mansfield

A–B ratio   used in pregnancy ultrasound scans to assess the amount of blood through the umbilical cord; a low ratio is normal, a high ratio may indicate intrauterine growth retardation.

abdomen   the largest body cavity.

abdominal   associated with the abdomen.

abdominal aorta   that part of the aorta within the abdomen. Smaller arteries branch from it to supply oxygenated blood to abdominal structures, for example, kidneys.

abdominal aortic aneurysm (AAA)   a swelling in the abdominal aorta. *See also* **aneurysm**.

abdominal breathing   more than usual use of the diaphragm and abdominal muscles to increase the input of air to, and output from, the lungs. It can be done voluntarily. When it occurs in disease it is a compensatory mechanism for inadequate oxygenation.

abdominal cavity   that area below the diaphragm; the abdomen (see figure on p. 2).

abdominal excision (of the rectum)   an operation sometimes performed for rectal cancer. The rectum is mobilized via an abdominal approach. The bowel is divided well proximal to the cancer. The proximal end is brought out as a permanent colostomy. Excision of the distal bowel, containing the cancer and the anal canal, is completed through a perineal incision.

abdominal reflex   a superficial reflex where the abdominal muscles contract when the skin is lightly stroked.

abdominal regions   where the surface anatomy is divided into nine regions; used to describe the location of organs or symptoms, such as pain.

abdominal thrust (Heimlich's manoeuvre)   a technique for removing foreign matter from the trachea of a choking person. Performed by holding the patient from behind and jerking the operator's clenched fist into the victim's epigastrium. Do not practice on volunteers.

abdominopelvic   associated with the abdomen and pelvis or pelvic cavity.

abdominoperineal   associated with the abdomen and perineum.

abdominoplasty (tummy tuck)   plastic surgical procedure used to tighten the abdominal muscles.

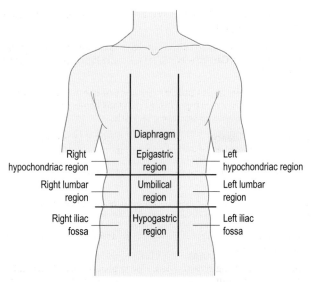

Regions of the abdominal cavity. From Ross and Wilson's anatomy and physiology in health and illness, 9th edn, Anne Waugh and Alison Grant (eds), 2001, Churchill Livingstone, Edinburgh, with permission.

abducens nerve the sixth pair of cranial nerves. They control the lateral rectus muscle of the eyeball, which turns the eyeball outwards.

abduct to draw away from the median line of the body. *See also* **adduct**.

abduction the act of moving, (or abducting) away from the midline. *See also* **adduction**.

abductor a muscle which, on contraction, draws a part away from the median line of the body. *See also* **adductor**.

aberrant abnormal; usually applied to a blood vessel or nerve which does not follow the normal course.

aberration a deviation from normal. *See also* **chromosomal aberration, optical aberration**.

ablation amputation, excision of part of the body or the removal of a growth or harmful substance.

abort to terminate before full development.

abortion abrupt termination of a process. The induced expulsion from the uterus of the product of conception before viability by medical or surgical means. N.B. The preferred term for unintentional loss of the product of conception prior to 24 weeks' gestation is miscarriage. ***criminal abortion***

intentional evacuation of the uterus by other than trained licensed personnel, or where abortion is prohibited by law.

abrasion   superficial injury to skin or mucous membrane from scraping or rubbing (excoriation). Can be used therapeutically for removal of scar tissue (dermabrasion).

abscess   localized collection of pus. May be acute or chronic. ***Brodie's abscess*** chronic osteomyelitis occurring without previous acute phase. In dentistry a common site is the apex of the root of a tooth.

absolute detector efficiency   the ability of a detector to measure the total events emitted by a source of ionizing radiation.

absorbed   when a photon interacts with an object and as a result loses all its energy.

absorbed dose   is the measure of the amount of radiation absorbed by an object.

absorbed fraction   the quantity of radiation absorbed by the tissues in radionuclide imaging.

absorption   in intensifying screens the incident photons are absorbed by the phosphor, 95% as a result of the photoelectric effect and 5% by the Compton effect. *See also* **photoelectric effect, Compton effect**.

absorption rate constant   a value describing the amount of a drug absorbed in a unit of time.

abuse   misuse of equipment, drugs and other substances, power and position. Deliberate injury to another person. It may be either physical, sexual, psychological or through neglect, such as failure to feed or keep clean. The term can apply to any group of individuals, especially those most vulnerable such as children, older people, and those with mental health problems or learning disabilities. *See also* **child abuse, elder abuse**.

accelerated fractionation   in radiotherapy it is the method of delivering small doses of radiation several times a day, over a reduced number of days compared with a standard course of treatment.

accelerating voltage   the kVp determining the minimum wavelength in the spectrum, in a constant potential unit it will be present throughout the exposure.

acceleration   change in velocity in unit time, unit metre/second/second.

accelerator   a chemical that controls activity by assuring the correct pH values are maintained; in developer sodium or potassium hydroxide is used.

acceptance tests   tests done on newly installed radiotherapy equipment and include checking that the agreed specification has been met with regard to the radiotherapy beam, movement of the tube stand, electrical aspects, radiation safety requirements and accessories.

accessory motion   sliding, gliding or rolling motion that occurs within and between joint surfaces during active or passive joint movement.

access time   the time taken for the computer to get information from a storage device, e.g. disk or tape.

Access to Health Records Act (1990)   allows access to both paper and computerized health records made after 1991, with certain exceptions, such as where they may cause serious physical or mental harm to a person.

acclimatization   the body's ability to adapt physiologically to a variation in environment such as climate or altitude.

accommodation   ability of the lens of the eye to increase its refractive power in order to focus on near objects. Decreased sensitivity to stimuli demonstrated by neurons that have been exposed to subthreshold stimuli for long periods of time.

accommodation reflex   constriction of the pupils and convergence of the eyes for near vision.

accountability   health professionals have a duty to care according to law. In some countries the statutory body, and/or the professional organization, develop a code of conduct via which each practitioner can accept responsibility and accountability for the professional service delivered to each patient/client. *See also* **duty of care, malpractice, negligence**.

accretion   an increase of substance or deposit round a central object.

accuracy   the ability of a detector to correctly indicate dose.

ACE inhibitors   angiotensin-converting enzyme inhibitors allow blood vessels to dilate by preventing the formation of angiotensin II, an artery constrictor. Used in the treatment of heart failure, hypotension, diabetic nephropathy and post-myocardial infarction.

acephalous   without a head.

acetabuloplasty   an operation to improve the depth and shape of the hip socket (acetabulum); necessary in such conditions as developmental dysplasia of the hip and osteoarthritis of the hip.

acetabulum   a cup-like socket on the external lateral surface of the pelvis into which the head of the femur fits to form the hip joint.

acetic acid   present as the acid in fixing solutions and is used in combination with aluminium chloride as the hardener.

acetoacetate   an acidic ketone produced during an interim stage of fat oxidation in the body. Some can be utilized as a fuel by tissues, such as the kidney. In situations where carbohydrate molecules are not available for metabolism, such as in diabetes mellitus or starvation, excess is produced and the high levels in the blood result in ketoacidosis with severe disturbances of pH, fluid and electrolytes.

acetonuria   acetone and other ketones in the urine. *See also* **ketonuria**.

achalasia an abnormal condition where the muscles are unable to relax, particularly the lower oesophageal sphincter.

Achilles tendinitis inflammation of the Achilles tendon.

Achilles tendon the tendinous termination of the soleus and gastrocnemius muscles inserted into the heel bone (os calcis or calcaneus).

acholia the absence of bile.

acholuria the absence of bile pigments from the urine. *See also* **jaundice**.

achondroplasia without cartilage. A disorder of the growth of cartilage in the epiphyses of the long bones and skull.

acid any substance that has an excess of hydrogen ions over hydroxyl ions, for example, hydrochloric acid. They have a pH below 7 and turn blue litmus red and react with alkalis to form salts plus water. The chemical in the fixer solution that neutralizes the alkaline developer as soon as the film reaches the fixing tank and therefore prevents further development, the acid used is either acetic acid or sulphuric acid and depends on the hardener used.

acidaemia a high level of acid (hydrogen ions) in the blood resulting in a below normal blood pH < 7.35 (hydrogen ion concentration >44 mmol/L). *See also* **acidosis**.

acid–base balance equilibrium between the acid and base elements of the blood and body fluids.

acidity the state of being acid or sour. The degree of acidity can be measured on the pH scale where a pH below 7 is acid and pH 6 denotes a weak acid and pH 1 a strong acid.

acidosis process leading to the accumulation of excess acid in the body. *respiratory acidosis* due to hypoventilation and the accumulation of carbon dioxide. *metabolic acidosis* due to the generation of excess acid (lactic acidosis) or depletion of alkali (for example, diarrhoea). *See also* **acidaemia**.

acid phosphatase an enzyme which synthesizes phosphate esters of carbohydrates in an acid medium. An increase of this enzyme in the blood is indicative of cancer of the prostate gland.

Acinetobacter a genus of Gram-negative aerobic bacteria causing infections that include wound infection, pneumonia and meningitis. The microorganism has developed antibiotic resistance and is a particular danger to critically ill patients having intensive or high-dependency care.

acini minute saccules or alveoli, lined or filled with secreting cells. Several acini combine to form a lobule.

acoustic sound or hearing.

acoustic cavitation a potential biological effect of ultrasound imaging, marked by large amplitude oscillations of microscopic gas bubbles.

acoustic enhancement   an artefact that occurs in ultrasound imaging when an object with a low level of absorption causes objects which are further away from the probe to be brighter than they should be.

acoustic impedance   a value given to a substance and is calculated by multiplying the density of the medium by the velocity of the ultrasound travelling through the medium and is independent of frequency.

acoustic neuroma   a benign tumour (schwannoma) affecting the eighth cranial nerve (vestibulocochlear nerve) as it passes through the skull into the brainstem, causing problems in hearing and balance.

acoustic shadow   in ultrasound imaging, the absence of echoes produced by a dense structure such as a calculus which prevents the transmission of ultrasound waves by reflection.

acoustic shadowing   tissues which reflect or absorb ultrasound, for example, gall stones, will cast a shadow on the image. The tissue interface has to be similar to or larger than the ultrasound beam to cause shadowing.

acoustic window   an area of the body used to allow imaging of underlying structures, for example, the spaces between the ribs, the liver.

acquired immune deficiency syndrome (AIDS)   a term used to denote a particular stage of infection with human immunodeficiency virus (HIV). The Centers for Disease Control and Prevention (CDC) define AIDS as the development of an AIDS-defining illness in a patient with HIV infection.A low CD4$^+$ T cell count of less than 200 per mL (or less than 14% of lymphocytes) in an HIV-positive person is also regarded as AIDS-defining, regardless of symptoms or opportunistic infections.

acrocephalia (acrocephaly)   a congenital malformation whereby the top of the head is pointed and the eyes protrude, due to premature closure of sagittal and coronal skull sutures.

acrocephalosyndactyly   a congenital malformation consisting of a pointed top of head, with fusion of fingers and/or toes. *See also* **Apert's syndrome**.

acrocyanosis   coldness and blueness of the extremities due to circulatory disorder.

acrodynia   acute, painful reddening of the extremities such as occurs in erythroedema polyneuropathy.

acromegaly   enlargement of the hands, face, feet, and the bones of the head and chest occurring due to excess growth hormone in an adult, almost always from overactivity of the anterior lobe of the pituitary gland due to a pituitary adenoma.

acromicria   smallness of the hands, face and feet.

acromioclavicular   associated with the acromion process (of scapula) and the clavicle.

acromion   the point or summit of the shoulder: the triangular process at the extreme outer end of the spine of the scapula.

acropacy   thickening of the extremities.

acrosome   structure surrounding the nucleus of a spermatozoon. It contains lytic enzymes which, when released by many spermatozoa (during the acrosome reaction), facilitate the penetration of an oocyte by a single spermatozoon.

actin   one of the contractile proteins in a muscle myofibril; it reacts with myosin to cause contraction.

actinobiology   study of the effects of radiation on living organisms.

action   the activity or function of any part of the body.

action potential   change in electrical potential and charge that occurs across excitable cell membranes during nerve impulse conduction or when muscles contract.

active   energetic. ***active principle*** an ingredient which gives a complex drug its chief therapeutic value, for example, atropine is the active principle in belladonna. ***active range of motion*** the movement of a joint without assistance through a range of motion. Those produced by patients using their own neuromuscular mechanisms. *See also* **immunity**.

activators   impurities which stimulate the phosphor of an intensifying screen to emit light.

actual scores   each score has a real value.

acuity   clearness, sharpness, keenness. *See also* **auditory acuity, visual acuity**.

acute   short and severe; not long drawn out or chronic.

acute abdomen   a pathological condition within the abdomen requiring immediate surgical intervention.

acute coronary syndromes   describes the spectrum of events ranging from the partial occlusion of a coronary artery resulting in unstable angina through to the complete occlusion of a coronary artery resulting in myocardial infarction.

acute dilatation of the stomach   sudden enlargement of this organ due to paralysis of the muscular wall *See also* **paralytic ileus**.

acute heart failure   cessation or impairment of heart action, in previously undiagnosed heart disease, or in the course of another disease.

acute injury   an injury that presents with a rapid onset and has a short duration, due to a traumatic episode. Term used to describe the first 24–48 hours after onset of an injury such as that sustained during a sporting activity.

acute respiratory distress syndrome (ARDS)   characterized by difficulty breathing, poor oxygenation, stiff lungs and typical changes on a chest X-ray, following a recognized cause of acute lung injury. Analysis of arterial blood gases reveals a fall in PaO_2 and eventually an increased $PaCO_2$ and a fall in pH.

acute tubular necrosis (ATN)   rapid onset necrosis of the renal tubules. It is usually caused by renal ischaemia due to shock, but may be due to the nephrotoxic effects of bacterial or chemical toxins. *See also* **renal failure**.

acute yellow atrophy   acute diffuse necrosis of the liver; icterus gravis; malignant jaundice.

acyesis   absence of pregnancy.

acystia   congenital absence of the bladder.

adactyly   absence of fingers.

Addison's disease   deficient secretion of cortisol and aldosterone due to primary failure of the adrenal cortex, causing electrolyte imbalance, diminished blood volume, hypotension, weight loss, hypoglycaemia, muscular weakness, gastrointestinal upsets and pigmentation of skin.

address   a number which designates a particular storage area in the memory of the computer.

adduct   to draw towards the midline of the body. *See also* **abduct**.

adduction   the act of adducting, drawing towards the midline of the body. *See also* **abduction**.

adductor   any muscle which moves a part toward the median axis of the body. *See also* **abductor**.

adenectomy   surgical removal of a gland.

adenitis   inflammation of a gland, or lymph node. ***hilar adenitis*** inflammation of bronchial lymph nodes.

adenoacanthoma   a tumour of glandular tissue which may be benign or malignant and is identified by changes in the squamous cells.

adenocarcinoma   a malignant epithelial cell tumour of glandular tissue.

adenofibroma   *see* **fibroadenoma**.

adenoid   resembling a gland. *See also* **adenoids**.

adenoidectomy   surgical removal from the nasopharynx of enlarged pharyngeal tonsil (adenoid tissue).

adenoids   abnormally enlarged pharyngeal tonsils. Lymphoid tissue situated in the nasopharynx which can obstruct breathing and impede hearing.

adenoma   a benign, premalignant tumour of glandular epithelial tissue.

adenomatous polyp   a benign tumour of the large intestine which may develop into a malignant tumour.

adenomyoma   a non-malignant tumour composed of muscle and glandular elements, usually applied to benign growths of the uterus.

adenopathy   any disease of a gland.

adenosine diphosphate (ADP) an important cellular metabolite involved in energy exchange within the cell. Chemical energy is conserved in the cell, by the phosphorylation of ADP to ATP primarily in the mitochondrion, as a high-energy phosphate bond.

adenosine monophosphate (AMP) an important cellular metabolite involved in energy release for cell use.

adenosine triphosphate (ATP) an intermediate high-energy compound which on hydrolysis to ADP releases chemically useful energy. ATP is generated during catabolism and utilized during anabolism.

adenotonsillectomy surgical removal of the pharyngeal tonsil (adenoid tissue) and palatine tonsils.

adenovirus a group of DNA-containing viruses. They cause upper respiratory and gastrointestinal infections and conjunctivitis.

adhesion abnormal union of two parts, occurring after inflammation; a band of fibrous tissue which joins such parts. In the abdomen such a band may cause intestinal obstruction; in joints it restricts movement; between two surfaces of pleura it prevents complete pneumothorax.

adipose fat; of a fatty nature. The cells constituting adipose tissue contain either white or brown fat.

adiposity excessive accumulation of fat in the body.

aditus in anatomy, an entrance or opening.

adjustable template a large number of parallel rods or pins which can be adjusted to the patient shape and clamped into position to show the patient contour.

adjuvant a treatment or drug used alongside another to increase its efficiency or effectiveness.

adjuvant therapy a treatment given together with another. It is usually applied to the treatment of cancer where cytotoxic drugs are used after removal of the tumour by surgery or radiotherapy. The purpose of treatment is to enhance the chance of cure and prevent recurrence. *See also* **neoadjuvant therapy**.

adnexa structures that are in close proximity to a part.

adnexa oculi the lacrimal apparatus.

adnexa uteri the ovaries and uterine (fallopian) tubes.

adrenal near the kidney. *adrenal glands* endocrine glands, one situated on the upper pole of each kidney. The *adrenal cortex* secretes glucocorticoids, mineralocorticoids and sex hormones which control metabolism, the chemical constitution of body fluids and secondary sexual characteristics. Under the control of the pituitary gland via the secretion of adrenocorticotrophic hormone. The *adrenal medulla* secretes noradrenaline (norepinephrine) and adrenaline (epinephrine). *See also* **adrenalectomy**.

adrenalectomy removal of an adrenal gland, usually for tumour. If both adrenal glands are removed, replacement administration of cortical hormones is required.

adrenaline (epinephrine)   a catecholamine hormone, produced by the adrenal medulla. It enhances the effects of the sympathetic nervous system during times of physiological stress by preparing the body for 'fight or flight' responses. These include increased heart rate, bronchodilation and increased respiratory rate and glucose release. Adrenaline (epinephrine) is used therapeutically as a sympathomimetic in situations that include acute allergic reactions, and in local anaesthetic to prolong the anaesthetic effects.

adrenergic   describes nerves which liberate the catecholamine noradrenaline (norepinephrine) from their terminations. Most sympathetic nerves release noradrenaline as a neurotransmitter.

adrenoceptor (adrenergic receptor)   receptor sites on the effector structures innervated by sympathetic nerves. Two main types: alpha (α) and beta (β). Both receptor types, which respond differently to neurotransmitters, have further subdivisions.

adrenocorticotrophic hormone (ACTH, corticotrophin)   secreted by the anterior lobe of the pituitary gland it stimulates the production of hormones by the adrenal cortex.

adrenogenital syndrome   an endocrine disorder, usually congenital, resulting from abnormal activity of the adrenal cortex. A female child will show enlarged clitoris and possibly labial fusion, perhaps being confused with a male. The male child may show pubic hair and enlarged penis. In both male and female there is rapid growth, muscularity and advanced bone age.

adrenoleucodystrophy (ALD)   a group of neurodegenerative disorders associated with adrenocortical insufficiency.

adult polycystic kidney diseases (APKD)   *see* **polycystic kidney disease**.

advance directive   a written declaration made by a mentally competent person setting out their wishes regarding life-prolonging medical interventions if they are incapacitated by an irreversible disease or are terminally ill, which prevents them making their wishes known to health professionals at the time. An advance directive is legally binding if it is in the form of an advanced refusal and the maker is competent at the time. Also known as a *living will*.

advanced life support (ALS)   the use of drugs, artificial aids and advanced skills to save or preserve life during resuscitation procedures. *See also* **cardiopulmonary resuscitation**.

advancement   surgical detachment of a tendon or muscle followed by re-attachment at an advanced point.

adventitia   the external coat, especially of an artery or vein.

adverse drug reactions (ADRs)   a term describing any unwanted effects of a drug. They range from very minor through to extremely unpleasant or life-threatening. They are classified into five types: A (augmented effects), B (bizarre effects), C (chronic effects), D (delayed effects) and E (ending effects, which occur when administration is stopped suddenly).

advocacy process by which a person supports or argues for the needs of another. Healthcare professionals may act as advocate for their patients or clients, or assist individuals to develop the skills needed for self-advocacy.

aerobe a microorganism that requires oxygen to maintain life.

aerobic requiring free oxygen or air to support life or a specific process. *aerobic energy* the production of adenosine triphosphate (ATP) by oxidative phosphorylation.

aerogenous gas producing.

aerophagia (aerophagy) excessive air swallowing.

aetiology (etiology) the study of the cause of disease.

afebrile without fever.

afferent conducting inward to a part or organ; used to describe nerves, blood and lymphatic vessels. *See also* **efferent**.

afferent degeneration that which spreads up sensory nerves.

afferent nerve one conveying impulses from the tissues to the nerve centres. Also known as *sensory nerves*.

affinity describes the chemical attraction between two substances, for example, oxygen and haemoglobin.

afibrinogenaemia a lack of fibrinogen resulting in a serious disorder of blood coagulation.

aflatoxin carcinogenic metabolites of certain strains of *Aspergillus flavus* that can affect peanuts and carbohydrate foods stored in warm humid climates. Hepatic enzymes produce the metabolites of aflatoxins which predispose to liver cancer.

aftercare the care given during convalescence and rehabilitation. It may be within the remit of health professionals such as therapists or nurses, or may be provided by social care staff or family members.

after-glow the production of light from a crystal after the irradiation of the crystal stops. *See also* **phosphorescence**.

afterload the pressure of blood in the pulmonary artery and aorta that forms the resistance that ventricular contraction must overcome to pump blood into the circulation. *See also* **preload**.

afterloading the method of inserting a number of guides into a body cavity and then mechanically inserting radioactive source over the guides. This technique reduces the radiation dose to the hands of the operator.

agammaglobulinaemia absence of gammaglobulin in the blood, with consequent inability to produce immunity to infection. *See also* **Bruton's agammaglobulinaemia**.

aganglionosis absence of ganglia, as those of the distal bowel. *See also* **Hirschsprung's disease, megacolon**.

agar a gelatinous substance obtained from certain seaweeds. It is used as a bulk-increasing laxative and for solidifying bacterial culture media.

ageism stereotyping people according to chronological age: over-emphasizing negative aspects to the disadvantage of more positive points. Discriminatory attitudes in society disadvantage older people on the basis of age alone. However, ageist views can impact on people of any age.

agenesis incomplete and imperfect development.

age-specific death rate is the ratio of the number of deaths in a specific age group to the mean population of that age group multiplied by 100.

agglutinins antibodies that agglutinate or clump organisms or particles.

agility the ability to control the direction of the body or body part during rapid movement.

aglossia absence of the tongue.

aglutition difficulty in swallowing (dysphagia).

agnathia absence or incomplete development of the jaw.

agonist a muscle that shortens to perform a movement. Also describes a drug or other chemical that imitates the response of the natural chemical at a receptor site. *See also* **antagonist**.

agoraphobia morbid fear of being alone in large open places.

agranulocyte a non-granular leucocyte.

agranulocytosis marked reduction in or complete absence of granulocytes (polymorphonuclear leucocytes). Usually results from bone marrow depression caused by (a) hypersensitivity to drugs, (b) cytotoxic drugs or (c) irradiation. Symptoms include fever, ulceration of the mouth and throat. If untreated, prostration and death may ensue. *See also* **neutropenia**.

agraphia loss of language facility. *See also* **motor agraphia, sensory agraphia**.

AIDS-defining illness criteria for AIDS in a patient infected with HIV. Examples include candidiasis of bronchus, trachea, lungs or oesophagus, invasive cervical cancer, Kaposi's sarcoma, pulmonary tuberculosis or other mycobacterial infection, and *Pneumocystis carinii* pneumonia.

air the gaseous mixture which makes up the atmosphere surrounding the earth. It consists of approximately 78% nitrogen, 20% oxygen, 0.04% carbon dioxide, 1% argon, and traces of ozone, neon, helium, etc. and a variable amount of water vapour.

air embolism results from an air bubble entering the circulation.

air hunger a deep indrawing of breath which characterizes the late stages of uncontrolled haemorrhage.

air knives are used in the drier section of automatic film processors to increase the velocity of the air as it strikes the film surface.

air swallowing (aerophagia) swallowing of excessive air particularly when eating: it may result in belching or the passage of flatus from the anus.

airway   used to describe the entry to the larynx from the pharynx. *See also* **Brook airway, oropharyngeal airway**.

alactacid (alactic) anaerobic system   a series of chemical reactions occurring within the cells whereby adenosine triphosphate for energy use is produced, without oxygen, from adenosine diphosphate (ADP) and creatine phosphate (phosphocreatine).

alactacid oxygen debt component   the amount of oxygen required to replace the adenosine triphosphate (ATP) and creatine phosphate (phosphocreatine) stores in cells during the process of recovery from exercise.

ALARA   a principle which states that the radiation dosage to patients and staff should be kept *a*s *l*ow *a*s *r*easonably *a*chievable.

Albers–Schönberg disease   *see* **osteopetrosis**.

albinism   a congenital hypopigmentation of the hair, skin and eyes. It is caused by a deficiency of melanin pigment in skin and/or the eye. Other associated eye and neurological defects can contribute to poor vision.

albino   a person affected with albinism.

albumin   a protein found in animal and vegetable material. It is soluble in water and coagulates on heating. Serum albumin is the main protein of blood plasma.

albuminuria   the presence of albumin in the urine. The condition may be temporary and clear up completely, may indicate serious kidney disease.

aldolase   an enzyme present in muscle tissue.

aldolase test   increased levels of aldolase and other enzymes in the blood are indicative of some muscle diseases, for example, severe muscular dystrophy.

aldosterone   mineralocorticoid hormone secreted by the adrenal cortex. Secretion is regulated by the action of renin and angiotensin. It enhances the reabsorption of sodium accompanied by water and the excretion of potassium by the renal tubules.

aldosterone antagonist   a drug that blocks the action of aldosterone.

Alexander technique   a series of techniques used to improve the functioning of mind and body in movement known as 'psychophysical' re-education. It is based on the belief that poor posture can lead to ill health, injury and chronic pain. The technique aims to promote postural improvement through self-awareness.

alexia   word blindness; an inability to interpret the significance of the printed or written word, but without loss of visual power. Can be due to a brain lesion or insufficient/inappropriate sensory experience during an 'ab initio' stage of learning.

alginates   seaweed derivatives used in some wound dressings. They have high absorbency, haemostatic properties and can be removed without damaging delicate tissues.

algorithm logical steps which define how a problem can be solved. A step by step procedure for the solution of a problem by computer by using specific mathematical or logical operations. In CT the mathematical process used in image reconstruction, different algorithms may be used to produce differing images to better demonstrate particular structures.

aliasing in ultrasound when high velocities in one direction appear as high velocities in the opposite direction. It occurs when an analogue signal is sampled at a frequency which is lower than half its maximum frequency. All the frequency above half of the sampling frequency is projected below the base line (backfolded) in the low frequency region causing artefacts on the image. An artefact that occurs in magnetic resonance imaging due to the image encoding process, it occurs when the field of view is smaller than the area being imaged.

alimentary associated with food.

alimentary tract comprises the mouth, oesophagus, stomach, small intestine, ascending colon, transverse colon, descending colon, sigmoid colon, rectum and anal canal.

alkali also called a ***base***. Substances that have an excess of hydroxyl ions over hydrogen ions, for example, sodium bicarbonate. They have a pH greater than 7 and turn red litmus blue. Alkalis react with acids to produce salts plus water, and with fats to form soaps. ***alkaline reserve*** a biochemical term denoting the amount of buffered alkali (normally bicarbonate) available in the blood for buffering acids (normally dissolved CO_2) formed in or introduced into the body and limiting pH changes in the blood.

alkaline relating to or possessing the properties of an alkali. Containing an excess of hydroxyl over hydrogen ions.

alkaline phosphatase an enzyme present in several tissues, for example, bone, liver and kidney. An increase of this enzyme in the blood is indicative of obstructive jaundice and increased osteoblast activity associated with some bone disease.

alkalinuria alkalinity of urine.

alkaloid similar to an alkali. Also describes a large group of organic bases present in plants and which have important physiological actions, for example, morphine, atropine, quinine and caffeine.

allergen an antigen which produces an allergic, or immediate-type hypersensitivity response.

allergy hypersensitivity to a foreign substance that is normally harmless but causes a violent action in the patient, for example, asthma, hay fever, migraine, iodine-based contrast agents. *See also* **anaphylaxis, sensitization**.

allogenic transplant a transplant, usually of bone marrow, from an immunologically compatible sibling.

allograft grafting or transplanting an organ or tissue from one person to another who does not share the same transplantation antigens. Also known as a homograft.

alloy blocks shielding blocks of an alloy of lead, bismuth or cadmium placed on a tray on the radiotherapy accessory mount to shape the radiation beam so that it accurately covers the treatment area. Blocks can be individually made for each patient, accounting for beam divergence and pre-mounted on a tray.

alopecia partial or complete loss of hair which can be premature, congenital or senile.

alpha (α)-antitrypsin a liver protein that normally opposes trypsin. Reduced blood levels are linked with a genetic predisposition to emphysema and liver disease.

alpha decay the spontaneous emission of an alpha particle from the nucleus of an atom, resulting in the atomic number of the element decreasing by 2 and the mass number decreasing by 4.

alphafetoprotein (AFP) a protein produced by fetal gut and liver cells and by adult liver cancer cells. Raised levels are seen in maternal serum and amniotic fluid in fetal abnormalities including neural tube defects. May be used as a tumour marker for cancers of the liver and the testes affecting adults.

alpha particle the nucleus of a helium-4 atom consisting of two protons and two neutrons.

alternating current when electrons flow through a circuit in one direction and then the other.

altitudinal when describing a visual field defect implies loss of vision in superior or inferior half of field.

aluminium chloride used as a hardener in fixing solutions which contain acetic acid as the acid.

aluminium sulphate used as a hardener in fixing solutions which contain sulphuric acid as the acid.

alveolar ridge the part of the mandible and maxilla in which the teeth are embedded.

alveolitis inflammation of alveoli. When caused by inhalation of an allergen it is termed *extrinsic allergic alveolitis*.

alveolus an air sac of the lung. In dentistry, a bony tooth socket within the jaw bone. A gland follicle or acinus.

Alzheimer's disease a progressive form of neuronal degeneration in the brain, a common case of dementia in older people which is irreversible. Can affect younger patients (i.e. under 65 years of age), often when there is a family history of the disease.

A-mode used in early ultrasound machines, the voltage was produced across the transducer as a vertical deflection on the face of the oscilloscope. The horizontal sweep was calibrated to indicate the distance from the transducer to the reflecting surface. Demonstrates only the position and length of a reflecting structure.

amalgam   any of a group of alloys containing mercury. *See also* **dental amalgam**.

amastia   congenital absence of the breasts.

amaurosis   partial or total blindness.

amaurosis fugax   temporary loss of vision in an eye due to interruption of arterial supply.

ambient light   the light in the room where a film is being viewed.

ambulant   able to walk.

ambulatory   mobile, walking about.

ambulatory ECG (Holter monitoring)   recording heart rhythm and rate over a 24-hour period to detect transient ischaemia or arrhythmias. The person continues with their normal activities and keeps a record of times and activities. *See also* **electrocardiogram**.

ambulatory surgery (day surgery)   surgery carried out on the day of admission and, in the absence of problems, the person is discharged the same day to the care of the primary care team.

ambulatory treatment   interventions such as blood product transfusion or chemotherapy, provided for patients on a day care basis. *See also* **continuous ambulatory peritoneal dialysis**.

amelia   congenital absence of a limb or limbs. *complete amelia* absence of both arms and legs.

amelioration   a reduction in the severity of symptoms.

amenorrhoea   absence of menstruation. When menstruation has not been established at the time when it should have been, it is termed *primary amenorrhoea*; absence of menstruation after they have commenced is referred to as *secondary amenorrhoea*.

ametria   congenital absence of the uterus.

amino acids   organic acids in which one or more of the hydrogen atoms are replaced by the amino group, NH_2. They are the end product of protein hydrolysis and from them the body synthesizes its own proteins. They are classified as either essential (indispensable) or non-essential (dispensable). Ten (eight in adults and a further two during childhood) cannot be synthesized in sufficient quantities in the body and are therefore essential (indispensable) in the diet – arginine, histidine, isoleucine, leucine, lysine, methionine, phenylalanine, threonine, tryptophan and valine. The remainder, which can be synthesized in the body if the diet contains sufficient amounts of the precursor amino acids, are designated non-essential (dispensable) amino acids. However, some of these are conditionally essential and depend upon adequate amounts of their precursor.

aminoaciduria   the abnormal presence of amino acids in the urine; it usually indicates an inborn error of metabolism as in cystinosis and Fanconi syndrome.

aminopeptidases intestinal enzymes that act upon the amine end of the peptide chain during the digestion of protein.

ammonia a compound of nitrogen and hydrogen. Several inherited errors of ammonia metabolism can cause learning disability, seizures and other neurological manifestations.

ammonium thiosulphate used as a fixing agent in fixer solutions.

amnesia complete loss of memory; can be divided into organic (true) amnesia (for example, delirium, dementia), and psychogenic amnesia (for example dissociative states). The term **anterograde amnesia** is used when there is poor recall of events following an accident or brain injury, and **retrograde amnesia** when the loss of memory is prior to the injury.

amnesic syndrome chronic profound impairment of recent memory with preserved immediate recall. Often accompanied by disorientation for time and confabulation (the creation of false memory to fill the gaps in memory). Commonly caused by thiamin(e) deficiency, which can be secondary to chronic alcohol use, dietary deficiency, gastric cancer, etc.

amniocentesis a diagnostic procedure for detecting chromosomal, metabolic and haematological abnormalities of the fetus. It involves inserting a needle under ultrasound guidance through the abdominal wall into the amniotic sac to obtain a sample of amniotic fluid.

amnion membrane of embryonic origin lining the cavity of the uterus during pregnancy containing amniotic fluid and the fetus.

amnionitis inflammation of the inner fetal membrane (the amnion).

amnioscopy an instrument that when passed through the abdominal wall enables viewing of the fetus and amniotic fluid. Clear, colourless fluid is normal; yellow or green staining is due to meconium and occurs in cases of fetal hypoxia. **cervical amnioscopy** can be performed late in pregnancy. A different instrument is inserted via the vagina and cervix for the same reasons.

amniotic cavity the fluid-filled cavity between the fetus and the inner fetal membrane (amnion).

amniotic fluid fluid produced by the inner fetal membrane (amnion) and the fetus, which surrounds the fetus throughout pregnancy. It protects the fetus from temperature variations and physical trauma, and permits fetal movement. It is secreted and reabsorbed by cells lining the amniotic cavity and is swallowed by the fetus and excreted as urine. *See also* **amniocentesis, amnioscopy**.

amniotic fluid embolism an embolus caused by amniotic fluid entering the maternal circulation. An extremely rare but very serious complication of pregnancy.

amoeba a unicellular (single cell) protozoon. Strains that are human parasites include *Entamoeba histolytica*, which causes amoebic dysentery (intestinal amoebiasis).

amoebiasis infestation of large intestine by the protozoon *Entamoeba histolytica*, where it causes mucosal ulceration leading to pain, diarrhoea alternating with constipation and blood and mucus passed rectally, hence the term 'amoebic dysentery'. If the amoebae enter the hepatic portal circulation they may cause a liver abscess. Diagnosis is by isolating the amoeba in the stools. Cutaneous amoebiasis may cause perianal or genital ulceration in homosexual men.

amoeboid   resembling an amoeba in shape or in mode of movement such as leucocytes.

amoeboma   a tumour in the caecum or rectum caused by *Entamoeba histolytica*. Fibrosis may occur and obstruct the bowel.

amorph   a gene that is inactive, i.e. does not express a trait.

amorphous   not having a regular shape.

ampere (A)   one of the seven base units of the International System of Units (SI). A measurement of electrical current.

amphiarthroses   cartilagenous joints which either have no movement or minimal movement, for example the joint between the epiphysis and diaphysis of a growing long bone, symphysis pubis.

amplification gain   is the measure of the extent to which developer increases the initial effect of exposure on the silver halide grains.

amplitude   the maximum value of either positive or negative current or voltage that occurs on an alternating current waveform. In ultrasound, the magnitude (height) of the ultrasound beam, the ultrasound pulse is very brief so the power values arranged over a period of time will be low compared to peak intensity. *See also* **peak value**.

ampoule   a sealed glass or plastic phial containing a single sterile dose of a drug.

ampulla   any flask-like dilatation such as that in the uterine (fallopian) tube.

ampulla of Vater   the enlargement formed by the union of the common bile duct with the pancreatic duct where they enter the duodenum.

amputation   removal of an appending part, for example, limb.

amputee   a person who has had amputation of one or more limbs.

amylase   any enzyme that converts starches into sugars. Found in saliva and pancreatic juice; it converts starchy foods to maltose. The amount of amylase in the blood is increased in disorders of the pancreas such as pancreatitis.

amyloidosis   formation and deposit of amyloid in any organ, notably the liver and kidney. ***primary amyloidosis*** has no apparent cause. ***secondary amyloidosis*** can occur in any prolonged toxic condition such as Hodgkin's disease, tuberculosis and leprosy. It is common in the genetic disease familial Mediterranean fever.

amyotrophic lateral sclerosis (ALS)   a form of motor neuron disease in which there is a loss of the upper motor neurons from the cortex to the brainstem and spinal cord as well as the loss of the lower motor neurons from the brainstem and spinal cord to the muscles.

anacrotic a wave in the ascending curve of an arterial tracing, indicating the opening of the aortic valve (that between the left ventricle and the aorta). An abnormality of this occurs in aortic stenosis. *See also* **dicrotic**.

anaemia a deficiency in either the quantity or quality of red corpuscles in the blood. Produces clinical manifestations arising from hypoxaemia, such as lassitude and breathlessness on exertion. There are very many possible causes, for example, haemolytic disease of the newborn, megaloblastic anaemia, thalassaemia. *See also* **aplastic anaemia, haemolytic anaemia, pernicious anaemia**.

anaemia of chronic disease anaemia associated with chronic inflammatory diseases, infection or cancer.

anaerobe a microorganism that is unable to grow in the presence of molecular oxygen for example gangrene.

anaerobic relating to the absence of oxygen. Describes processes that occur without oxygen, and certain microorganisms that survive without free oxygen or air. *anaerobic energy* energy that is produced without using oxygen via two energy systems: alactacid and lactacid.

anaesthesia loss of sensation. *general anaesthesia* loss of sensation with loss of consciousness. In *local anaesthesia* injection of a drug that inhibits peripheral nerve conduction so that painful stimuli fail to reach the brain. *Spinal anaesthesia* loss of sensation by the injection of local anaesthetic into the cerebrospinal fluid between the vertebrae usually of the lower back, causing loss of sensation but no loss of consciousness. Also used to describe the loss of feeling produced by a spinal lesion. *See also* **caudal anaesthesia, epidural anaesthesia**.

anaesthesiology the science dealing with anaesthetics, their administration and effect.

anaesthetic a drug that induces general or local loss of sensation. *general anaesthetic* a drug that produces unconsciousness by inhalation or injection. *local anaesthetic* a drug that injected into the tissues or applied topically causes local insensibility to pain. *See also* **spinal anaesthetic**.

anaesthetist a doctor with specialist training to administer general anaesthesia.

anaesthetize to administer drugs or gases to produce general anaesthesia.

analeptic restorative.

analgesia the relief of pain without causing unconsciousness. Loss of sensation of pain without loss of touch.

analgesic a drug used to relieve pain without causing unconsciousness.

analogue represents a quantity changing in steps which are continuous, as opposed to *digital* which is in discrete steps.

analogue signal   a continuous electrical signal used to transmit images to a computer, television.

analogue to digital converter   a device which converts analogue signals into digital signals which can be understood and manipulated by a computer.

analysis of variance (ANOVA)   a statistical method of comparing sample means.

analytical epidemiology   the study of the relationship between different risk factors and the development of disease.

anaphylactic shock   shock caused by an allergic reaction.

anaphylaxis   a severe reaction, often fatal occurring in response to drugs, bee stings and food allergies. The symptoms are, severe difficulty in breathing, rapid pulse, sweating and collapse. *See also* **allergy, sensitization**.

anaplasia   loss of the distinctive characteristics of a cell, associated with proliferative activity as in cancer.

anaplastic carcinoma   a malignant tumour of the thyroid gland which grows rapidly and is more common in the elderly. It is relatively resistant to radiotherapy.

anarthria   a severe form of dysarthria. The affected person is unable to produce the motor movements required for speech. The muscle weakness is apparent in the phonatory, articulatory, respiratory and resonatory speech systems. *See also* **dysarthria**.

anastomosis   the anatomical intercommunication of the branches of two or more tubular structures, for example, arteries or veins. In surgery, the establishment of an intercommunication between two hollow organs, vessels or nerves.

anatomical position   for the purpose of accurate description the anterior view is of the upright body facing forward, hands by the sides with palms facing forwards. The posterior view is of the back of the upright body in that position (see figure on p. 21).

ancylostomiasis (hookworm disease, miners' anaemia)   infestation of the human intestine with *Ancylostoma*, giving rise to malnutrition and severe anaemia.

androblastoma (arrhenoblastoma)   a tumour of the ovary; can produce male or female hormones and can cause masculinization in women or precocious puberty in girls.

androgens   steroid hormones secreted by the testes (testosterone) and adrenal cortex in both sexes. They have widespread anabolic effects, produce the male secondary sex characteristics, for example, male hair distribution and stimulate spermatogenesis.

anechoic   without echoes.

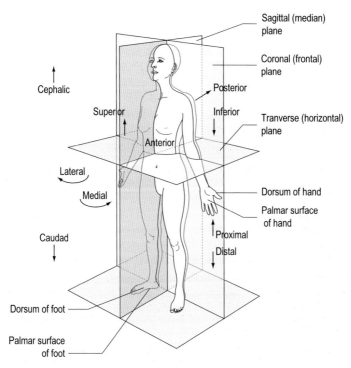

Anatomical position showing cardinal planes and directional terminology. From The physiotherapist's pocket book, J Kenyon and K Kenyon, 2004, Churchill Livingstone, Edinburgh, with permission.

anencephaly   absence of the cranial skull, which begins to ossify at 10 weeks interuterine life, and the brain. The condition is incompatible with life. It can be detected by raised levels of alphafetoprotein in the amniotic fluid.

aneuploidy   any variation in the number of chromosomes, refers to individual chromosomes rather than sets of chromosomes, for example, more chromosomes are present in Down syndrome.

aneurysm   local dilatation of a blood vessel, usually an artery, due to a local fault in the wall through defect, disease or injury, producing a swelling, often pulsating, over which a murmur may be heard. The pressure of blood can cause the swelling to increase in size and rupture. *See also* **dissecting aneurysm, fusiform aneurysm, saccular aneurysm**.

Angelman syndrome   an inherited condition that arises from mutations in the maternal chromosome 15 during formation of the gamete. Features include: 'puppet-like' gait, learning disability, brachycephaly (short, broad skull), inappropriate emotional outbursts, tongue protrusion and hooked nose.

angiectasis   abnormal dilatation of blood vessels. *See also* **telangiectasis**.

angiitis   inflammation of a blood or lymph vessel. *See also* **vasculitis**.

angina   sense of constriction.

angina pectoris   severe but temporary attack of cardiac pain that may radiate to the arms, throat, lower jaw or the back. Results from myocardial ischaemia. Often the attack is induced by exercise (angina of effort).

angiocardiography   the radiographic demonstration of the heart and great vessels by injecting a contrast agent via a catheter in the brachial or femoral arteries.

angiodysplasia   vascular malformation initially involving the large bowel, which may cause lower gastrointestinal bleeding.

angiogenesis   the formation of new blood vessels (vascularization), for example, during wound healing, or the development of new blood vessels supplying a tumour.

angiography   demonstration of the blood vessels of the arterial system after injection of a contrast agent into an artery.

angiology   the science dealing with blood and lymphatic vessels.

angioma   any bengin tumour with blood or lymph vessels.

angio-oedema (angioneurotic oedema)   a severe form of urticaria which may involve the skin of the face, hands or genitalia and the mucous membrane of the mouth and throat; oedema of the glottis may be fatal. Immediately there is an abrupt local increase in vascular permeability, as a result of which fluid escapes from blood vessels into surrounding tissues. Swelling may be due to an allergic hypersensitivity reaction to drugs, pollens or other known allergens, but in many cases no cause can be found.

angioplasty   surgery on a narrow artery to increase the blood flow through the vessel. *See also* **percutaneous transluminal angioplasty, transluminal angioplasty**.

angiosarcoma   a malignant tumour arising from blood vessels.

angiospasm   spasm of blood vessels.

angiotensin   a substance formed by the action of renin on a precursor protein in the blood plasma. In the lungs *angiotensin I* is converted into *angiotensin II*, a highly active substance which constricts blood vessels and causes release of aldosterone from the adrenal cortex in the angiotensin-aldosterone response.

angle of insonation   this is important in pulsed Doppler ultrasound examinations to obtain an accurate representation of blood flow and should be 60° or less.

angular frequency   in magnetic resonance is the frequency of oscillation or rotation.

anhydraemia   deficient fluid content of blood.

anhydrous   entirely without water, dry.

anicteric   without jaundice.

anion   a negatively charged ion, for example chloride (Cl^-). They move towards the positive electrode (anode) during electrolysis.

anion gap   the difference between the amount of anions and cations in the blood. *See also* **cation**.

aniridia   congenital absence of the iris.

anisomelia   unequal length of limbs.

ankle   the synovial saddle joint formed between the talus, fibula and tibia.

ankle equinus   a congenital or acquired condition or deformity, which is characterized by deficient dorsiflexion at the ankle joint. During the stance phase of normal gait a minimum 10° of ankle joint dorsiflexion is needed for normal walking. *See also* **talipes**.

alkylating agent   organic molecules that disrupt cell division by binding to the DNA in the nucleus. *See also* **cytotoxic**.

ankyloblepharon   adhesion of the eyelid margins, usually lateral, often secondary to chronic inflammation.

ankylosing spondylitis   an inflammatory condition affecting the spine and sacroiliac joints and characterized (in its later stages) by ossification of the spinal ligaments and ankylosis of sacroiliac joints. It occurs most commonly in young men. *See also* **spondylitis**.

ankylosis   stiffness or fixation of a joint. *See also* **spondylitis**.

annular   ring-shaped. ***annular ligaments*** hold in proximity two long bones, as in the wrist and ankle joints.

annular array   in ultrasound, using crystals of the same frequency which are arranged in a circle and are electronically focussed at several depths.

anode   part of an X-ray tube that is made of either copper with a tungsten target embedded in it, or molybdenum with a tungsten/rhenium target; the positive anode can be either stationary or rotating. The target is at an angle to produce a larger effective focal spot.

anode heel effect   due to the angle of the target on the anode of an X-ray tube, some of the radiation produced is absorbed by the target and therefore the intensity of the emergent X-ray beam is greater at the cathode end of the tube than at the anode end.

anogenital   associated with the anus and the genital region.

anomaly   that which is unusual or differs from the normal.

anomaly scan   an ultrasound scan undertaken in the second trimester, usually between 20 and 22 weeks, to look for any fetal abnormalities and the position of the placenta.

anoplasty   surgical repair or reconstruction of the anus.

anorchism   congenital absence of one or both testes.

anorectal   associated with the anus and rectum, for example, a fissure.

anorexia   lack of appetite for food. ***anorexia nervosa*** a psychological illness, most common in female adolescents. There is avoidance of carbohydrate intake leading to weight loss. There is associated over-exercising, purging and disturbance of body image. Can lead to mortality by starvation in severe cases. *See also* **eating disorders**.

anosmia   absence of the sense of smell.

anovular   relating to absence of ovulation.

anovular bleeding   occurs in dysfunctional uterine bleeding associated with hormone disturbance.

anovular menstruation   is bleeding as the result of taking oral contraceptives.

anoxaemia   literally, no oxygen in the blood. Usually used to indicate hypoxaemia.

anoxia   literally, no oxygen in the tissues. Usually used to signify hypoxia.

antagonist   a muscle that reverses or opposes the action of an agonist muscle. Also describes a drug or chemical that blocks the action of another molecule at a cell receptor site, for example, the narcotic antagonist naloxone reverses the action of opioid drugs. *See also* **agonist**.

antagonistic action   action performed by those muscles that limit the movement of an opposing group.

antegrade pyelography   the radiographic examination of the renal tract following the infusion of contrast agent directly into the renal pelvis.

anteflexion   the bending forward of an organ, commonly applied to the position of the uterus. *See also* **retroflexion**.

antemortem   before death. *See also* **postmortem**.

antenatal   before birth (prenatal). *See also* **postnatal**.

antepartum   before birth. From 24 weeks' gestation to full term. *See also* **postpartum**.

anterior   in front of; the front surface of; ventral. *See also* **posterior**.

anterior chamber   of the eye the space between the poster-ior surface of the cornea and the anterior surface of the iris. *See also* **aqueous**.

anterior tibial syndrome   severe pain and inflammation over anterior tibial muscle group, with inability to dorsiflex the foot.

anterograde   proceeding forward. *See also* **retrograde**.

anteroposterior radiograph   a radiograph taken from the front to the back of the body (see Figure on p. 25).

anteversion   the normal forward tilting, or displacement forward, of an organ or part. *See also* **retroversion**.

anthracosis accumulation of carbon in the lungs due to inhalation of coal dust; may cause fibrotic reaction. A form of pneumoconiosis.

anthrax a contagious disease of domestic animals such as cattle, which may be transmitted to humans by inoculation, inhalation and ingestion, causing malignant pustule (skin lesion) with septicaemia, inhalation anthrax or woolsorter's disease (haemorrhagic bronchopneumonia), meningitis and severe gastroenteritis. Causative organism is the bacterium *Bacillus anthracis*. Preventive measures include immunization of humans and animals, postexposure prophylaxis with antibiotics, for example, ciprofloxacin, and proper disposal of infected animals. Occupations at high risk include veterinary surgeons, livestock farmers, butchers, and those handling hides and wool.

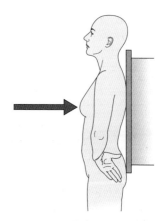

Anteroposterior (AP). From Pocketbook of radiographic positioning, 2nd edn, Ruth Sutherland, 2003, Churchill Livingstone, Edinburgh, with permission.

anthropoid resembling man. The word is also used to describe a pelvis that is narrow from side to side, a form of contracted pelvis.

anthropological baseline a line joining the infraorbital margin to the superior border of the external auditory meatus (see Figure below).

anthropology the study of humankind. Subdivided into several specialties. *See also* **ethnography**.

anthropometry measurement of the human body and its parts for the purposes of comparison and establishing norms for sex, age, weight, race and so on.

anti-anabolic preventing the synthesis of body protein.

antibacterial describes an agent that destroys bacteria or inhibits their growth. *See also* **antibiotics, antiseptics, bactericidal, bacteriostatic, disinfectants**.

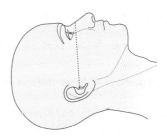

Anthropological baseline. From Pocketbook of radiographic positioning, 2nd edn, Churchill Livingstone, Ruth Sutherland, 2003, Edinburgh, with permission.

antibiotic the term generally used for all drugs that act against bacteria. Some have a narrow spectrum of activity whereas others act against a wide range of bacteria (broad spectrum).

antibodies   a substance, either natural or introduced, that helps to protect the body against infection.

anticoagulant   an agent that reduces the propensity of blood to clot. Uses: (a) to obtain specimens suitable for pathological examination and chemical analyses where whole blood or plasma is required instead of serum; (b) during the collection of blood for transfusion, the anticoagulant usually being sodium citrate; (c) as therapy in the prophylaxis and treatment of thromboembolic conditions, for example, heparin.

anticoagulation   the process of suppressing or reducing blood coagulation.

anti-curl backing   used for single emulsion films and coat the opposite side of the base from the emulsion to prevent the film from curling.

anti-D   an antibody directed against the Rhesus D blood group antigen. Given to RhD-negative women who have RhD-positive babies to prevent subsequent immune-mediated disease such as haemolytic disease of the newborn.

antidiuretic   reducing the volume of urine.

antidiuretic hormone (ADH)   vasopressin.

antiemetic   any agent such as a drug that prevents or treats nausea and vomiting.

antienzyme   a substance that exerts a specific inhibiting action on an enzyme. Found in the digestive tract to prevent autodigestion of the mucosa, and in blood where they act as immunoglobulins.

anti-frothant   a chemical added to the developer to reduce foaming due to agitation of the developer by the rollers.

anti-GBM disease   disease caused by specific antibodies to the glomerular basement membranes. It features rapidly progressive glomerulonephritis and pulmonary haemorrhage. Previously known as *Goodpasture's disease.*

antigen   substance that stimulates the production of a specific immune response.

antihaemophilic factor (AHF)   factor VIII in the blood coagulation cascade, present in plasma. A deficiency causes haemophilia A (classical).

anti-halation layer   a coloured dye in the anti-curl backing of a film to absorb any reflected light and therefore prevent unsharpness on the film.

antihistamine   a drug which suppresses some of the effects of histamine released in the body as a result of an allergic reaction.

antihypertensive   describes any agent that reduces high blood pressure.

anti-infective   describes any agent which prevents infection.

anti-inflammatory   tending to prevent or relieve inflammation.

antilymphocyte globulin (ALG)   an immunoglobulin which binds to antigens on T cells and inhibits T cell-dependent immune responses; occasionally used in preventing graft rejection during organ transplantation.

antimetabolites   one of a group of chemical compounds which prevent the effective use of the corresponding metabolite, and interfere with normal growth or cell mitosis if the process requires that metabolite.

antimitochondrial antibody (AMA)   autoantibodies against mitochondrial components. Certain types are a marker for primary biliary cirrhosis.

antineoplastic   describes any substance or procedure that kills or slows the growth of cancerous/neoplastic cells, such as cytotoxic chemotherapy, radiotherapy, or hormonal or biological response modification therapy.

anti-neutrophil cytoplasmic antibody (ANCA)   a group of autoantibodies directed against cytoplasmic components of neutrophils and associated with a range of pathological conditions such as polyarteritis.

antinuclear antibody (ANA)   a family of many types of autoantibody directed against cell nuclei that are found in connective tissue disorders, particularly systemic lupus erythematosus (SLE) and Sjögren syndrome. The many types recognized can be used to categorize rheumatological disorders.

antioxidants   substances that delay the process of oxidation. Some minerals, for example, zinc, and vitamins A, C and E, contained in a balanced diet, function as antioxidants and help to minimize free radical oxidative damage to cells.

antiperistalsis   reversal of the normal peristaltic action.

antiprothrombin (anticoagulant)   stops blood coagulation by preventing conversion of prothrombin into thrombin.

antisepsis   prevention of sepsis (tissue infection); introduced into surgical procedures in 1880 by Lord Lister.

antiseptics   chemical substances that destroy or inhibit the growth of microorganisms. They can be applied to living tissues, for example, chlorhexidine used for skin preparation before invasive procedures and hand decontamination.

antiserum   serum prepared from the blood of an animal immunized by the requisite antigen, containing a high concentration of polyclonal antibodies against that antigen.

antispasmodic (spasmolytic)   describes any measure or drugs used to relieve spasm in muscle.

antistatic   preventing the accumulation of static electricity.

antistreptolysin   against streptolysins. A raised antistreptolysin titre in the blood is indicative of recent streptococcal infection.

antithrombin III   substance that inhibits blood coagulation. It is synthesized in the liver and is normally present in the blood, where it restricts coagulation to areas where it is needed. *See also* **thrombin**.

antithyroid   any agent used to decrease the activity of the thyroid gland.

antitoxin   an antibody which neutralizes a given toxin. Made in response to the invasion by toxin-producing bacteria, or the injection of toxoids.

antituberculosis drugs   drugs used in the treatment of tuberculosis.

antitumour antibiotics   cytotoxic antibiotics that act against tumour cells by disrupting cell membranes and DNA. *See also* **cytotoxic**.

antitussive   describes any measures which suppress a cough.

antiviral   acting against viruses.

antrectomy   surgical excision of the antrum of the stomach.

antro-oral   associated with the maxillary antrum and the mouth.

antrostomy   surgical opening from nasal cavity to antrum of Highmore (maxillary sinus).

antrum   a cavity, especially in bone.

anuria   complete absence of urine output by the kidneys.

anus   the end of the alimentary canal, at the extreme termination of the rectum. It is formed of a sphincter muscle which relaxes to allow faecal matter to pass through. *See also* **artificial anus, imperforate anus**.

aorta   the main artery arising out of the left ventricle of the heart.

aortic   associated with the aorta.

aortic incompetence   regurgitation of blood from the aorta back into the left ventricle.

aortic murmur   abnormal heart sound heard over aortic area; a ***systolic murmur*** alone is the murmur of aortic stenosis, a ***diastolic murmur*** denotes aortic regurgitation.

aortic regurgitation (incompetence)   regurgitation of blood from aorta back into the left ventricle.

aortic stenosis   narrowing of aortic valve. This is usually due to rheumatic heart disease or a congenital bicuspid valve which predisposes to the deposit of calcium.

aortitis   inflammation of the aorta.

aortography   demonstration of the aorta after introduction of a radiographic contrast agent, either via a catheter passed along the femoral or brachial artery or by direct translumbar injection.

aperient   a mild drug given to produce peristaltic action in the bowel and therefore emptying. *See also* **laxative**.

aperistalsis   absence of peristaltic movement in the bowel. Characterizes the condition of paralytic ileus.

Apert's syndrome   congenital craniosynostosis accompanied by deformities of the hands. *See also* **acrocephalosyndactyly, syndactyly**.

apex   the summit or top of anything which is cone-shaped, for example, the tip of a lung. In a heart of normal size the ***apex beat*** (systolic impulse) can be seen or felt in the 5th left intercostal space in the mid-clavicular line. It is the lowest and most lateral point at which an impulse can be detected and provides a rough indication of the size of the heart.

Apgar score   a measure used to evaluate the general condition of a newborn baby, developed by an American anaesthetist, Dr Virginia Apgar. A score of 0, 1 or 2 is given for the criteria of heart rate, respiratory effort, skin colour, muscle tone and response to stimulation. A score between 8 and 10 indicates a baby in good condition.

aphagia   inability to swallow.

aphakia   absence of the lens. Describes the eye after removal of a cataract without artificial lens implantation.

aphasia   a language disorder that follows brain damage, due primarily to an impaired linguistic system. The term does not describe language disorders that involve problems with expression or comprehension caused by mental health problems, including psychoses, confusion and dementia, or muscle weakness, or problems with hearing. There are several classifications but generally aphasia is described as being expressive (motor) aphasia or receptive (sensory) aphasia. However, many people exhibit problems with both language expression and comprehension. *See also* **dysarthria**.

aphonia   inability to make sound due to neurological, behavioural, psychogenic or organic causes. *See also* **dysarthria**.

aphthae   small ulcers of the gastrointestinal mucosa surrounded by a ring of erythema.

apical   the summit or apex.

apical projection   a radiographic examination of the lung apices, using an angled beam to project the clavicles away from the lung tissue.

apical foramen   a hole at the base of the root of a tooth which allows the passage of blood vessels and nerves.

apicectomy   excision of the apex of the root of a tooth.

aplasia   incomplete development of tissue or an organ; absence of growth.

aplastic   without structure or form. Incapable of forming new tissue. ***aplastic anaemia*** is the result of complete bone marrow failure.

apnoea   absence of breathing for short periods as seen in Cheyne–Stokes respiration. It is due to lack of the necessary CO_2 tension in the blood for stimulation of the respiratory centre. *See also* **periodic breathing**.

apocrine glands   modified sweat glands, especially in axillae, genital and perineal regions. Responsible after puberty for body odour. *See also* **eccrine**.

apodia   congenital absence of the feet.

aponeurosis   a broad glistening sheet of tendon-like tissue which serves to invest and attach muscles, for example, abdominal muscles, to each other, and also to the parts that they move.

aponeurositis   inflammation of an aponeurosis.

apophysis   a projection, protuberance or outgrowth. Usually used in connection with bone.

apoplexy   obsolete term for cerebrovascular accident (stroke).

apoptosis   programmed cell death.

apparent focal spot   the target of an X-ray tube is at an angle to allow a larger area to be struck by electrons while still maintaining the smaller, apparent, focal spot when viewing from the tube port.

appendectomy   *see* **appendicectomy**.

appendicectomy   excision of the veriform appendix.

appendicitis   inflammation of the veriform appendix.

appendicular skeleton   the bones forming the pectoral girdle, upper limbs, pelvic girdle and lower limbs.

appendix   an appendage. ***veriform appendix*** a worm-like appendage of the caecum about the thickness of a pencil and usually measuring from 2.5 to 15 cm in length. It contains lymphoid tissue and its position is variable.

appetite   the desire for food, influenced by physical activity, metabolic, dietary, psychological and behavioural factors. It may be increased or decreased pharmacologically. Appetite is also influenced by health status. *See also* **anorexia, bulimia, eating disorders**.

applicator   an instrument used for local application of remedies, for example, vaginal medication applicator. In radiotherapy attached to the tube housing to provide an accurate means of setting up the source–skin distance and is a form of secondary collimation. *See also* **Fulfield applicator**.

apposition   the approximation or bringing together of two surfaces or edges.

appraisal   making a valuation. ***performance appraisal*** or ***review*** a formal procedure whereby an appraiser (manager) systematically reviews the role performance of the appraisee and they jointly set goals for the future.

approved name   the generic or non-proprietary name of a drug, such as salbutamol. Should be used in prescribing except in the case of drugs where bioavailability differs between brands.

apraxia   inability to perform a motor act or use an object normally, due typically to damage in the parietal lobe of the brain.

apyrexia   absence of fever.

aqueduct   a canal. ***aqueduct of Sylvius*** the canal connecting the 3rd and 4th ventricles of the brain; aqueductus cerebri.

aqueous watery.

aqueous humour the fluid contained in the anterior and posterior chambers of the eye.

arachnodactyly congenital abnormality resulting in long, slender fingers. Said to resemble spider legs (hence 'spider fingers').

arachnoid resembling a spider's web.

arachnoid mater (membrane) a delicate membrane enveloping the brain and spinal cord, lying between the pia mater internally and the dura mater externally; the middle membrane of the meninges.

arborization an arrangement resembling the branching of a tree. Characterizes both ends of a neuron, i.e. the dendrites and the axon as it supplies each muscle fibre.

arboviruses abbreviation for ARthropod-BOrne viruses. Include various RNA viruses transmitted by arthropods: mosquitoes, ticks, sandflies, etc. They cause diseases such as yellow fever, dengue, sandfly fever and several types of encephalitis.

arch aortography the radiographic examination of the aorta and its major branches by injecting a contrast agent via femoral or axillary catheterization.

arch of aorta the proximal one of the four portions of the aorta giving rise to the three arterial branches called the innominate (brachiocephalic) left common carotid and left subclavian arteries.

archival permanence the length of time a radiographic film can be stored without significant deterioration of image quality.

arc therapy when a source of radiation moves through a prescribed angle during treatment.

arcus senilis an opaque ring round the edge of the cornea, seen in old people.

areola the pigmented area round the nipple of the breast. A ***secondary areola*** surrounds the primary areola in pregnancy.

areolar tissue a loose connective tissue consisting of cells and fibres in a semisolid matrix.

arginase an enzyme present in the liver, kidney and spleen. It converts arginine into ornithine and urea.

ariboflavinosis a deficiency state caused by lack of riboflavin and other members of the vitamin B complex. Characterized by cheilosis, seborrhoea, angular stomatitis, glossitis and photophobia.

Arnold–Chiari malformation a group of disorders affecting the base of the brain. Commonly occurs in hydrocephalus associated with meningocele and myelomeningocele. There are degrees of severity but usually there is some 'kinking' or 'buckling' of the brainstem with cerebellar tissue herniating through the foramen magnum at the base of the skull.

array   an arrangement of components. *See also* **annular array, linear array, curved array, phased array**.

arrectores pilorum   internal, plain, involuntary muscles attached to hair follicles, which, by contraction, erect the hair follicles, causing 'gooseflesh'.

arrhythmia   any deviation from the normal rhythm, usually referring to the heart beat. *See also* **asystole, extrasystole, fibrillation, heart, tachycardia**.

artefact   in magnetic resonance where an additional image occurs in the reconstructed image which does not match the anatomy or pathology in the patient. In ultrasound an abnormality on an image which is due to data acquisition, processing or the nature of the ultrasound beam.

arterial blood gases (ABGs)   measurement of the oxygen (PaO_2), carbon dioxide ($PaCO_2$) and acid–base (pH or hydrogen ion concentration) content of the arterial blood.

arterial haemorrhage   the loss of blood from an artery.

arterial line   cannula placed in an artery to sample blood for gas analysis and for continuous blood pressure monitoring. Usually used only in specialist units (ITU, HDU and theatre) because of the potential risk of severe blood loss. They should always be attached to a pressure transducer and monitor, and have an alarm that indicates any disconnection. *See also* **arterial blood gases, blood pressure**.

arterial ulcer   a leg ulcer caused by a defect in arterial blood supply. They are found on the foot, usually between the toes or close to the ankle; the adjacent skin is discoloured, shiny and hairless; and the ulcer is small and deep with some exudate. They are often associated with a history of cardiovascular disease or diabetes mellitus.

arteriography   demonstration of the arterial system after injection of a radiographic contrast agent.

arteriole   a small artery, joining an artery to a capillary network. They control the amount of blood entering the capillary network. They are able to constrict and dilate to change peripheral resistance thereby influencing blood pressure.

arteriopathy   disease of any artery.

arterioplasty   reconstructive surgery applied to an artery.

arteriosclerosis   degenerative arterial change associated with advancing age. Primarily a thickening of the media (middle) layer and usually associated with some degree of atheroma.

arteriotomy   incision or needle puncture of an artery.

arteriovenous   associated with an artery and a vein.

arteriovenous fistula   the artificial connection of an artery to a vein to promote the enlargement of the latter, to facilitate the removal and replacement of blood during haemodialysis.

arteriovenous shunt   the direct connection between an artery and a vein.

arteritis   an inflammatory disease affecting the media (middle) layer of arteries. It may be due to an infection such as syphilis or it may be part of a collagen disease. The arteries may become swollen and tender and the blood may clot in them.

artery   a vessel carrying blood from the heart to the various tissues. The internal endothelial lining provides a smooth surface to prevent clotting of blood. The middle layer of plain muscle and elastic fibres allows for distension as blood is pumped from the heart. The outer, mainly connective tissue layer prevents overdistension. The lumen is largest nearest to the heart; it gradually decreases in size.

artery forceps   forceps used to produce the arrest of bleeding or the slowing of blood flow (haemostasis).

arthralgia (articular neuralgia, arthrodynia)   pain in a joint, used especially when there is no inflammation. *Intermittent* or *periodic arthralgia* is the term used when there is pain, usually accompanied by swelling of the knee at regular intervals.

arthritis   inflammation of one or more joints which swell, become warm to touch, and are tender and painful on movement. There are many causes and the treatment varies according to the cause. *See also* **gout, osteoarthritis, rheumatoid arthritis, Still's disease**.

arthroclasis   breaking down of adhesions within the joint cavity to produce a wider range of movement.

arthrodesis   the stiffening of a joint by surgical means.

arthrodynia   painful joints. *See also* **arthralgia**.

arthrography   a radiographic examination to determine the internal structure of a joint, outlined by contrast agent – either a gas or a liquid contrast agent, or both.

arthrology   the science that studies the structure and function of joints, their diseases and treatment.

arthropathy   any joint disease. The condition is currently classified as: *enteropathic arthropathies* resulting from chronic diarrhoeal disease; *psoriatic arthropathies* psoriasis; *seronegative arthropathies* include all other instances of inflammatory arthritis other than rheumatoid arthritis; *seropositive arthropathies* include all instances of rheumatoid arthritis.

arthroplasty   surgical remodelling of a joint, replacement arthroplasty of the hip, insertion of an inert prosthesis of similar shape, total replacement arthroplasty of the hip, replacement of the head of femur and the acetabulum, both being cemented into the bone.

arthroscope   an instrument used for the visualization of the interior of a joint cavity.

arthroscopy   the act of visualizing the interior of a joint. Uses an intra-articular camera to assess, repair or reconstruct various tissues within and around joints.

arthrosis   degeneration in a joint.

arthrotomy   incision into a joint.

articular   associated with a joint or articulation. Applied to cartilage, surface, capsule, etc.

articulation   the junction of two or more bones; a joint. Enunciation of speech.

artificial anus   *see* **colostomy**.

artificial blood   a fluid able to transport O_2.

artificial kidney   *see* **dialyser**.

artificial limb   *see* **orthosis, prosthesis**.

artificial lung   *see* **respirator**.

artificial menopause   an earlier menopause caused by surgery or radiotherapy.

artificial pacemaker   cardiac pacemaker. *See also* **cardiac**.

artificial pneumothorax   *see* **pneumothorax**.

artificial respiration   *see* **cardiopulmonary resuscitation**.

asbestos   a fibrous, mineral substance which does not conduct heat and is incombustible. It has many uses, including brake linings, asbestos textiles and asbestos-cement sheeting.

asbestosis   a form of pneumoconiosis from inhalation of asbestos dust and fibre. *See also* **mesothelioma**.

ascariasis   infestation by nematodes (roundworms). The ova are ingested and hatch in the duodenum. The larvae pass to the lungs in the blood, from where they ascend to be swallowed and returned to the bowel. They may occasionally obstruct the intestine or the bile ducts.

Aschoff's nodules   nodules present in the myocardium in myocarditis caused by rheumatic fever.

ASCII (American Standard Code for Information Interchange)   defines the decimal and binary code of all the characters stored in a computer.

ascites (hydroperitoneum)   free fluid in the peritoneal cavity, well demonstrated by using ultrasound.

asepsis   the condition of being free from living pathogenic micro-organisms.

aseptic technique   describes procedures used to exclude pathogenic micro-organisms from an environment. It includes the use of sterile gloves and gowns in theatre, non-touch technique and the use of sterilized equipment.

Used where there is a possibility of introducing microorganisms into the patient's body.

Askin tumour   highly malignant tumour of the chest wall.

asomatogosia   loss of awareness of parts of the body (soma) and their position in space, a perceptual sequela of cerebrovascular accident (stroke) affecting the right parietal lobe of the cerebrum, which may lead to lack of awareness, even denial, of the presence of disability.

asparaginase   an enzyme derived from microorganisms. In the form of crisantaspase, used pharmacologically to treat cancers, for example, acute lymphoblastic leukaemia. *See also* **cytotoxic**.

asparagine   a conditionally essential (indispensable) amino acid.

aspartate (aspartic acid)   a non-essential (dispensable) amino acid.

Asperger's syndrome   a pervasive developmental disorder sharing characteristics with autism, without delayed language or cognitive development. The relationship of Asperger's syndrome to autism remains unclear.

aspergillosis   opportunist infection, most frequently of lungs, caused by any species of *Aspergillus*. *See also* **bronchomycosis**.

Aspergillus   a genus of fungi, found in soil, manure and on various grains. Some species are pathogenic.

asphyxia   a deficiency of oxygen in the blood and an increase in carbon dioxide in the blood and tissues. Common causes are drowning, electric shock, a foreign body in the air passages, inhalation of smoke or poisonous gasses, trauma or disease of the lungs or air passages.

aspiration (paracentesis, tapping)   the removal of fluids from a body cavity by means of suction or siphonage such as fluid from the peritoneal cavity, postoperative gastric aspiration, etc. Describes the entry of fluids or food into the airway.

aspiration pneumonia   inflammation of lung from inhalation of foreign body, most often food particles or fluids. *See also* **Heimlich's manoeuvre**.

aspirator   a negative pressure device used for withdrawing fluids from body cavities.

assault   threat of unlawful contact. Constitutes trespass against the person. *See also* **battery**.

assay   a quantitative test used to measure the amount of a substance present or its level of activity, for example, hormones or drugs. The analysis of the purity or effectiveness of a substance.

assimilation   the process whereby digested foodstuffs are absorbed and used by the cells and tissues.

assisted conception   techniques used when normal methods of conception have failed. They include in vitro fertilization (IVF) and transcervical embryo transfer or gamete intrafallopian tube transfer (GIFT), zygote intrafallopian transfer (ZIFT), preimplantation genetic diagnosis (PGD) and intracytoplasmic sperm injection (ICSI).

asthenia   lack of strength; weakness, debility.

asthma   gasping for breath, wheezing and difficulty in expiration because of muscular spasm in the bronchi. Inhaled or oral corticosteroids reduce the acute immune reaction, while inhaled β_2 receptor-agonists relieve bronchial spasm.

astigmatism   light from one point not focussing on another point.

astringent   describes an agent which contracts organic tissue, thus lessening secretion. May be used in the management of heavily exuding wounds.

astrocyte   a star-shaped neuroglial cell.

astrocytoma   a slowly invasive primary tumour of the brain.

asymmetry   lack of similarity of the organs or parts on each side.

asymptomatic   symptomless.

asystole   absence of heart beat. One type of cardiac arrest.

ataxia (ataxy)   failure of voluntary muscle coordination resulting in irregular jerky movements and unsteadiness.

atelectasis   numbers of pulmonary alveoli do not contain air due to failure of expansion (***congenital atelectasis***) or resorption of air from the alveoli (collapse).

atheroma   fatty deposits in an artery wall.

atherosclerosis   coexisting atheroma and arteriosclerosis.

athletic trainer   a term used in North America for an individual who is trained in the prevention, evaluation, treatment and rehabilitation of athletic injuries.

atlanto-axial joint   a joint between the odontoid process of the axis (second cervical vertebra) and a facet on the arch of the atlas (the first cervical vertebra).

atlas   the first cervical vertebra.

ATM (Asynchronous Transfer Mode)   a computer circuit which is made when a computer is connected to the internet to enable the transfer of data at speeds of up to 155 Mb/s.

atom   a particle with a nucleus which contains protons which carry a positive charge, surrounded by orbiting electrons which carry a negative charge. The smallest particle of an element capable of existing individually, or in combination with one or more atoms of the same or another element.

atomic mass number (A)   the total number of nucleons in the nucleus of an atom.

atomic mass unit (amu) or Dalton   a relative weight used to measure atoms and subatomic particles. Protons and neutrons have both been designated as being 1 amu. ***atomic number*** the number of protons in the atomic nucleus or the number of electrons, such as hydrogen which, with one of each, has the atomic number 1.

atomic number (Z)   the number of protons in the nucleus of an atom.

atomic weight (mass) (or relative atomic mass)   the relative average mass of an atom based on the mass of an atom of carbon-12.

atomizer   nebulizer.

atonia   total flaccidity or no muscle tone caused by complete loss of motor supply to a muscle.

atopic dermatitis   that variety of infantile eczema that may be associated with asthma or hay fever.

atopic syndrome   a hereditary predisposition to develop hypersensitivity disorders, such as eczema, asthma, hay fever and allergic rhinitis. Associated with excess IgE production.

atresia   closure, or lack of a normal body opening, duct or canal such as the bowel or bile duct.

atrial fibrillation   a cardiac arrhythmia. Chaotic irregularity of atrial rhythm with an irregular ventricular response. Commonly associated with mitral stenosis, hyperthyroidism (thyrotoxicosis) or heart failure.

atrial flutter   a cardiac arrhythmia caused by irritable focus in atrial muscle and usually associated with coronary heart disease. Speed of atrial beats is between 260 and 340 per minute. The ventricular response is slower and may respond to every four atrial beats.

atrial septal defect   a hole in the atrial septum. Most commonly due to a congenital defect. Types include: ***ostium secundum defect***, which is most common and is situated around the site of the foramen ovale; and ***ostium primum defects*** situated lower down on the atrial septum.

atrioventricular (A-V)   associated with the atria and the ventricles of the heart. Applied to a node, tract and valves.

atrioventricular bundle   part of the conducting system of the heart. Carries impulses from the atrioventricular node to the ventricles. Divides into right and left bundle branches that transmit the impulses to the apex of each ventricle. ***atrioventricular node*** part of the conducting system of the heart. Situated at the bottom of the right atrium, it transmits impulses from the sinus node to the atrioventricular bundle. Also known as the ***bundle of His***

atrium   cavity, entrance or passage. One of the two upper receiving chambers of the heart.

atrophy   loss of substance of cells, tissues or organs. There is wasting and a decrease in size and function. The process may be physiological such as that occurring as part of normal ageing, or pathological, as in disuse atrophy when a limb is immobilized. *See also* **motor neuron disease**.

atropine   the principal alkaloid of belladonna.

attachment   a document sent with an e-mail. In psychology a term describing the dependent relationship which one individual forms with another, emanating from the unique bonding between infant and parent figure.

attenuation   absorption. The process by which pathogenic micro-organisms are induced to develop or show less virulent characteristics, they can then be used in the preparation of vaccines. It is a measure of the absorption of an X-ray beam along a specific path through a substance. Of ultrasound at diagnostic frequencies, attenuation is approximately proportional to frequency, with the higher frequencies being absorbed more than the lower frequencies, the weakening of ultrasound as it goes through tissue due to absorption, reflection and scattering of the sound wave, measured in decibels. *See also* **linear attenuation coefficient**.

attenuation coefficient   is a measure of the attenuation of an X-ray beam along a specific path through a substance. *See also* **linear attenuation coefficient**.

atypical   not typical; unusual, irregular; not conforming to type, for example, atypical pneumonia.

audiology   the scientific study of hearing.

audit   investigative methods used to systematically measure outcomes and review performance. *See also* **medical audit**.

Audit Commission   within the NHS the main role of the Audit Commission is to promote 'best practice' in terms of economy, effectiveness and efficiency.

audit trail   a way of working and record keeping that allows the processes to be transparent and clear.

auditory   associated with the sense of hearing.

auditory acuity   ability to hear clearly and distinctly. Tests include the use of tuning fork, whispered voice and audiometer. Hearing can be tested in babies by otoacoustic emission testing (OAE).

auditory area   that portion of the temporal lobe of the cerebral cortex which interprets sound.

auditory canal (external auditory meatus)   the canal between the pinna and eardrum.

auditory nerves   the eighth pair of cranial nerves. Also called the ***vestibulo-cochlear nerve***.

auditory ossicles   three small bones – malleus, incus and stapes – located within the middle ear.

auger electrons   are ejected during radioactive decay and have discrete energy levels equal to the photon energy minus the binding energy of the electron.

aura   a premonition; a peculiar sensation or warning of an impending attack, such as occurs in epilepsy or migraine.

aural   associated with the ear.

auricle   the pinna of the external ear. An appendage to the cardiac atrium. Obsolete term for atrium.

auricular   ear shaped.

auricular line   a line perpendicular to the anthropological base line through the centre of the external auditory meatus. *See also* **anthropological base line**.

auriculoventricular   obsolete term. *See* **atrioventricular**.

auriscope   *see* **otoscope**.

auscultation   examination of the internal organs by listening to the sounds they produce.

autoantibody   an antibody which binds self-antigen expressed in normal tissue.

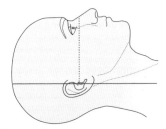

Auricular line. From Pocketbook of radiographic positioning, 2nd edn, Ruth Sutherland, 2003, Churchill Livingstone, Edinburgh, with permission.

autoantigen   a self-antigen, expressed in normal tissue, which is the target of autoantibodies or self-reactive T cells.

autoclave   apparatus for high-pressure steam sterilization, to sterilize in an autoclave.

autodigestion   self-digestion of body tissue during life.

autogenic   describes a process or condition that originates from within the organism.

autogenic facilitation   reflex activation of a muscle through activation of its own sensory receptors; self-generated excitation of muscle, for example, the stretch reflex.

autogenic inhibition reflex   inhibition of a muscle through activation of stretch receptors, the Golgi tendon organs, in its own tendons; self-generated relaxation of muscle that normally prevents build-up of too much, potentially injurious, tension in a muscle.

autogenic therapy   a complementary therapy that employs a combination of self-hypnosis and relaxation.

autograft   tissue grafted from one part of the body to another.

autoimmune disease   an illness caused by, or associated with, the development of an immune response to normal body tissues.

autoimmunity   the production of antibodies against the subjects own tissue.

autoinfection   self-infection or pathogens transferred from one part of the body to another, for example by the hands or towels etc.

autointoxication   poisoning from abnormal or excessive metabolic products produced in the body, some of which may originate from infected or necrotic tissue.

autologous   when a patient acts as the source of cells. This may include a patient donating blood or blood products prior to elective surgery to be transfused postoperatively. Cross-matching and compatibility problems are avoided, as is the risk of blood-borne infections.

autologous bone marrow transplant   when a patient is in remission their bone marrow or peripheral blood stem cells are harvested and then reinfused to reinforce the bone marrow. May be performed for patients with leukaemia. Their bone marrow or peripheral blood stem cells are harvested, stored and replaced after leukaemic cells have been destroyed with cytotoxic chemotherapy or radiotherapy.

autologous implants   implants using tissue obtained from the same patient.

automated peritoneal dialysis (APD)   a type of peritoneal dialysis where the fluid exchanges are performed at night by the use of a mechanical device.

automatic   occurring without the influence of the will; spontaneous; without volition; involuntary acts.

automatic chemical mixers   equipment to mix the processing chemicals used to minimize the handling of chemicals by the staff, to promote even mixing and reduce chemical fumes.

automatic shuttering   in digital imaging, the automatic blackening of the film outside the collimated image to increase the subjective contrast of the image. *See also* **subjective contrast**.

autonomic   independent; self-governing.

autonomic nervous system (ANS)   is divided into parasympathetic and sympathetic portions. They are made up of nerve cells and fibres which cannot be controlled at will. They are concerned with the control of glandular secretion and involuntary muscle.

autopsy   the examination of a dead body (cadaver) for diagnostic purposes.

autosome   in humans one of 44 (22 pairs) non-sex chromosomes. The full chromosome complement of 46 (23 pairs) found in somatic cells comprises 44 autosomes and two sex chromosomes.

autosomal inheritance   is determined by the expression or not of genes on the autosomes. It may be dominant or recessive.

autotransformer   a type of transformer where the primary and secondary coils are wound round a single core; it is used when only low-voltage changes are required.

avascular   bloodless; not vascular, i.e. without blood supply.

avascular necrosis   death of tissue due to complete depletion of its blood supply. Usually applied to that of bone tissue following injury or possibly through disease. Commonly seen with fractures of the femoral neck, leading to death of the femoral head. Also seen in scaphoid and head of humerus fractures. Often a precursor of osteoarthritis.

average dose in radiotherapy the value of dose calculated by adding together all the individual radiation doses in the area and then dividing the total by the number of doses.

average gradient a method of measuring the straight line portion of a characteristic curve to determine the contrast of a film. A right angle triangle is drawn on the characteristic curve with the hypotenuse of the triangle extending from density 0.25 and 2 on the straight line portion of the curve. The angle between the hypotenuse and the horizontal line of the triangle is calculated, therefore the tangent of the angle the slope makes equals the average gradient. *See also* **contrast**.

averaging a method of improving the signal-to-noise ratio in magnetic resonance imaging. The same magnetic resonance signal is added up and the total is divided by the number of signals.

avian relating to birds.

avian tuberculosis is caused by *Mycobacterium avium* complex (MAC) or *M. avium-intracellulare* (MAI), which also cause atypical tuberculosis in humans, especially in immunocompromised individuals.

avitaminosis any disease resulting from a deficiency of vitamins.

Avogadro's number is 6×10^{23} molecules which is the number of molecules in a mole.

avulsion a forcible wrenching away of a structure or part of the body.

avulsion fracture a fracture caused by the tearing away of a fragment of bone by a ligament or tendon.

axes the vertical (y axis) and horizontal (x axis) lines on a graph.

axial projection a radiograph taken when either a joint is flexed and/or the beam angled.

axial resolution in ultrasound, the ability to see small structures along the beam; this is dependent on the pulse length which is determined by the wavelength. When the distance between two reflecting surfaces of the object is half the pulse length or less the object will not be demonstrated.

axial skeleton the bones forming the head and trunk.

axilla the armpit.

axillary applied to nerves, blood and lymphatic vessels, of the axilla.

axis the second cervical vertebra. An imaginary line passing through the centre; the median line of the body.

axon the long process of a nerve cell conveying impulses away from the cell body.

axonotmesis (neuronotmesis, neurotmesis) peripheral degeneration as a result of damage to the axons of a nerve, through pinching, crushing or prolonged pressure. The internal architecture is preserved and recovery depends upon regeneration of the axons, and may take many months.

axon reflex   reflex dilatation of the arterioles occurring when sensory nerves in the skin are stimulated by massage manipulations or trauma.

azoospermia   absence of spermatozoa in the semen.

azygos   occurring singly, not paired.

azygos veins   three unpaired veins of the abdomen and thorax which empty into the inferior vena cava.

B

. . . .

B₀ the symbol used for the static main magnetic field, in magnetic resonance imaging, which is orientated along the x axis and measured in Tesla.

B₁ the symbol used for radiofrequency magnetic field, in a magnetic resonance imaging system, and measured in Tesla.

Babinski's reflex or sign movement of the great toe upwards (dorsiflexion) instead of downwards (plantar flexion) on stroking the sole of the foot. It is indicative of disease or injury to upper motor neurons. Babies exhibit dorsiflexion, but after learning to walk they show the normal plantar flexion response.

bacillaemia the presence of bacilli in the blood.

bacille Calmette–Guérin a form of tubercle bacilli; it has lost its power to cause tuberculosis, but retains its antigenic function; it is the base of a vaccine used for immunization against tuberculosis. Also used in urology for the treatment of high-risk superficial bladder cancer.

bacillus colloquial term for any rod-shaped microorganism.

Bacillus a type of bacteria consisting of aerobic, Gram-positive, rod-shaped cells that produce endospores. The majority have flagella and are motile. The spores are common in soil and dust.

Bacillus anthracis bacteria which cause anthrax in humans and domestic animals.

Bacillus cereus bacteria which produce exotoxins and cause food poisoning. It can occur after eating cooked food, for example, rice, that has been stored prior to reheating.

back pointer used in radiotherapy to indicate the central exit point of the radiation. *See also* **front pointer**.

back projection mathematical basis for tomographic imaging. In CT scanning in order to overcome the blurring inherent in this method a filtered back projection is used, resulting in a sharper image.

back scatter radiation that having passed through the object hits a surface, for example the couch, and is reflected back onto the original object.

bacteraemia the presence of bacteria in the blood.

bacteria microscopic unicellular organisms widely distributed in the environment. Pathogens may be virulent and always cause infection, whereas others, known as opportunists, usually only cause infection when the host defences are impaired, such as during cancer chemotherapy. Non-pathogenic bacteria may become pathogenic if they move from their normal site, for example, intestinal bacteria causing a wound infection. Bacteria are classified and identified by features that include: shape and staining characteristics with Gram stain (positive or negative). Bacteria may be: (a) round (cocci), paired (diplococci), in bunches (staphylococci) or in chains (streptococci); (b) rod-shaped (bacilli); or (c) curved or spiral (vibrios, spirilla and spirochaetes).

bacterial   associated with bacteria.

bactericidal   describes agents that kill bacteria, for example, some antibiotics.

bactericidin   antibody that kills bacteria.

bacteriologist   an expert in bacteriology.

bacteriology   the scientific study of bacteria.

bacteriolysin   a specific antibody formed in the blood that causes bacteria to break up.

bacteriolysis   the disintegration and dissolution of bacteria.

bacteriophage   a virus parasitic on bacteria. Some of these are used in phage-typing staphylococci, etc.

bacteriostatic   describes an agent that inhibits bacterial growth, for example, some antibiotics.

bacteriuria   the presence of bacteria in the urine (100 000 or more pathogenic microorganisms per millilitre). Acute cystitis may be preceded by, and active pyelonephritis may be associated with, asymptomatic bacteriuria.

Bainbridge reflex   stretch receptors in the heart (right atrium) can increase heart rate through sympathetic stimulation when venous return increases.

Baker's cyst   a cyst that forms at the back of the knee. Often associated with rheumatoid arthritis and may appear only when the leg is straightened.

balance of probabilities   the standard of proof required in civil proceedings.

balanitis   inflammation of the glans penis.

balanitis xerotica obliterans (BXO)   inflammatory condition involving the glans and prepuce.

balanoposthitis   inflammation of the glans penis and prepuce.

balanus   the glans of the penis or clitoris.

ball and socket joint   a type of synovial joint with a wide range of movement, for example shoulder joint.

ball catcher's projection   an anteroposterior oblique projection of both hands.

bandage material applied to a wound or used to bind an injured part of the body. May be used to: (a) retain a dressing or splint; (b) support, compress, immobilize; (c) prevent or correct deformity. Available in strips or circular form in a range of different materials and applying varying levels of pressure. *compression bandages* are widely used in the management of venous leg ulceration.

bandwidth the difference between the maximum and minimum frequency in a system. A range of frequencies in magnetic resonance. *See also* **receiver bandwidth, transmitter bandwidth**.

Bankart's operation for recurrent dislocation of the shoulder joint: the defect of the glenoid cavity of the scapula is repaired.

barbiturates a group of sedative/hypnotic drugs. They are associated with serious problems of dependence and tolerance, and sudden withdrawal may cause a serious withdrawal syndrome that includes anxiety, convulsions and even death. They have been replaced by safer drugs and their use is limited to anaesthesia and sometimes for epilepsy.

barbotage a method of extending the spread of spinal anaesthesia whereby local anaesthetic is directly mixed with aspirated cerebrospinal fluid and reinjected into the subarachnoid space.

bar chart a graph displaying the data in columns, which are separate from each other.

barium enema a radiographic examination of the large bowel using barium sulphate as the contrast agent. Barium sulphate liquid, followed by a quantity of air, is introduced into the large bowel by means of a rectal tube, during fluoroscopy. It is used for diagnostic purposes, for example, for colon cancers, in conjunction with endoscopy. *See also* **barium sulphate, colonoscopy**.

barium meal (barium swallow) a radiographic examination of the upper gastrointestinal tract (oesophagus and stomach) and the small intestine with follow-through radiographs, using barium sulphate as the contrast agent. The barium sulphate suspension is swallowed and radiographs are taken of the gastrointestinal tract. Pre-examination fasting is required and medicines, for example, some antacids, that may interfere with the examination should be stopped. Further fasting may be required until follow-through radiographs are completed.

barium sulphate a heavy insoluble powder used, in an aqueous suspension, as a contrast agent in radiographic visualization of the alimentary tract by either being introduced orally, via the rectum or via a colostomy.

Barlow's test a manoeuvre designed to test for congenitally dislocatable hips in the neonate. Often used in association with the Ortolani test. *See also* **developmental dysplasia of the hip**.

barn a unit of measure used in atomic physics to measure cross sections which equal $10^{-28}\,\mathrm{m}^2$. *See also* **scattered cross-section**.

barroceptors sensory nerve endings which respond to pressure changes. They are present in the cardiac atria, aortic arch, venae cavae, carotid sinus and the internal ear.

Barrett's oesophagus benign, ulcer-like lesions in columnar epithelium of the lower oesophagus often resulting from chronic irritation by the acid from gastric reflux. Predisposes to oesophageal cancer.

barrier nursing a method of preventing the spread of infection from an infectious individual to other people. It is achieved by isolation techniques.

Bartholin's glands (greater vestibular glands) two small glands situated at each side of the external orifice of the vagina. Their ducts open into the vestibule. They produce lubricating mucus that facilitates coitus.

bartholinitis inflammation of Bartholin's (greater vestibular) glands.

Barton's fracture a break in the distal articular surface of the radius which may be associated with dorsal dislocation of the carpus on the radius.

basal cell carcinoma a tumour of the basal aspect of the epidermis which accounts for 80% of all skin tumours.

basal dose rate used in brachytherapy and is the average of all dose rates calculated at the minimum dose point in the central transverse plane of a brachytherapy dose distribution. Used in the Paris system of dosimetry.

basal ganglia structures in the peripheral nervous system. *See also* **basal nuclei**.

basal metabolic rate (BMR) the energy consumed at complete rest for essential physiological functions. It is influenced by nutritional status, age, gender, physiological status, disease, certain drugs and ambient temperature. It is determined by measuring the oxygen consumption when the energy output has been reduced to a basal minimum, that is the person is fasting and is physically and mentally at rest, and is expressed per kilogram body weight. In clinical practice it is usually estimated by prediction equations and used to estimate energy requirements.

basal metabolism the minimum energy expended in the maintenance of essential physiological processes such as respiration.

basal nuclei a collection of interconnected structures (grey cells) deep within the cerebral hemispheres concerned with cognition, and modifying and coordinating voluntary muscle movement. Their proper functioning requires the release of the neurotransmitter dopamine. Sometimes erroneously referred to as ganglia, which more properly describes structures in the peripheral nervous system. Site of degeneration in Parkinson's disease. *See also* **dopamine**.

base the lowest part such as the lung. The major part of a compound. An alkali. A supporting medium for other layers of either a film or intensifying screens. *See also* **blue-based films, clear-based films**.

basement membrane   a thin layer beneath the epithelium of mucous surfaces.

BASIC (Beginners All-purpose Symbolic Instruction Code)   a high level language for computers and almost universally used for home computers.

basic fog   the recorded density of a radiographic film base plus the recorded density of chemical blackening on an unexposed part of a film.

basic life support (BLS)   a term that describes the application of artificial respiration (usually by mouth-to-mouth breathing) and external cardiac massage to save life without the use of artificial aids or equipment.

basilic   prominent.

basilic vein   on the inner side of the arm.

basophil   a cell which has an affinity for basic dyes. A polymorphonuclear granulocyte (white blood cell) which takes up a particular dye: it is phagocytic and has granules containing heparin and histamine.

basophilia   increase in the number of basophils in the blood. Basophilic staining of red blood cells.

Batchelor plaster   a type of double abduction plaster, with the legs encased from groins to ankles, in full abduction and medial rotation. The feet are then attached to a wooden pole or 'broomstick'. Alternative to frog plaster, but the hips are free. *See also* **developmental dysplasia of the hip**.

battery   legal term. An unlawful touching. Constitutes a trespass against the person. *See also* **assault**.

Battle's sign   bruising over the mastoid process indicative of a skull fracture.

baud   the unit for measuring the rate at which data are transmitted or received.

B cells   *see* **lymphocytes**.

BCG (bacille Calmette–Guérin)   an attenuated form of tubercle bacilli: it has lost its power to cause tuberculosis, but retains its antigenic function; it is the base of a vaccine used for immunization against tuberculosis. Also used in urology for the treatment of high-risk superficial bladder cancer.

beam   metal pole attached to a hospital bed to facilitate the use of traction. For example, a Thomas' splint can be slung up, with pulleys and weights attached, to allow movement and provide counterbalance to the weight of the splint and leg.

beam direction device   pointers, light sources or laser beams used to indicate the beam direction, the centre of the beam and the source skin distance.

beam direction shell   a device worn by the patient to enable accurate and reproducible treatment localization, patient positioning, patient contour, beam exit and entry points and a base for additional build-up material. Produced using either clear Perspex or a thermoplastic material.

beam's eye view   when an observer looks directly at the planning target volume from the position of the central ray from the X-ray tube, this gives the extent of the beam coverage.

beam hardening   when the total intensity of the X-ray beam is reduced by the addition of filters, as the reduction is much greater at lower energies. An increase in the average energy of an X-ray spectrum caused by greater absorption of the low-energy component by filtration.

beam hardening filters   addition of pieces of metal to improve the relative penetration of the X-ray beam, they are not effective at megavoltages. *See also* **compound filters**.

beam intensity modulation   linear accelerator beam intensity is varied during treatment by altering the collimation leaves to create a better dose distribution over the field.

beam profile   the dose of the X-ray beam including any scattered radiation which is added to the primary beam as it passes through the patient. The variation of dose along a line at right angles to the central axis of a radiation beam.

beam quality   is the penetrating ability of primary radiation and is influenced by: the accelerating voltage (kVp) across the tube, the voltage waveform, the target material, the inherent filtration and the additional filtration.

beam width   the width of an ultrasound beam at a given depth in the patient.

beat   pulsation of the blood in the heart and blood vessels. ***dropped beat*** refers to the loss of an occasional ventricular beat as occurs in extrasystoles. ***premature beat*** an extrasystole.

Beau's lines   transverse ridges or grooves which reflect a temporary retardation of the normal nail growth following a debilitating illness. They first appear towards the proximal nail fold and move towards the free edge as the nail grows. The distance the groove has moved indicates quite accurately the length of time since the illness or trauma (nail growth being about 1 mm per week).

becquerel (Bq)   the derived SI unit (International System of Units) for radioactivity. Equals the amount of a radioactive substance undergoing one nuclear disintegration per second. Has replaced the curie.

bed cradle   a frame placed over a patient's body to relieve the weight of bedding over the injured part of the body.

bed elevator   a wedge used to raise either end of a bed, for example, to aid breathing or to treat shock.

bedpan   a shallow vessel used for defecation or urination by patients who are confined to bed.

bedsore   obsolete term for **decubitus ulcer** or **pressure sore**. A breakdown of the skin due to pressure or immobility; usual sites are buttocks, heels, elbows, shoulders.

bedwetting   *see* **enuresis**.

Beer Lambert Law   the greater the distance a ray of light travels in a coloured medium the more it is absorbed.

Behçet syndrome   a form of systemic vasculitis. There is stomatitis, genital ulceration and uveitis. There may also be skin nodules, thrombophlebitis and arthritis of one or more of the large joints. Gastrointestinal and neurological complications may occur. The syndrome is associated with the presence of a certain human leukocyte antigen (HLA). Treatment is with non-steroidal anti-inflammatory drugs (NSAIDs), corticosteroids and immunosuppressant drugs.

bejel   a non-venereal form of syphilis mainly affecting children in the Middle East and sub-Saharan Africa. The causative organism is *Treponema pallidum*. It usually starts in the mouth and affects mucosae, skin and bones.

Bell's palsy   usually non-permanent facial hemiparesis due to idiopathic (cause unknown) lesion of the seventh (facial) cranial nerve.

Bence Jones protein   protein that is excreted in the urine of some patients with multiple myeloma; composed of fragments of immunoglobulin molecules.

benchmarking   part of quality assurance. Involves the identification of examples of best practice from others engaged in similar practice. From this, best practice benchmark scores in agreed areas of care are identified, against which individual units can compare their own performance.

bends (Caisson disease)   results from sudden reduction in atmospheric pressure, as experienced by divers on return to surface, aircrew ascending to great heights. Caused by bubbles of nitrogen which are released from solution in the blood; symptoms vary according to the site of these. The condition is largely preventable by proper and gradual decompression technique. *See also* **decompression illness**.

benign   benign, simple or innocent tumours are encapsulated, do not infiltrate adjacent tissue and are unlikely to recur if removed. They are non-malignant (of a growth), non-invasive (no capacity to metastasize), non-cancerous (of a growth). Describes a condition or illness which is not serious and does not usually have harmful consequences.

benign hypotonia   describes infants who are initially floppy but otherwise healthy. Improvement occurs and the infant regains normal tone and motor development.

benign intracranial hypertension (BIH)   a condition in which there is raised intracranial pressure with papilloedema and which can lead to the loss of vision, typically in young, obese women. Often associated with thrombosis in the sagittal sinus.

benign myalgic encephalomyelitis (BME)   a flu-like illness with varied symptoms including dizziness, muscle fatigue and spasm, headaches and other neurological pain. A high percentage of BME sufferers have a higher level of coxsackie B antibodies in their blood than the rest of the population.

benign tumour   a localized growth which is not malignant and does not metastasize but may be dangerous by virtue of its position.

Bennett's fracture   fracture/dislocation of proximal end of first metacarpal involving the first carpo-metacarpal joint.

benzene   a colourless inflammable liquid obtained from coal tar. Extensively used as a solvent. Continued occupational exposure to it results in aplastic anaemia and, rarely, leukaemia.

benzodiazepines   a group of anxiolytic/hypnotic drugs. Dependence and withdrawal problems may occur. They may be misused.

benzotriazole   a radiographic developer restrainer.

beri-beri   a deficiency disease caused by lack of vitamin B_1 (thiamin). It occurs mainly in those countries where the staple diet is polished rice. Beri-beri is usually described as either 'wet' (cardiac) or 'dry' (neurological) depending on the symptoms. The symptoms are pain from neuritis, paralysis, muscular wasting, progressive oedema, mental deterioration and, finally, heart failure.

berylliosis   an industrial disease: there is impaired lung function because of interstitial fibrosis from inhalation of beryllium. Corticosteroids are used in treatment.

beta decay   the process of ejecting a beta particle from the nucleus of an atom; if the particle is negative (negatron) the atomic number will increase by one, if the particle is positive (positron) the atomic number will decrease by one.

beta particle   a mass, equal to that of an electron, which is ejected from the nucleus of an atom and has either a positive or a negative charge.

biaxial joint   a joint that allows movement round two axes for example, flexion, extension, abduction and adduction.

bibliographical databases   details of papers, etc., but sometimes abstracts and full articles, are available electronically via CD-ROM or the internet, for example, Medline.

bicellular   composed of two cells.

biceps   two-headed muscle of the upper arm.

biconcave   concave or hollow on both surfaces.

biconvex   convex on both surfaces.

bicornate   having two horns; generally applied to a double uterus or a single uterus possessing two horns.

bicuspid   having two cusps or points. ***bicuspid teeth*** the premolars. ***bicuspid valve*** the mitral valve between the left atrium and ventricle of the heart.

bifid   divided into two parts. Cleft or forked.

bifurcation   division into two branches.

bilateral associated with both sides.

bile a bitter, alkaline, viscid, greenish-yellow fluid secreted by the liver and stored in the gallbladder. 500–1000 mL is produced each day. It contains water, mucin, lecithin, cholesterol, bile salts, bile acids, the pigments bilirubin and biliverdin and substances for excretion. Bile is needed for the absorption of fat-soluble vitamins, stimulates peristalsis and deodorizes faeces.

bile acids organic acids; cholic and chenodeoxycholic, present in bile.

bile ducts the hepatic and cystic, which join to form the common bile duct that empties into the duodenum.

bile pigments made up of bilirubin and biliverdin, produced by haemolysis in the spleen. Normally these colour the faeces only but in jaundice the skin and urine may also become coloured. *See also* **bilirubin, biliverdin**.

bile salts emulsifying agents, sodium glycocholate and taurocholate. Conjugated bile acids (with taurine and glycine) form these sodium salts.

biliary associated with bile.

biliary colic pain in the right upper quadrant of abdomen, due to obstruction of the gallbladder or common bile duct, usually by a stone; it may last several hours and is usually steady, which differentiates it from other forms of colic. Vomiting may occur.

biliary fistula an abnormal track conveying bile to the surface or to some other organ.

bilious a word usually used to signify vomit containing bile. A non-medical term, usually meaning 'suffering from indigestion'.

bilirubin a red pigment derived mostly from haemoglobin during red blood cell breakdown. Unconjugated fat-soluble bilirubin, which gives an indirect reaction with Van den Bergh's test, is potentially toxic to metabolically active tissues, particularly the basal nuclei of the immature brain. Unconjugated bile is transported to the blood attached to albumen to make it less likely to enter and damage brain cells. In the liver the enzyme glucuronyl transferase conjugates fat-soluble bilirubin with glucuronic acid to make it water-soluble, in which state it is relatively non-toxic (reacts directly with Van den Bergh's test) and can be excreted in the bile. *See also* **haemolytic disease of the newborn, jaundice**.

bilirubinaemia the presence of bilirubin in the blood. Sometimes used (incorrectly) for an excess of bilirubin in the blood.

bilirubinuria the presence of the bile pigment bilirubin in the urine.

biliverdin the green pigment formed by oxidation of bilirubin.

bilobate having two lobes.

bilobular having two little lobes or lobules.

binary a system of counting to base two, i.e. generating figures with only 1 or 0.

binary fission   a method of reproduction common among the bacteria and protozoa. The cell divides into two equal 'daughter' cells.

binder   an agent used to suspend the phosphors in the phosphor layer of an intensifying screen, acetate acrylate is often used and contains a dye to control screen speed and unsharpness.

binocular vision   the focusing of both eyes on one object at the same time, in such a way that only one image of the object is seen.

binovular   derived from two separate ova. Binovular twins may be of different sexes.

bioavailability   the amount of a drug (or nutrient) that enters the circulation in the active form. It is dependent on the route of administration and the degree to which the drug is metabolized before it reaches the bloodstream. Drugs administered intravenously will have 100% bioavailability, whereas those given orally may not be fully absorbed and are subject to first-pass metabolism in the liver. Some drugs are totally metabolized in the liver, so other routes of administration must be used such as sublingually.

biochemistry   the chemistry of life and organic molecules.

bioethics   the application of ethical principles to biological problems.

biofeedback   presentation of immediate visual or auditory information about usually unconscious body functions such as blood pressure, heart rate and muscle tension. Either by trial and error or by operant conditioning a person can learn to repeat behaviour which results in a satisfactory level of body functions.

biofilm   collection of microorganisms and their products that stick to a surface, for example, a urinary catheter.

bioflavonoids   a large group of coloured substances that occur naturally in many vegetables and fruit (for example, tomatoes, broccoli, cherries, plums, etc.). Bioflavonoids are also present in tea and wine. Many are antibacterial and some may offer protection against heart disease and cancer.

biohazard   anything that presents a hazard to life. Some specimens for the pathological laboratory are so labelled.

biological effect   when a body is irradiated changes can occur which can include, skin reddening, loss of hair, radiation-induced cancers, genetic changes, changes in blood count and, if sufficiently high radiation dose is received to the whole body, death.

biological engineering   designing microelectronic or mechanical equipment for external use by patients: for attachment to patients, or placement inside patients.

biological half-life   the time taken for the concentration of a certain chemical in an organ to be reduced to half its original concentration.

biological response modifier (BRM)   cancer treatment that manipulates the patient's immune response in order to destroy cancer cells. They include colony stimulating factors, interleukins and interferons.

biologically effective dose a comparison between the total radiation dose given during a fractionated treatment and a single dose of the same quantity of radiation. A quantity used in the radiobiology of radiotherapy to compare the effects of different fractionation schedules. The total dose given in very small fractions required to produce a particular effect.

biology the science of life, concerned with the structure, function and organization of all living organisms.

biophysical profile used in the third trimester to assess fetal well being using measurable parameters of: fetal breathing, fetal movement, fetal tone, amniotic fluid volume and heart rate.

biopsy removal of tissue to provide a sample for microscopic examination to establish a precise diagnosis.

biopsy forceps long, metal forceps with a scissor action of the end blade, used for taking tissue samples from narrow passages.

biorhythm the cyclical patterns of biological functions unique to each person, for example, sleep–wake cycles, body temperature, etc.

biosensors non-invasive devices that measure the result of biological processes, for example, skin temperature or blood oxygen saturation.

biotechnology the use of biology in the scientific study of technology and vice versa.

biparietal diameter the transverse distance between the two parietal bones of the skull. A measurement used in ultrasound imaging to assess the gestational age of a fetus in the second and third trimesters.

biparous producing two offspring at one birth.

biphasic positive airways pressure (BIPAP) mode of ventilatory (respiratory) support in which the airway pressure alternates between two levels. The higher pressure ventilates the patient or provides pressure support, while the lower pressure acts as positive end expiratory pressure/continuous positive airway pressure. Can be delivered non-invasively (without intubation) by mask to patients with chronic lung disease or as an aid to weaning from ventilatory support.

bipolar having two poles.

bisexual having some of the physical genital characteristics of both sexes; a hermaphrodite. When there is gonadal tissue of both sexes in the same person that person is a true hermaphrodite. Describes a person who is sexually attracted to both men and women.

bisphosphonates drugs that reduce bone turnover. Used in the management of bone diseases and the hypercalcaemia associated with cancer.

bit the smallest unit of data in a computer, a contraction of **BI**nary digi**T**.

bite block   a dental impression suspended from a gantry which the patient bites to enable accurate head position to be maintained during treatment.

bivalve   having two blades such as in the vaginal speculum. In orthopaedics, the division of a plaster of Paris splint into two portions – an anterior and posterior half.

bivariate statistics   descriptive statistics that compare the relationship between two variables, such as correlations. Can be used to decide whether multivariate statistics are needed.

black body   a body which will absorb 100% of all radiations falling on it.

bladder   a membranous sac containing fluid or gas. A hollow organ for receiving fluid. *See also* **gallbladder, urinary bladder**.

bladder outflow obstruction   pathophysiological obstruction to the lower urinary tract commonly due to benign prostatic hyperplasia in older males.

Blalock–Taussig procedure   a temporary measure to improve pulmonary blood flow in congenital heart abnormalities, such as tetralogy of Fallot. A shunt is constructed by anastomosing the subclavian artery to the pulmonary artery to divert blood from the systemic circulation to the lungs.

blastocyst (blastula)   stage in early embryonic development that follows the morula, which becomes cystic and enfolds. Comprises a fluid-filled cavity and inner cell mass surrounded by trophoblast cells.

blastoderm   a cell layer of the blastocyst. Eventually becomes the three primary germ layers, ectoderm, endoderm and mesoderm, from which the embryo will form.

blastomycosis   granulomatous condition caused by *Blastomyces dermatitidis*; infection starts in the lungs and lymph nodes. May affect the skin, viscera, bones and joints.

'bleeding time'   the time required for the spontaneous arrest of bleeding from a skin puncture: under controlled conditions this forms a clinical test.

blepharon   the eyelid.

blind loop syndrome   a condition resulting from sluggish movement of faeces (stasis) in the small intestine leading to bacterial growth, thus producing diarrhoea and malabsorption (for example, due to surgical anastomosis or dysmotility).

blind spot   the spot at which the optic nerve leaves the retina. Without any cones or rods it is insensitive to light.

blink mode   the comparison of two images in quick succession to identify minute changes between the images.

blood   the red viscid fluid filling the heart and blood vessels. It consists of a colourless fluid, plasma, in which are suspended the red blood cells (erythrocytes), the white cells (leucocytes), and the platelets (thrombocytes). The plasma contains a great many substances in solution including factors which enable the blood to clot.

blood-borne viruses (BBV)   viruses transmitted via blood to cause infection. Include: HIV and several hepatitis viruses.

blood–brain barrier (BBB)   the protective arrangement that prevents many substances crossing from the blood to the brain. It consists of capillary endothelial cells and astrocytes that ensure that the capillary wall is relatively impermeable. The barrier allows the passage of nutrients and metabolic waste. However, some drugs, alcohol and other toxic substances, for example, lead in young children, can pass from the blood through this barrier to the cerebrospinal fluid.

blood count   calculation of the number of red or white cells per cubic millimetre of blood, using a haemocytometer. *See also* **differential** blood count.

blood culture   a sample of venous blood is incubated in a suitable medium at an optimum temperature, so that any microorganisms can multiply and so be isolated and identified microscopically. *See also* **septicaemia**.

blood formation   haemopoiesis.

blood gases (arterial blood gases)   measurement of the oxygen (PaO_2), carbon dioxide ($PaCO_2$) and acid–base (pH or hydrogen ion concentration) content of the arterial blood.

blood-letting   venesection.

blood plasma   the fluid part of blood.

blood pressure   the pressure exerted by the blood on the blood vessel walls. Usually refers to the pressure within the arteries, which may be measured in millimetres of mercury (mmHg) using a sphygmomanometer. The arterial blood pressure fluctuates with each heart beat, having a maximum value (the *systolic pressure*) which is related to the ejection of blood from the heart into the arteries and a minimum value (*diastolic pressure*) when the aortic and pulmonary valves are closed and the heart is relaxed. Usually values for both systolic and diastolic pressures are recorded (for example, 120/70). *See also* **hypertension, hypotension**.

blood sugar   the amount of glucose in the blood; varies within the normal range. It is regulated by hormones, for example, insulin. *See also* **hyperglycaemia, hypoglycaemia**.

blood transfusion   the intravenous replacement of lost or destroyed blood by compatible citrated human blood.

blood urea   the amount of urea (the end product of protein metabolism) in the blood; varies within the normal range. This is virtually unaffected by the amount of protein in the diet when the kidneys, which are the main organs of urea excretion, are functioning normally. When they are diseased the blood urea quickly rises.

blood volume   the amount of blood circulating in the body. In an adult male equal to 5.5 litres.

blow-out fracture   fracture of the orbital wall due to blunt trauma.

'blue baby'   cyanotic appearance at birth, often attributed to congenital cyanotic heart defects.

blue-based films   have a blue dye in the base and produce a slightly higher visual contrast.

B-mode   brightness modulation in ultrasound techniques. When the ultrasound reflections are recorded as dots of varying brightness on an oscilloscope, which is converted into a grey scale picture by a scan converter and a two-dimensional image is formed showing a section through the organ being examined.

Bobath concept   the concept of treatment of abnormal muscle tone and movement disorder, seen in children with cerebral palsy and adults after a stroke, and now widely applied to similar dysfunction caused by multiple sclerosis and other neurological conditions.

body mass index (BMI)   used as an index of adiposity. It is calculated by dividing an individual's weight (kg) by their height (m) squared. Separate charts are available for adults and children, adult charts should not be used for children. The WHO (1998) classification for BMI is: less than 18.5 underweight, 18.6–24.9 normal weight, 25–29.9 pre-obese, 30–34.9 obese class 1, 35–39.9 obese class 2 and greater than 40 obese class 3.

body temperature   the balance between heat produced and heat lost in the body. It is maintained around 37°C throughout the 24 hours but varies between 0.5 and 1.0°C during that period. Most heat is produced by metabolism, voluntary and involuntary muscular activities, and heat loss occurs through convection, conduction and evaporation of sweat; small amounts are lost during expiration, urination and defaecation. *See also* **core body temperature, shell body temperature**.

Bohler's angle   two lines drawn on a lateral radiograph of a calcaneum. Line one is from the posterior aspect of the calcaneum to its highest midpoint. The second line is from the highest midpoint to the highest anterior point. The normal angle is 25–40°, any other angle indicating an injury to the calcaneum.

boil (furuncle)   an acute inflammatory condition, surrounding a hair follicle; often caused by *Staphylococcus aureus*. Usually attended by suppuration; it has one opening for drainage in contrast to a carbuncle.

Bolam test   the test laid down in the case of Bolam versus Friern HMC on the standard of care expected of a professional in cases of alleged negligence.

bolus   a chewed lump of food ready to be swallowed. A large dose of medication, contrast agent or radioactive isotope injected all at once intravenously to raise the blood concentration rapidly. A tissue equivalent material used in radiotherapy when irradiating irregular body shapes, to attenuate the primary beam and absorb scattered radiation to maintain accurate treatment dosage or to increase the dose to the skin when high-energy photon beams are used.

bone   connective tissue in which salts, such as calcium carbonate and calcium phosphate, are deposited in an organic matrix to make it hard and dense. Bone tissue is of two types, hard dense compact bone and spongy cancellous bone. The separate bones make up the skeleton.

bone death   occurs when there is a loss of blood supply to the bone, can happen following a fracture.

bone density   a description of bone mass. It is decreased in osteoporosis. *See also* **peak bone density**.

bone graft   the transplantation of a piece of bone from one part of the body to another, or from one person to another. Used to repair bone defects or to supply osteogenic tissue.

bone marrow   the substance contained within bone cavities. At birth the cavities are filled with blood-forming *red marrow* but later in life, deposition of fat in the long bones converts the red into yellow bone marrow.

bone marrow biopsy (sampling)   an investigation of blood cell production whereby a sample of marrow is obtained by aspiration or trephine. Usually the site used is the iliac crest or sometimes the sternum.

bone marrow transplantation (BMT, stem cell transplant)   the infusion of bone marrow into a patient's vein. The bone marrow may be obtained either on an earlier occasion from the patient (*autologous transplantation*) or from a suitable donor (*allogeneic transplantation*). Usually follows myeloablative doses of chemotherapy or radiotherapy as therapy for (most commonly) haematological cancers although also used therapeutically and experimentally for some solid tumours.

booting Bps   **b**its **p**er **s**econd, the rate information is transferred between computers. Starting up a computer by loading it with its starting instructions.

borborygmi   rumbling noises caused by the movement of gas in the intestines.

botulism   an intoxication with the preformed exotoxin of *Clostridium botulinum*. Vomiting, respiratory, ocular and pharyngeal paralysis occur within 24–72 hours of eating food contaminated with the spores, which require anaerobic conditions to produce the toxin. Associated with home preserving of vegetables and meat and improperly treated tinned food.

bounce   the automatic return of email.

bovine   relating to the cow or ox.

bovine spongiform encephalopathy (BSE)   a fatal, infective (prion) neurological disease of cattle. *See also* **Creutzfeldt–Jakob disease**.

bovine tuberculosis   is endemic in cattle and transmitted to humans by drinking infected milk. Pasteurization of milk and monitoring of dairy herds are the mainstays of disease control. *M. avium intracellulare* (MAI) is an atypical mycobacterium which may infect severely immunocompromised individuals (such as those with advanced AIDS). Tuberculosis causes systemic effects such as pyrexia, night sweats and weight loss, plus those dependent upon the site, for example, cough in lung disease, haematuria in renal TB.

bowel   the large intestine.

Bowen's disease   a form of carcinoma in situ, which may progress to invasive malignancy, characterized by red-brown scaly or crusted lesions that resemble a patch of psoriasis or dermatitis.

box technique   in radiotherapy when two intersecting parallel pairs produce a uniform distribution of dose over the centrally placed volume enclosed by all four fields.

Boyle's anaesthetic machine   apparatus for delivering anaesthetic agents mixed with oxygen and nitrous oxide or air.

Bps (Bits per second)   the rate information is transferred between computers.

brachial   associated with the arm. Applied to vessels in this region (***brachial artery, brachial vein***) and a nerve plexus at the root of the neck.

brachialis   a muscle of the upper arm.

brachiocephalic   associated with the arm and head.

brachiocephalic (innominate) artery   large artery branching from the aortic arch which forms the right common carotid and right subclavian arteries.

brachiocephalic (innominate) veins   two large veins derived from the internal jugular and subclavian veins. Convey blood to the heart via the superior vena cava.

brachioradialis   a muscle of the forearm.

brachium   the arm (especially from shoulder to elbow), or any arm-like appendage.

brachydactyly   short phalanges.

brachytherapy   when a sealed radioactive source is placed in a body cavity, or inserted into tissue to deliver a large radiation dose to a tumour with a smaller dose to the surrounding tissue. The technique may be used to treat cancers of the anus, breast, cervix, lung, oesophagus and the tongue.

brachymesophalangy   short middle phalanges.

Bradford frame   a stretcher type of bed used for: (a) immobilizing the spine; (b) resting trunk and back muscles; (c) preventing deformity. It is a tubular steel frame fitted with two canvas slings allowing a 100–150 mm gap to facilitate personal care.

bradycardia   slow rate of heart contraction, resulting in a pulse rate less than 60 beats per minute. Can occur during sleep/old age/hypothermia or as a result of treatment with certain drugs.

bradykinesia abnormally slow or retarded movement associated with difficulty initiating and then stopping a movement; typically seen in Parkinson's disease.

bradypnoea an abnormally low rate of breathing.

brain (encephalon) the largest part of the central nervous system: it is contained in the cranial cavity and is surrounded by three membranes called meninges. It comprises the cerebral hemispheres, brainstem (midbrain, pons varolii and medulla oblongata) and the cerebellum. The *brainstem* connects the cerebral hemispheres to the cerebellum and the spinal cord. The cerebrospinal fluid inside the brain is contained in the ventricles, and outside in the subarachnoid space acts as a shock absorber to the delicate nerve tissue.

brain death a situation where the brainstem is fatally and irreversibly damaged. The brainstem is responsible for maintaining vital functions including breathing. Strict criteria must be met before the patient is declared dead. These include testing certain reflexes, for example, gag and pupillary, and the absence of factors that could depress brainstem activity. Suitable patients may become organ donors if this coincides with the wishes of the family and those of the patient if known.

branchial relating to the gills. Embryonic clefts or fissures either side of the neck from which the nose, ears and mouth will eventually develop.

branchial cyst a cyst in the neck resulting from a developmental abnormality of the branchial clefts.

Braun's frame a metal frame, bandaged for use, and equally useful for drying a lower leg plaster and for applying skeletal traction (Steinmann's pin or Kirschner wire inserted through the calcaneus) to a fractured tibia, after reduction.

breast the anterior upper part of the thorax. The mammary gland.

breast board an immobilization device used to aid and maintain patient positioning during treatment. The patient's shoulders may be raised while providing arm support and/or handgrips.

breast bone the sternum.

breast care nurse specialized nurse who provides counselling and support to patients with breast cancer including advice on prostheses available to patients who have had a mastectomy.

breast jig a support which raises the patient's shoulders and provides arm support and/or handgrip to enable the patient to maintain the position during radiotherapy treatment.

breech/birth presentation refers to the position of a baby in the uterus such that the buttocks would be born first: the normal position is head first.

bregma the anterior fontanelle.

Bremsstrahlung radiation electromagnetic radiation produced by the rapid deceleration of an electron during a close approach to the atomic nucleus, e.g. the X-ray quanta produced when electrons from the filament of the X-ray tube interact with the nuclei of the target.

bridge   in dentistry, restoration to replace one or more teeth using artificial crowns connected to natural teeth.

British sign language (BSL)   a type of sign language (signing) used in the UK.

broadband   a transmission technique which uses a number of frequencies to allow a number of computer and/or telephone messages to be sent together.

broad focus   the selection of a large filament to enable a larger area of the anode to be bombarded with electrons.

broad ligaments   lateral ligaments; double fold of parietal peritoneum which hangs over the uterus and outstretched uterine (fallopian) tubes, forming a lateral partition across the pelvic cavity.

Broca's area   the motor speech area, situated in the dominant cerebral hemisphere (usually the left). Injury to this centre can result in an inability to speak.

Brodie's abscess   chronic abscess in bone.

bronchi   the two tubes into which the trachea divides at its lower end.

bronchial   associated with the bronchi.

bronchial alveolar lavage (BAL)   irrigation of the lungs with small volumes of saline which are then aspirated and examined for infection; occasionally large volume lavage may be therapeutic.

bronchial cancer   *see* **non-small cell carcinoma, oat cell carcinoma**.

bronchial tree   network of bronchi as they subdivide within the lungs.

bronchial asthma   *see* **asthma**.

bronchiectasis   abnormal dilatation of the bronchi which, when localized, is usually the result of pneumonia or lobar collapse in childhood, but when generalized is due to some inherent disorder of the bronchial mucous membrane as in cystic fibrosis. Characterized by recurrent respiratory infections with profuse purulent sputum and digital clubbing. Eventually leads to respiratory failure. Treatment is with appropriate antibiotics and regular physiotherapy to optimize sputum clearance.

bronchiole   one of the minute subdivisions of the bronchi which terminate in the alveoli (air sacs) of the lungs.

bronchiolitis   inflammation of the bronchioles, usually due to viral infection in children in the first year of life.

bronchiolitis obliterans syndrome (BOS)   progressive scarring and loss of function seen in the lungs, in part as a result of chronic rejection of a transplanted lung over time.

bronchitis   inflammation of the bronchi. *acute bronchitis* as an isolated incident is usually a primary viral infection occurring in children as a complication of the common cold, influenza, whooping cough, measles or rubella. Secondary infection occurs with bacteria, commonly *Streptococcus pneumoniae* or *Haemophilus influenzae*. **acute bronchitis** in adults is usually an acute exacerbation of chronic bronchitis precipitated by a viral infection but sometimes by a sudden increase in atmospheric pollution. **chronic bronchitis** is defined as a cough productive of sputum for at least 3 consecutive months in 2 consecutive years. The bronchial mucus-secreting glands are hypertrophied with an increase in goblet cells and loss of ciliated cells due to irritation from tobacco smoke, or atmospheric pollutants. *See also* **chronic obstructive pulmonary disease (COPD), pulmonary emphysema**.

bronchoconstrictor   any agent which constricts the bronchi.

bronchodilator   any agent which dilates the bronchi.

bronchogenic   arising from one of the bronchi.

bronchography   radiological demonstration of the bronchial tree following the introduction of contrast agent via the trachea.

bronchomycosis   general term describing a variety of fungal infections of the bronchi and lungs, for example, pulmonary candidiasis.

bronchophony   abnormal transmission of voice sounds heard over consolidated lung or over a thin layer of pleural fluid.

bronchopleural fistula   pathological communication between the pleural cavity and one of the bronchi.

bronchopneumonia   describes a type of pneumonia in which areas of consolidation are distributed widely around bronchi and not in a lobar pattern. Generally affects patients at the extremes of age, those who are debilitated or secondary to existing condition.

bronchopulmonary   associated with the bronchi and the lungs.

bronchorrhoea   an excessive discharge of mucus from the bronchial mucosa.

bronchoscope   an endoscope used for examining and taking biopsies from the interior of the bronchi. Also used for removal of inhaled foreign bodies. Bronchoscopes are either flexible fibreoptic instruments or rigid tubes.

bronchoscopy   visual examination of the tracheobronchial tree using a bronchoscope.

bronchospasm   sudden constriction of the bronchial tubes due to contraction of involuntary smooth muscle in their walls.

bronchostenosis   narrowing of one of the bronchi.

bronchotracheal   associated with the bronchi and trachea.

bronchus   one of the two tubes into which the trachea divides at its lower end.

Brook airway   used in expired air ventilation to avoid direct contact with the patient.

brought in dead (BID)   describes a situation where the person has died prior to arriving at the hospital.

brow   the forehead; the region above the supraorbital ridge.

Brown-Séquard syndrome   the compression of the spinal cord, usually by a tumour, resulting in a loss of pain and temperature sensation on the opposite side of the body from the compression.

brucellosis   a disease contracted by drinking contaminated milk which may affect the spine with the appearance of osteomyelitis.

Brudzinski's sign   immediate flexion of knees and hips on raising head from pillow. Seen in meningitis.

bruise (contusion, ecchymosis)   a discoloration of the skin due to an extravasation of blood into the underlying tissues; there is no break of the skin.

bruit   *see* **murmur**.

Bruton's agammaglobulinaemia   a congenital condition in boys, in which B lymphocytes are absent but cellular immunity remains intact. *See also* **dysgammaglobulinaemia**.

bruxism   abnormal grinding of teeth, often producing wearing down (attrition) of the surface.

Bryant's 'gallows' traction   skin traction applied to the lower limbs; the legs are then suspended vertically (from an overhead beam), so that the buttocks are lifted just clear of the bed. Used for fractures of the femur in children up to 4 years. Now largely replaced with hoop traction.

bubo   enlargement of lymph nodes, especially in the groin. A feature of chancroid, lymphogranuloma venereum and bubonic plague.

buccal   relating to the cheek or mouth.

buccal cavity   the mouth.

bucket handle tear   a description given to a type of tear of the meniscus of the knee joint that extends along the length of the meniscus.

bucky   a device for holding a cassette beneath an X-ray table which contains a grid which moves during the radiographic exposure.

Buerger's disease (thromboangiitis obliterans)   a chronic obliterative vascular disease of peripheral vessels that results in ischaemia, intermittent limping (claudication), skin changes and gangrene. The incidence is associated with the presence of HLA-A9 and HLA-B5. It affects young and middle-aged men. *Buerger's exercises* were designed to treat this condition. The legs are placed alternately in elevation and dependence to assist perfusion of the extremities with blood.

buffer   substances that limit pH change by their ability to accept or donate hydrogen ions as appropriate. Radiographic film processing, in developer boric acid and sodium hydroxide are used to absorb the products of development and therefore maintain the pH of the solution. In biological systems they limit pH changes that would inhibit cell functioning. The important buffer systems in the body include: bicarbonate (hydrogen carbonate) system, hydrogen phosphates and proteins, for example, haemoglobin. Any agent that reduces shock or jarring due to contact. In computing an area which stores information at one rate and releases it at a slower rate to another device.

bug a problem in the computer or (usually) in the program.

bulbar associated with the medulla oblongata. ***bulbar palsy or paralysis*** paralysis which involves the labioglossopharyngeal (lips, tongue and pharynx) region and results from degeneration of the motor nuclei in the medulla oblongata. There are problems with swallowing and speech. Individuals are at risk of inhaling fluids and food, with the development of pneumonia.

bulbourethral (Cowper's) glands two mucus-secreting glands which open into the bulb of the male urethra. Their secretion is part of seminal fluid.

bulimia abnormal increase in the sensation of hunger.

bulimia nervosa a pattern of binge eating occurring in response to stress.

bunion *see* **hallux valgus**.

Burkitt's lymphoma a lymphosarcoma, usually of the jaw, predominantly occurring in African children living in low-lying moist areas.

burn tissue damage (necrosis) due to chemicals, moist heat, dry heat, electricity, flame, friction or radiation; classified as partial or full thickness according to the depth of skin destroyed: the latter usually requiring skin graft(s). Analgesia and the prevention of shock, infection and malnutrition are important aspects of treatment.

burr an attachment for a surgical drill which is used for cutting into tooth or bone.

bursa a fibrous sac lined with synovial membrane and containing a small quantity of synovial fluid. Bursae are found between (a) tendon and bone, (b) skin and bone, (c) muscle and muscle. Their function is to facilitate movement by reducing friction between these surfaces.

bursitis inflammation of a bursa. ***olecranon bursitis*** inflammation of the bursa over the point of the elbow. ***prepatellar bursitis*** (housemaid's knee) a fluid-filled swelling of the bursa in front of the kneecap (patella). It is frequently associated with excessive kneeling. A blow can result in bleeding into the bursa and there can be infection with pyogenic pathogens. ***retrocalcaneal bursitis*** inflammation of an anatomical bursa located between the posterior angle of the calcaneus and the Achilles tendon near to its insertion. There is a fluctuant soft tissue swelling both sides of the tendon.

bus a semi-standard connector to the computer through which all data are passed to an external device.

buttock   one of the two projections posterior to the hip joints. Formed mainly of the gluteal muscles.

byssinosis   a form of pneumoconiosis caused by inhalation of cotton or linen dust.

byte   the number of bits which are needed to form a single character, usually 8. *See also* **bit**.

C

CA-125 a glycoprotein found in the blood serum of patients with ovarian or other glandular cell carcinomas. Increasing levels of the antigen mean increasing tumour growths which may indicate poor prognosis. Also known as *cancer cell surface antigen 125*.

cachexia a condition of extreme debility typical of the late stages of chronic disease, symptoms include weight loss and general bodily deterioration.

cadaver a corpse. In a medical context it implies a dead body which is dissected in a medical school, or in a mortuary at a postmortem examination.

caecum the blind, pouch-like commencement of the colon in the right iliac fossa. To it is attached the vermiform appendix; it is separated from the ileum by the ileocaecal valve.

caesium-137 (^{137}Cs) a radioactive substance which, when sealed in needles or tubes, can be used for interstitial and surface applications. It can also be employed as a source for treatment by Selectron. Historically has been used for external beam therapy.

caesium iodide crystal a crystal which used to be used in the detector of a CT scanner to detect any radiation passing through the patient. Now obsolete. *See also* **ceramic detectors**.

caisson disease results from sudden reduction in atmospheric pressure, as experienced by divers on return to surface, aircrew ascending to great heights. Caused by bubbles of nitrogen which are released from solution in the blood; symptoms vary according to the site of these. The condition is largely preventable by proper and gradual decompression technique. *See also* **decompression illness**.

calamine zinc carbonate with ferric oxide. Used in lotions and creams for the relief of itching; however, it is not generally effective.

calcaneus (calcaneum, os calcis) the heel bone.

calcareous chalky. Relating to lime or calcium.

calcification the hardening of an organic substance by a deposit of calcium salts within it. May be physiological, as in bone, or pathological, as in arteries.

calcitonin (thyrocalcitonin) hormone secreted by the thyroid gland. It has a fine-tuning role in calcium homeostasis. It opposes the action of parathyroid hormone and reduces levels of calcium and phosphate in the serum by its action on the kidneys and bone. It inhibits calcium reabsorption from bone and stimulates the excretion of calcium and phosphate in the urine. Calcitonin is released when the serum calcium level rises. Synthetic calcitonin is used in the management of metastatic bone cancer, Paget's disease and osteoporosis.

calcitriol (1,25-dehydroxycholecalciferol)   the active form of vitamin D concerned with calcium homeostasis.

calcium (Ca)   a metallic element. Needed by the body for neuromuscular conduction and blood coagulation and as an important component of the skeleton and teeth. An essential nutrient.

calcium carbonate   a calcium salt used in many antacid medicines.

calcium gluconate   a calcium salt used to treat calcium deficiencies and disorders such as rickets.

calcium tungstate   the main phosphor used in conventional intensifying screens now superseded by rare earth phosphors.

calculus   a stone, small mineral deposits. Examples include gallstones and renal calculi. ***dental calculus*** a hard calcified deposit that forms on the surface of the teeth, also known as tartar.

Caldwell–Luc operation (radical antrostomy)   a radical operation previously used for sinusitis.

calibrated stepwedge   a piece of equipment which is made up of different thickness of aluminium with a layer of copper on the base, wedges are calibrated so that when radiographed each step produces an exact increase or decrease in density on the film. *See also* **stepwedge**.

caliper   a two-pronged instrument for measuring the diameter of a round body, used chiefly in pelvimetry. A two-pronged instrument with sharp points which are inserted into the lower end of a fractured long bone, a weight is attached to the other end of the caliper, which maintains a steady pull on the distal end of the bone. ***Thomas' walking caliper*** is similar to the Thomas' splint, but the W-shaped junction at the lower end is replaced by two small iron rods which slot into holes made in the heel of the boot, the ring should fit the groin perfectly, and all weight is then borne by the ischial tuberosity.

callus   the partly calcified tissue which forms about the ends of a broken bone and ultimately accomplishes repair of the fracture, when this is complete the bony thickening is known as permanent callus. ***corn (callosity, keratoma, mechanically induced hyperkeratosis)*** a yellowish plaque of hard skin caused by pressure or friction, the stratum corneum becomes hypertrophied, most commonly seen on the feet and palms of the hands. A painful, cone-shaped overgrowth and hardening of the epidermis, with the point of the cone in the deeper layers. Corns on the sole of the foot and over joints are often described as hard corns, and those occurring between the toes are described as soft corns.

calor   heat: one of the five classic local signs and symptoms of inflammation, the others are dolor, loss of function, rubor and tumor.

calorie   a unit of heat. In practice the calorie is too small a unit to be useful and the **kilocalorie** (kcal) is the preferred unit in studies in metabolism. A kcal is the amount of heat required to raise the temperature of 1 kg of water by 1°C. In medicine, science and technology generally, the calorie has been replaced by the **joule** (derived SI unit) as a unit of energy, work and heat. For approximate conversion: 4.2 kJ=1 kcal.

calorific   describes any phenomena that relate to heat production.

calorimetry   the precise method of measuring the absorbed dose of radiation in a body by calculating the temperature rise when the body is irradiated.

Campylobacter   a genus of Gram-negative motile bacteria. *Campylobacter jejuni* is a common cause of bacterial food poisoning. It causes abdominal pain and bloodstained diarrhoea that may last for 10–14 days. The microorganism is associated with raw meat and poultry, the fur of infected pet animals and unpasteurized milk. No reported person-to-person spread.

canal   a bony tunnel.

canaliculus   a minute capillary passage. Any small canal, such as the passage leading from the edge of the eyelid to the lacrimal sac or one of the numerous small canals leading from the Haversian canals and terminating in the lacunae of bone.

canal of Schlemm   a canal in the inner part of the sclera, close to its junction with the cornea, which it encircles. It drains excess aqueous humour to maintain normal intraocular pressure. Impaired drainage results in raised intraocular pressure.

cancellous   resembling latticework; light and spongy; like a honeycomb. Describes a type of bone tissue.

cancer   a general term which covers any malignant growth in any part of the body. The growth is purposeless, parasitic, and flourishes at the expense of the human host. Characteristics are the tendency to cause local destruction, to invade adjacent tissues and to spread by metastasis. Frequently recurs after removal. **carcinoma** refers to malignant tumours of epithelial tissue, **sarcoma** to malignant tumours of connective tissue.

cancerophobia   obsessive fear of cancer.

candela (cd)   one of the seven base units of the International System of Units (SI). Measures luminous intensity.

candida (Monilia)   a type of fungi which is widespread in nature.

candidiasis (candidosis, moniliasis, thrush)   infection caused by a species of *Candida*, usually *Candida albicans*. Infection may involve the mouth, gastrointestinal tract, skin, nails, respiratory tract or genitourinary tract (vulvovaginitis, balanitis), especially in individuals who are debilitated, for example, by cancer or diabetes mellitus, or immunosuppressed and after long-term or extensive treatment with antibiotics, which upsets the microbial flora, and other drugs, for example, corticosteroids. Oral infection can be caused by poor oral hygiene, including carious teeth and ill-fitting dentures.

canine   of or resembling a dog.

canine tooth   pointed tooth with a single cusp (cuspid) and root, placed third from the midline in both primary and secondary dentitions. A lay term for the upper permanent canine is 'eye tooth'. There are four in all.

cannula   a hollow tube, usually plastic, for the introduction or withdrawal of fluid from the body. In some types the lumen is fitted with a sharp-pointed trocar to facilitate insertion, which is withdrawn when the cannula is in situ.

cannulation   insertion of a cannula, such as into a vein to facilitate the administration of intravenous fluids.

cans   the container for the sodium iodide crystals of scintillation counters to prevent the absorption of moisture by the crystal which would make it cloudy.

canthus   the angle formed by the junction of the eyelids. The inner one is known as the nasal canthus and the outer as the outer (temporal) canthus.

capacitance   is the amount of charge a body can hold per unit potential difference. In a sphere the capacitance is the ratio of the total charge on the body to its potential. If there are two surfaces the capacitance is the ratio of the total charge of one sign on the body to the potential difference between the surfaces.

capacitor   an electrical component consisting of two plates separated by a dielectric, when it receives a potential difference across the plates a charge is stored.

capelline bandage (divergent spica)   a bandage applied in a circular fashion to the head or an amputated limb.

capillary   literally, hair-like; any tiny thin-walled vessel forming part of a network which facilitates rapid exchange of substances between the contained fluid and the surrounding tissues. ***bile capillary*** begins in a space in the liver and joins others, eventually forming a bile duct. ***blood capillary*** unites an arteriole and a venule. ***capillary fragility*** an expression of the ease with which blood capillaries may rupture. ***lymph capillary*** begins in the tissue spaces throughout the body and joins others, eventually forming a lymphatic vessel.

capillary blockade   the injection of large radioactive particles (20–50 μm) that are unable to pass through capillaries and therefore block the first capillary bed they reach. Used in radionuclide imaging to see the vascular bed of the lungs.

capital budget   financial allocation for the purchase of items, such as equipment, that will last longer than 12 months, or items that cost more than an agreed level. *See also* **revenue budget**.

capitate   forms one of the carpal bones of the wrist.

capitation funding   method of allocating money and other resources based on the number of people living in a geographical area. *See also* **weighted capitation**.

capsule   the ligaments which surround a joint. A gelatinous or rice paper container for a drug. The outer membranous covering of certain organs, such as the kidney, liver.

capsulectomy   the surgical excision of a capsule. Refers to a joint or lens; less often to the kidney.

capsulitis   inflammation of a capsule. Sometimes used as a synonym for frozen shoulder.

carbaminohaemoglobin   a compound formed between carbon dioxide and haemoglobin. Some carbon dioxide in the blood is carried in this form.

carbohydrate   an organic compound containing carbon, hydrogen and oxygen. Formed in nature by photosynthesis in plants. Carbohydrates are the major source of energy in most diets, on average 1 g of carbohydrate is metabolized to produce 16 kJ heat. They include starches, sugars and non-starch polysaccharides (NSP), and are classified in three groups – monosaccharides, disaccharides and polysaccharides.

carbon   a non-metallic element found in all organic molecules and living matter. Carbon can bond with four other atoms and is able to form a huge number of complex molecules.

carbon dioxide   a gas; a waste product of many forms of combustion and metabolism, excreted via the lungs. Builds up in respiratory insufficiency or failure and carbon dioxide tension in arterial blood ($PaCO_2$) rises above normal levels.

carbon monoxide   a poisonous gas that combines with haemoglobin to form a stable compound. This blocks the normal reversible oxygen-carrying function and leads to hypoxia. The onset of hypoxia may be insidious but it is associated with confusion, headache, increasing respiratory rate, flushed appearance, changes in conscious level, seizures and cardiac arrhythmias.

carbon tetrachloride   colourless volatile liquid used in dry cleaning and some types of antifreeze. Exposure may result in toxicity and liver damage.

carbonic anhydrase   an enzyme that assists the transfer of carbon dioxide from tissues to blood and to alveolar air by reversibly catalysing the decomposition of carbonic acid into carbon dioxide and water.

carbonic anhydrase inhibitors   drugs that reduce the production of aqueous humour, thereby reducing intraocular pressure. They also have diuretic effects.

carboxyhaemoglobin   a stable compound formed by the union of carbon monoxide and haemoglobin; the red blood cells then lose their respiratory function.

carboxyhaemoglobinaemia   carboxyhaemoglobin in the blood.

carboxyhaemoglobinuria   carboxyhaemoglobin in the urine.

carbuncle   an acute inflammation (usually caused by *Staphylococcus*). There is a collection of boils causing necrosis in the skin and subcutaneous tissue.

carcinoembryonic antigen (CEA)   increased amounts in the serum of adults can be a tumour marker for colorectal cancers and for non-malignant conditions, such as liver cirrhosis caused by alcohol misuse.

carcinogen   agent, substance or environment causing cancer.

carcinogenesis   the production of cancer.

carcinoid syndrome   cluster of symptoms including flushing, palpitation, diarrhoea and bronchospasm from histological (usually low grade) malignancy; often originates in the appendix.

carcinoma   a malignant tumour of epithelial tissue (for example, mucous membrane) and derivatives such as glands.

carcinoma in situ   condition with cells closely resembling cancer cells. A very early cancer. Well described in uterus and prostate. Previously called **preinvasive carcinoma**.

carcinomatosis   widespread malignancy affecting many organs.

cardia   the oesophageal opening into the stomach.

cardiac   associated with the heart, associated with the cardia of the stomach.

cardiac arrest   complete cessation of effective output (of blood) from heart activity. Failure of the heart action to maintain an adequate circulation. The clinical picture of cessation of circulation in a patient who was not expected to die at the time.

cardiac bed   one which can be manipulated so that the patient is supported in a sitting position.

cardiac bypass   operation; the bypassing of atheromatous vessels supplying heart muscle (myocardium).

cardiac catheterization   a long plastic catheter or tubing is inserted into an artery or vein and moved under X-ray guidance until it reaches the heart. A catheter inserted into the brachial or femoral artery gives access to the left side of the heart and those inserted into the brachial or femoral vein can be guided into the right atrium, ventricle and the pulmonary artery. Cardiac catheterization can be used for: (a) recording pressures and cardiac output; (b) the introduction of radiopaque contrast agent for angiography; (c) treatments, such as angioplasty and stent insertion. *See also* **angioplasty**.

cardiac cycle   the series of movements through which the heart passes in performing one heart beat, which corresponds to one pulse beat and takes about one second. *See also* **diastole, systole**.

cardiac enzymes   released from damaged myocardial cells. Abnormal levels found in the blood are suggestive of a diagnosis of myocardial infarction.

Used to confirm or refute the diagnosis of myocardial infarction. The enzymes usually measured are troponins and creatine kinase (CK) but aspartate aminotransferase (AST) and lactate dehydrogenase (LDH) may also be measured.

cardiac massage performed during cardiac arrest. With the person lying on his or her back on a firm surface, the lower part of the sternum (breastbone) is depressed to compress the heart and force blood into the circulation. *See also* **cardiopulmonary resuscitation (CPR)**.

cardiac monitor equipment used to visually record the heart cycle and therefore monitor the activity of the heart.

cardiac oedema gravitational oedema. Such patients secrete excessive aldosterone which increases excretion of potassium and conserves sodium and chloride. Anti-aldosterone (aldosterone antagonists) drugs are useful, for example, spironolactone. *See also* **oedema**.

cardiac output (CO) the volume of blood ejected by the heart per minute, typically 4–5 L/min at rest. It can be expressed as the cardiac index (CI), cardiac output divided by body surface area.

cardiac pacemaker an electrical device for maintaining myocardial contraction by stimulating the heart muscle. A pacemaker may be permanent or temporary. They are programmed in a variety of modes. Nowadays pacemakers can be programmed to alter their rate in response to physical activity.

cardiac tamponade excessive fluid surrounding the heart, usually blood when the cause is traumatic, causes compression of the heart especially the right ventricle leading to impaired cardiac function. Can occur in surgery and penetrating wounds or cardiac rupture.

cardialgia literally, pain in the heart. Often used to mean heartburn (pyrosis).

cardiogenic of cardiac origin.

cardiogenic shock shock caused when the action of the heart is impaired, for example, in heart failure, cardiac injury, disease of the heart muscles.

cardiograph an instrument for recording graphically the force and form of the heart beat.

cardiologist a medically qualified person who specializes in diagnosing and treating diseases of the heart.

cardiology study of the structure, function and diseases of the heart.

cardiomegaly enlargement of the heart.

cardiomyopathy a disease of the myocardium associated with cardiac dysfunction. It is classified as dilated cardiomyopathy, hypertrophic cardiomyopathy, arrhythmogenic right ventricular cardiomyopathy or restrictive cardiomyopathy. Management includes treatment of the cause (if possible), treatment of heart failure and sometimes heart transplantation.

cardiophone a microphone strapped to a patient which allows audible and visual signal of heart sounds. By channelling pulses through an electrocardiograph, a graphic record can be made. Can be used for the fetus.

cardioplegia the use of an electrolyte solution to induce electromechanical cardiac arrest. *cold cardioplegia* combined with hypothermia to reduce the oxygen consumption of the myocardium during open heart surgery.

cardiopulmonary associated with the heart and lungs.

cardiopulmonary bypass used in open heart surgery. The heart and lungs are excluded from the circulation and replaced by a pump oxygenator.

cardiopulmonary resuscitation (CPR) the techniques used to maintain circulation and respiration following cardiopulmonary arrest. It involves (a) the maintenance of a clear airway, (b) artificial respiration using mouth-to-mouth or mouth-to-nose respiration, or with a bag and face mask, or by an endotracheal tube, and (c) maintenance of the circulation by external cardiac massage. *See also* **resuscitation**.

cardiorenal associated with the heart and kidney.

cardiorespiratory associated with the heart and the respiratory system.

cardiorrhaphy stitching of the heart wall: usually reserved for traumatic surgery.

cardiothoracic associated with the heart and thoracic cavity. A specialized branch of surgery.

cardiotocograph the instrument used in cardiotocography.

cardiotocography (CTG) a procedure whereby the fetal heart rate is measured either by an external microphone or by the application of an electrode to the fetal scalp, recording the fetal ECG and from it the fetal heart rate. An external transducer placed on the mother's abdomen measures the uterine contractions.

cardiotomy syndrome pyrexia, pericarditis and pleural effusion following heart surgery. It may develop weeks or months after the operation and is thought to be an autoimmune reaction.

cardiotoxic describes any agent that has an injurious effect on the heart.

cardiovascular associated with the heart and blood vessels.

cardiovascular endurance the ability to sustain exercise without undue fatigue, cardiac distress or respiratory distress.

cardioversion use of electrical countershock for restoring the heart rhythm to normal.

carditis inflammation of the heart. A word seldom used without the appropriate prefix, for example, endo-, myo-, peri-.

caries inflammatory decay of bone, usually associated with pus formation. In dentistry tooth decay. *See also* **dental caries**.

carina   a keel-like structure exemplified by the keel-shaped cartilage at the bifurcation of the trachea into two bronchi.

cariogenic   causing caries, by convention referring to dental caries.

carneous mole   a fleshy mass in the uterus comprising blood clot and a dead fetus or parts of a dead fetus that have not been expelled with miscarriage.

carotid   the principal artery on each side of the neck. At the bifurcation of the common carotid into the internal and external carotids there are: (a) the *carotid bodies* a collection of chemoreceptors which, being sensitive to chemical changes in the blood, protect the body against lack of O_2; (b) the *carotid sinus* a collection of baroreceptors; increased pressure causes slowing of the heart beat and lowering of blood pressure.

carotid angiography   the demonstration of the brain circulation by direct injection of a contrast agent into the carotid artery or via a catheter in the femoral vein which is passed to the carotid artery.

carpal   associated with the wrist.

carpal bones   the eight bones that lie between the distal end for the radius and ulna and the metacarpals.

carpal tunnel syndrome   nocturnal pain, numbness, weakness of the thumb and tingling in the area of distribution of the median nerve in the hand. Due to compression as the nerve passes under the fascial band. Most common in middle-aged women.

carpometacarpal   associated with the carpal and metacarpal bones.

carpopedal   associated with the hands and feet.

carpopedal spasm   painful spasm of hands and feet in tetany. *See also* **hypocalcaemia**.

carpus   the bones of the wrist.

carrier   a person who harbours microorganisms of an infectious disease without showing symptoms and who can transmit infection to others. A person who carries a recessive gene at a specific chromosome location (locus) and therefore passes on a hereditary abnormality.

cartesian co-ordinate   the point on a graph where the value of x meets the value of y.

cartilage   a dense connective tissue capable of withstanding pressure. There are several types according to the function it has to fulfil. There is relatively more cartilage in a child's skeleton but much of it has been converted into bone by adulthood.

cartilaginous joints (amphiarthroses)   joints with either no movement or minimal movement and joined by a layer of cartilage.

caruncle   a red fleshy projection. Hymenal caruncles surround the entrance to the vagina after rupture of the hymen. The *lacrimal caruncle* is the fleshy prominence at the inner angle of the eye.

case–control study   a retrospective research study that compares outcomes for a group with a particular condition with those of a control group who do not have the condition.

case study   research that studies data from one case, or a small group of cases.

caseation   the formation of a soft, cheese-like mass, as occurs in tuberculosis.

caseous degeneration   cheese-like tissue resulting from atrophy in a tuberculoma or gumma.

Casoni test   intradermal injection of fresh, sterile hydatid fluid. A white papule indicates a hydatid cyst.

cassette   a piece of equipment to hold either an imaging plate or radiographic film. It may also contain intensifying screens and a grid.

cast   material or exudate that has been moulded to the form of the cavity or tube in which it has collected. A rigid casing often made with plaster of Paris and applied to immobilize a part of the body.

castration   surgical removal of the testes in the male, or of the ovaries in the female. Castration can be part of the treatment for a hormone-dependent cancer.

CAT   computed axial tomography.

catabolism (katabolism)   the series of chemical reactions in the living body whereby complex substances are broken down into simpler ones accompanied by the release of energy. This energy is needed for converting simple compounds into complex compounds in the body (anabolism), and the other activities of the body.

catalyst   any substance that regulates or accelerates the rate of a chemical reaction without itself undergoing a permanent change.

cataplexy   a condition of muscular rigidity induced by severe mental shock or fear. The patient remains conscious.

cataract   opacity of the lens of the eye causing partial or complete blindness. Usually age-related, but many causes including congenital, traumatic or metabolic such as diabetes mellitus.

catarrh   chronic inflammation of a mucous membrane with constant flow of a thick sticky mucus.

catecholamines   a group of important physiological amines, such as adrenaline (epinephrine), noradrenaline (norepinephrine) and dopamine. They act as hormones and neurotransmitters and affect blood pressure, heart rate, respiratory rate and blood sugar. Abnormally high levels are secreted by adrenal and other tumours and can be detected in the urine. *See also* **phaeochromocytoma**.

categorical data   data that can be categorized, for example, hair colour. *See also* **nominal data, ordinal data**.

CAT scanner   computer assisted tomography or computed axial tomography. *See also* **CT scanner**.

cat scratch fever   a virus infection resulting from a cat scratch or bite. There is fever and lymph node swelling about a week after the incident. Recovery is usually complete, although an abscess may develop.

catheter   a hollow tube of variable length and bore, usually having one fluted end and a tip of varying size and shape according to function. Catheters are made of many substances including soft and hard rubber, gum elastic, glass, silver, other metals and plastic materials, some of which are radiopaque. They have many uses including: blowing gas, air or powder into a cavity, cardiac catheterization, introduction of contrast agent for angiography, withdrawal of fluid from body cavities, for example, urinary catheter and the administration of drugs, fluids and nutrients.

catheterization   insertion of a catheter, most usually into the urinary bladder. *See also* **cardiac catheterization**.

cathetron unit   a high-rate dose, remotely controlled, afterloading device for radiotherapy. Hollow steel catheters are placed in the desired position. They are then connected to a protective safe by hollow cables. The radioactive cobalt moves from the safe into the catheters. After delivery of the required dose, the cobalt returns to the safe, thus avoiding radiation hazard to staff. Currently superseded by units such as the Selectron.

cathode   is the assembly that contains the negatively charged filament, focussing cup, supporting wires and cathode support in an X-ray tube.

cathode rays   streams of electrons coming from the heat filament or cathode.

cathode ray tube   used in older computer monitors where an electron gun is focussed on a fluorescent screen, where electrons hit the screen light is produced and therefore an image is formed. *See also* **glass plasma display, liquid crystal display**.

cation   a positively charged ion which moves towards the cathode when an electric current is passed through an electrolytic solution. *See also* **anion**.

cauda   a tail or tail-like appendage.

cauda equina   lower part of the spinal cord where the nerves for the legs and bladder originate.

caudad   towards the feet.

caudal anaesthesia   injection of local anaesthetic into the epidural space at the level of the sacrum causing loss of sensation in the lower abdomen and pelvis.

cauterize   to cause tissue destruction by applying a heated instrument.

cautery   an agent or device, for example, electricity, chemicals or extremes of temperature, which destroys cells and tissues. Uses include the prevention of blood loss during surgery, or to remove abnormal tissue.

cavernous　having hollow spaces.

cavernous sinus　a channel for venous blood, on either side of the sphenoid bone. It drains blood from the cerebral hemispheres, orbits and the bones of the skull. Sepsis around the eyes or nose can cause cavernous sinus thrombosis.

cavitation　the formation of a cavity, as in pulmonary tuberculosis. When gas bubbles expand, contract, increase in pressure or temperature due to the passage of ultrasound.

cavity　a hollow; an enclosed area.

CDROM (Compact Disk Read-Only Memory)　an object for storing computer data; once the data have been stored they cannot be changed.

CDRW (Compact Disk Re-Writer)　an object for storing computer data; the data can be re-written if required.

celestin tube　a soft rubber intubation tube which is pulled through an oesophageal tumour by the use of a string or guidewire and is attached to the stomach with a suture. Used to maintain a free passage of food and fluid.

cell　basic structural unit of living organisms. A mass of protoplasm (cytoplasm) and usually a nucleus within a plasma or cell membrane. Some cells, for example, erythrocytes, are non-nucleated whereas others, such as voluntary muscle, may be multinucleated. The cytoplasm contains various subcellular organelles – mitochondria, ribosomes, etc. – that undertake the metabolic processes of the cell.

cell cycle　the events occurring within a cell from one mitotic division to the next. Comprises the dynamic course of division of normal and cancer cells incorporating phases of DNA synthesis (S-phase), growth phases (GI and GII), mitosis (M) and 'rest phase' (G0).

cell cycle phase non-specific　describes a cytotoxic drug that acts at any time in the cell cycle.

cell cycle phase specific　describes a cytotoxic drug that acts during a specific phase of the cell cycle.

Celsius　the derived SI unit (International System of Units) for temperature. Named after Anders Celsius (1701–1744) who constructed the first centigrade thermometer. *See also* **centigrade**.

cement　the outer layer covering the root of a tooth and continuous with the enamel.

cementum　calcified organic hard tissue forming on the surface of a root of a tooth, and providing attachment for the periodontal ligament.

Centers for Disease Control and Prevention (CDC)　a federal agency in the USA (Atlanta). Its functions include the investigation, identification, prevention and control of disease.

centigrade　a scale with one hundred divisions or degrees. Most often refers to the thermometric scale in which the freezing point of water is fixed at

0°C and the boiling point at 100°C. It is usually called Celsius for medical and scientific purposes. *See also* **Celsius**.

central limit theorem   in research: sampling distribution becomes more normal the more samples that are taken.

central sterile supplies department (CSSD)   designated an area where packets are prepared containing the equipment and/or swabs and dressings necessary to perform activities requiring aseptic technique. *See also* **hospital sterilization and disinfection unit (HSDU)**.

central tendency statistic   averages. The tendency for observations to centre around a specific value rather than across the entire range. *See also* **mean, median, mode**.

central venous catheter/line   specialized intravenous cannula placed in a large vein (jugular, subclavian or femoral). Used for the measurement of central venous pressure, and fluids and drugs. Also allows long-term vascular access for the administration of drugs, blood products or nutritional support.

central venous pressure (CVP)   the pressure of the blood within the right atrium. It is measured using a central venous catheter attached to a manometer or pressure transducer.

centralized daylight system   a system where the loading and unloading of a cassette or film magazine is directly linked to an automatic film processor.

centric occlusion   contact of the upper and lower teeth with maximum contact of the cusps.

centrifugal   efferent. Having a tendency to move outwards from the centre, as the nerve impulses from the brain to the peripheral structures.

centrifuge   an apparatus which subjects solutions to centrifugal forces by high-speed rotation, thereby separating substances of different densities into discrete bands within the liquid phase. It is usually used to separate ('spin down') particulate material (for example, subcellular particles) from a suspending liquid.

centriole   a subcellular organelle that aids spindle formation during nuclear division. *See also* **meiosis, mitosis**.

centronics   a type of standard interface between computer and peripheral.

cephalalgia   pain in the head; headache.

cephalic   associated with the head; near the head.

cephalocele   hernia of the brain; protrusion of part of the brain through the skull.

cephalometric radiograph   a lateral projection of the skull and mandible for making cranial measurements to estimate the degree of any facial abnormality.

cephalometry   measurement of the living human head.

ceramic detector   a modern device used in CT scanning to measure the amount of radiation transmitted through a patient, giving a reduction in noise compared with earlier detectors and in chest scans there is said to be a reduction in beam hardening artefacts.

cerebellar gait   a staggering, unsteady, wide-based walk seen in patients with damage to the cerebellum or its connections. *See also* **gait**.

cerebellum   that part of the brain which lies behind and below the cerebrum. Its chief functions are the coordination of fine voluntary movements and the control of posture.

cerebral   associated with the cerebrum.

cerebral cavity   the ventricles of the brain.

cerebral compression   arises from any space-occupying intracranial lesion.

cerebral cortex   the outer layer of cells (grey matter) in the cerebral hemispheres.

cerebral hemisphere   one side of the cerebrum, right or left.

cerebral palsy   non-progressive brain damage that typically occurs at, or shortly after, birth resulting in a range of mainly motor conditions ranging from clumsiness to severe spasticity.

cerebral function monitor (CFM)   equipment for continuous monitoring of brain wave activity, for example, to detect seizures in sedated and paralysed patients.

cerebral perfusion pressure (CPP)   the pressure which drives blood through the brain. It is the difference between the arterial blood pressure and the intracranial pressure. If CPP is too low the blood flow to the brain may be inadequate and the brain deprived of oxygen.

cerebrospinal   associated with the brain and spinal cord.

cerebrospinal fluid   the clear fluid found within the ventricles (cavities) of the brain, central canal of the spinal cord and beneath the cranial and spinal meninges in the subarachnoid space. Protects and nourishes the brain and spinal cord. It is formed by the choroid plexus in the ventricles and circulates around the brain and spinal cord before it is reabsorbed on the outside of the brain.

cerebrovascular   associated with the blood vessels of the brain.

cerebrovascular accident   (stroke) (CVA) interference with the cerebral blood flow due to embolism, haemorrhage or thrombosis. Signs and symptoms vary according to the duration, extent and site of tissue damage; there may be only a passing, even momentary inability to move a hand or foot; weakness or tingling in a limb; stertorous breathing; incontinence of urine and faeces; coma; paralysis of a limb or limbs; and speech deficiency (aphasia). *See also* **transient ischaemic attack**.

cerebrum the largest and uppermost part of the brain. The longitudinal fissure divides it into two hemispheres, each containing a lateral ventricle. A mass of nerve fibres (white matter) is covered by a thin layer of nerve cells (grey matter). It controls the higher functions and contains major motor and sensory areas. The outer surface is convoluted.

cerumen ear wax, sticky brown secretion from glands in the external auditory canal. Traps dust and other particles entering the ear.

cervical associated with the neck. Associated with the cervix (neck) of an organ.

cervical canal the lumen of the cervix uteri, from the internal to the external os.

cervical intraepithelial neoplasm (CIN) abnormal changes in the basal layer of the squamous epithelial layers of the uterus and is divided into three grades, CIN 1 is pre-malignant through to CIN3 which is early cancer.

cervical rib an additional rib articulating with the seventh cervical vertebra.

cervical smear *see* **cervical intraepithelial neoplasia**.

cervical vertebrae the seven bones that form the neck.

cervicectomy amputation of the uterine cervix.

cervicitis inflammation of the uterine cervix.

cervix a neck.

cervix uteri uterine cervix, the neck of the uterus.

cetrimide a disinfectant with detergent properties. Used for wound cleansing and skin preparation.

chancre the primary syphilitic ulcer developing at the site of infection with *Treponema pallidum*. It is associated with swelling of local lymph nodes. The chancre is painless, hard (indurated), solitary and highly infectious.

characteristic curve applies to a particular film or film/screen combination and is the curve which results when the density is plotted against the log of relative exposure. It is also called *D log E curve, a Hurter and Driffield curve, a log It curve*. The curve is used to determine the basic fog level, threshold, toe, straight line portion, shoulder and maximum density of the film. *See also* **basic fog level, threshold, toe, straight line portion, shoulder, maximum density**. (See figure on p. 80).

charcoal used therapeutically for its adsorptive and deodorant properties. Can be taken to absorb abdominal gas. Activated charcoal incorporated into dressings is used to reduce odour in discharging wounds.

Charcot's joint complete disorganization of a joint associated with fluid-filled cavities in the spinal cord (syringomyelia), diabetes mellitus, or advanced cases of wasting away of the posterior nerve roots of the spinal cord (tabes dorsalis, locomotor ataxia). The condition is painless.

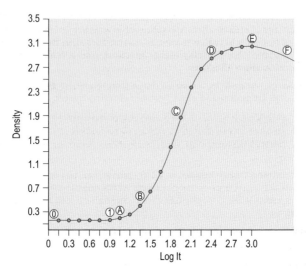

The characteristic curve. Basic Fog 0 to point 1. Threshold point A. Toe A to B. Straight line portion B to C. Shoulder D. Maximum density E. Region of solarization F onwards. From Radiographic imaging, 3rd edn, Chris Gunn, 2002, Churchill Livingstone, Edinburgh, with permission.

CHART   continuous hyperfractionated accelerated radiotherapy.

chelate   a compound composed of a central metal ion and an organic molecule with multiple bonds, formed in a ring formation.

chemonucleolysis   injection of an enzyme, usually into an intervertebral disc, for dissolution of same.

chemoradiation   giving chemotherapy and radiotherapy at the same time.

chemoreceptor   a sensory nerve ending or a cell having an affinity for, and capable of reacting to, a chemical stimuli, for example, taste, oxygen levels in the blood.

chemoresistant   describes a tumour that does not usually shrink with chemotherapy.

chemosensitive   describes a tumour that shrinks following chemotherapy administration.

chemotaxis   movements of a cell (for example, leucocyte) or a microorganism in response to chemical stimuli; attraction is termed positive chemotaxis, repulsion is negative.

chemotherapy   chemical agents of various types; prescribed to delay or arrest growth of cancer cells through interruption/inhibition of cell cycle; on a selective basis by impairing their ability to replicate. Usually given in combination rather than as single agents. They are non-selective and non-specific and therefore affect all cycling cells whether benign or malignant. Administration is by oral, intramuscular, intravenous, intracavitary, or intra-arterial routes. *See also* **alkylating agents, antimetabolites, antitumour antibiotics, vinca alkaloids**.

chenodeoxycholic acid   a bile acid. It can be taken orally to dissolve certain types of gallstones.

Cheyne–Stokes respiration   a cyclic pattern of irregular breathing followed by an absence of breathing for about 15 seconds, occurring in patients with cerebral disease, especially when there is increased intracranial pressure.

chi-square test   a statistical test used to compare groups to see if the behaviour of one of the groups is significant. A chi-square table is used and the results must be equal to or greater than the value given in the table to be significant.

chiasma   an X-shaped crossing or crossing of nerve fibres (decussation). *See also* **optic chiasma**.

child abuse   physical, sexual or emotional abuse or neglect of children by relatives or health and social care staff. *See also* **non-accidental injuries**.

chip   a piece of silicon or gallium arsenide which contains the microcircuitry which operates the computer.

chiropractic   a technique of spinal manipulation, based on the principle that defects in vertebral alignment may result in various problems caused by functional changes in the nervous system.

chiropractor   a person who uses chiropractic techniques.

chi-square statistic (χ^2)   a technique used to analyse the relationship between expected frequency and the actual frequency of data obtained. A test of statistical significance used to determine the probability of results occurring by chance. *See also* **non-parametric tests**.

chlorhexidine   a disinfectant solution which is effective against a wide range of bacteria. Used for general skin cleansing and disinfection, and hand decontamination, etc.

chloride   a salt of hydrochloric acid. A major anion in extracellular fluid.

chlorine   a greenish-yellow, irritating gaseous element. Powerful disinfectant, bleaching and deodorizing agent in the presence of moisture when nascent oxygen is liberated. Mainly used as hypochlorites, or other compounds which slowly liberate active chlorine.

chloroform   a heavy liquid, once used extensively as a general anaesthetic. Used as chloroform water as a flavouring and preservative in aqueous mixtures.

choanae   funnel-shaped openings. *See also* **nares**.

cholangiography   rarely performed radiographic examination of hepatic, cystic and bile ducts. Can be performed: (a) after oral or intravenous administration of a radiographic contrast agent, (b) by direct injection at operation to detect any further stones in the ducts, (c) during or after operation by way of a T-tube in the common bile duct, (d) by means of an injection via the skin on the anterior abdominal wall and the liver, when it is called percutaneous transhepatic cholangiography (PTC). *See also* **endoscopic retrograde cholangiopancreatography**.

cholangitis   inflammation of the bile ducts.

cholecystectomy   surgical removal of the gallbladder. *See also* **laparoscopic cholecystectomy**.

cholecystenterostomy   literally, the establishment of an artificial opening (anastomosis) between the gallbladder and the small intestine. Specific terminology more frequently used.

cholecystitis   inflammation of the gallbladder.

cholecystoduodenal   associated with the gallbladder and duodenum as an anastomosis between them.

cholecystoduodenostomy   the establishment of an artificial connection (anastomosis) between the gallbladder and the duodenum.

cholecystography   rarely performed radiographic examination of the gallbladder after administration of opaque contrast agent. Superseded by CT and MRI.

cholecystojejunostomy   an artificial connection (anastomosis) between the gallbladder and the jejunum.

cholecystokinin (CCK)   a hormone that contracts the gallbladder and relaxes the sphincter of Oddi thus allowing bile into the duodenum, and stimulates the secretion of pancreatic enzymes. Secreted by the duodenal mucosa.

cholecystolithiasis   the presence of stone or stones in the gallbladder.

cholecystostomy   a surgically established fistula between the gallbladder and the abdominal surface; used to provide drainage, in a collection of pus (empyema) in the gallbladder.

cholecystotomy   incision into the gallbladder.

choledochoduodenal   associated with the bile ducts and duodenum, for example, choledochoduodenal fistula.

choledochography   *see* **cholangiography**.

choledochojejunostomy   an anastomosis between the bile duct and the jejunum.

choledocholithiasis   the presence of a gallstone or gallstones in the extrahepatic bile ducts.

choledocholithotomy   surgical removal of a stone from the common bile duct.

choledochoscopy   endoscopic examination of the biliary tree.

choledochostomy   drainage of the common bile duct using a T-tube, usually after exploration for a stone.

choledochotomy   incision into the common bile duct.

cholelithiasis   the presence or formation of gallstones in the gallbladder or bile ducts.

cholestasis   an obstruction to the flow of bile. It produces jaundice, dark urine, pale stools, metallic taste and pruritus. *See also* **extrahepatic cholestasis, intrahepatic cholestasis**.

cholesteatoma   a benign encysted tumour containing squamous epithelial debris. Mainly occurs in the middle ear.

cholesterol   a sterol found in many tissues. It is an important component of cell membranes and is the precursor of many biological molecules, such as steroid hormones. High levels in the blood are linked with the development of arterial disease and some types of gallstones. *See also* **hypercholesterolaemia**.

cholesterosis   abnormal deposition of cholesterol.

cholic acid   a bile acid.

chondritis   inflammation of cartilage.

chondroblastoma   a benign tumour that usually develops in the epiphyses of the femur and humerus.

chondrocostal   associated with the costal cartilages and ribs.

chondrodynia   pain in a cartilage.

chondrolysis   dissolution of cartilage.

chondroma   a benign tumour of cartilage.

chondromalacia   softening of cartilage.

chondrosarcoma   malignant tumour of cartilage.

chondrosternal   associated with the costal cartilages and sternum.

chordoma   a rare tumour that develops in the fetal notochord.

choriocarcinoma (chorionepithelioma)   a malignant tumour of chorionic cells; develops following normal pregnancy (rarely), miscarriage or evacuation of a hydatidiform mole. A sensitive (though not specific) tumour marker is human chorionic gonadotrophin (HCG). Choriocarcinoma is usually chemosensitive and curable.

chorion   the outer membrane forming the sac that contains the amniotic fluid and the fetus.

chorion biopsy   *see* **amnion, chorionic villus sampling**.

chorionepithelioma   *see* **choriocarcinoma**.

chorionic   associated with the chorion. chorionic gonadotrophin. *See also* **human chorionic gonadotrophin**.

chorionic villi   vascular projections from the chorion from which the fetal part of the placenta is formed. Through which substances such as nutrients and waste diffuse between maternal and fetal blood and vice versa.

chorionic villus sampling (CVS)   also known as chorion biopsy or chorionic villus biopsy. A prenatal screening test for chromosomal and other inherited disorders. Samples of fetal tissue are obtained using the transabdominal or transcervical approach for the detection of genetic abnormalities during early pregnancy done after 10 weeks to avoid the potential risk of limb malformations.

choroid   the middle pigmented, vascular coat of the posterior five-sixths of the eyeball, continuous with the iris in front. It lies between the sclera externally and the retina internally, and prevents the passage of light rays.

choroid plexus   specialized capillaries in the cerebral ventricles that produce cerebrospinal fluid.

chromatic aberration   the non-convergence of different coloured rays in a lens.

chromatid   one of the strands that result from the duplication of chromosomes during nuclear division.

chromatid aberrations   caused when cells are irradiated after the DNA replication phase.

chromatin   the threads of DNA and protein that form the substance of chromosomes.

chromatography   a method of chemical analysis by which substances in solution can be separated from each other. Includes: *gel filtration chromatography*, *gas chromatography* and *ion exchange chromatography*.

chromosomal aberration   loss, gain or exchange of genetic material in the chromosomes of a cell resulting in deletion, duplication, inversion or translocation of genes.

chromosome   the genetic material present in the nucleus of the cell. During the preparation for cell division chromosomes appear as microscopic threads. They contain strands of DNA molecules or genes. Each species has a constant number; humans have 23 pairs (46) in each somatic cell: 22 pairs of autosomes and 1 pair of sex chromosomes (males have XY and females have XX). Mature gametes, however, have half the usual number (haploid) which results from the reduction division during meiosis. The 23 unpaired chromosomes inherited from each parent unite to produce an embryo with 46 chromosomes (diploid). Genetic sex is determined by the male gamete and depends on whether the oocyte is fertilized by a sperm that contributes a Y chromosome (genetic male) or an X chromosome (genetic female). Some genetic material is also present in organelles, such as the mitochondria. *See also* **meiosis, mitosis**.

chromosome aberrations   DNA damage caused when cells are irradiated in the G_1 phase of the cell cycle.

chronic   lingering, lasting, opposed to acute. The word does not imply any-thing about the severity of the condition.

chronic fatigue syndrome   *see* **benign myalgic encephalomyelitis**.

chronic heart failure   *see* **congestive heart failure**.

chronic leukaemia   *see* **leukaemia**.

chronic obstructive airways disease (COAD)   group of obstructive lung dis-eases in which airway resistance is increased with impaired airflow. *See also* **chronic obstructive pulmonary disease (COPD)**.

chronic obstructive pulmonary disease (COPD)   group of obstructive lung dis-eases where airway resistance is increased with impaired airflow, for exam-ple, pulmonary emphysema and chronic bronchitis. Defined on spirometric grounds as an $FEV_1 < 80\%$ and an FEV1:FVC ratio $< 70\%$. Usually seen as a long-term sequela of smoking. Genetic factors include α1-antitrypsin defi-ciency, and more recently, family clustering studies suggest other genetic susceptibility factors.

chronological age   a person's age in years.

chronotherapy   the administration of treatment, such as chemotherapy or radiotherapy, at the most effective time.

chyle   fatty, milky fluid formed from chylomicrons within the lymphatic lacteals of the intestinal villi.

chylomicron   tiny particles formed from triglycerides, lipoproteins and cho-lesterol and lipoproteins within the intestinal mucosa following the absorp-tion of digested fat. They form chyle within the lacteals.

chyme   partially digested food which is acidic passes from the stomach to the duodenum. Its acidity controls the pylorus to regulate the amount entering the duodenum.

chymotrypsin   an inactive proteolytic enzyme secreted by the pancreas: it is activated by trypsin.

cilia   the eyelashes. Microscopic hair-like projections from certain epithelial cells. Membranes containing such cells, for example, those lining the tra-chea and uterine (fallopian) tubes, are known as ciliated membranes.

ciliary   hair like.

ciliary body   a specialized structure in the eye connecting the anterior choroid to the iris, it is composed of the ciliary muscles and processes.

ciliary muscles   fine muscle fibres arranged in a circular manner. They con-trol accommodation.

ciliary processes   about 70 in number, they secrete aqueous humour.

circadian rhythm   any rhythm with a period of 24 hours.

circulation   passage in a circle. Usually means circulation of the blood. *See also* **pulmonary circulations, systemic circulation**.

circulation of bile   *see* **enterohepatic circulation**.

circulation of blood   the passage of blood from heart to arteries to capillaries to veins and back to heart.

circulation of cerebrospinal fluid   takes place from the ventricles of the brain to the cisterna magna, whence the fluid bathes the surface of the brain and the spinal cord, including its central canal. It is absorbed into the blood in the cerebral venous sinuses.

circulation of lymph   lymph is collected from the tissue spaces and passed in the lymphatic capillaries, vessels, nodes and ducts to be returned to the bloodstream.

circumduction   a combination of the movements of flexion, extension, abduction, adduction and internal and external rotation. For example the movement in the shoulder joint when the arm moves in a circle.

circumferential lamellae   rings of bone round the edge of a long bone.

circumvallate   surrounded by a raised ring, as the large circumvallate papillae at the base of the tongue.

cirrhosis   hardening of an organ. There are degenerative changes in the tissues with resulting fibrosis. Cirrhosis of liver is increasing in prosperous countries. Damage to liver cells can be from viruses, other microorganisms or toxic substances and dietary deficiencies interfering with the nutrition of liver cells, often the result of alcohol misuse. Associated developments include ascites, obstruction of the circulation through the hepatic portal vein with haematemesis, jaundice and enlargement of the spleen.

cisterna   any closed space serving as a reservoir for a body fluid.

cisterna chyli   the pear-shaped commencement of the thoracic duct. It receives lymph. ***cisterna magna*** is a subarachnoid space in the cleft between the cerebellum and medulla oblongata.

cisternal puncture   insertion of a special hollow needle with stylet between the occiput and atlas, into the cisterna magna. One method of obtaining cerebrospinal fluid but rarely used. *See also* **lumbar puncture**.

cisternography   the injection of a radionuclide into the subarachnoid space via a lumbar puncture. The radionuclide concentrates in the ventricles, demonstrates, communicating hydrocephalus, cerebrospinal fluid shunts and fistulae.

civil law   law relating to non-criminal matters. Civil action proceedings brought in the civil courts. Civil wrong act or omission which can be pursued in the civil courts by the person who has suffered the wrong.

classical scattering   *see* **coherent scattering**.

classified person   an employee who is likely to receive a dose of ionizing radiation which exceeds three-tenths of any relevant dose limit.

claustrophobia   fear of confined places.

clavicle   the collar bone.

clavus   a corn. *See also* **callus**.

claw-foot *see* **pes cavus**.

claw-hand the hand is flexed and contracted giving a claw-like appearance; the condition may be due to injury or disease.

cleanser (describes) agents that have cleansing properties. Drugs such as cetrimide are both disinfectant and cleansing. Used to remove dirt, grease, etc., from the skin or wounds, and for removing crusts and other debris from skin lesions.

clearance the ability of the kidney to remove a specific substance from the blood. *renal clearance* used to measure glomerular filtration rate and kidney function by calculating the volume of blood cleared of a substance such as creatinine, in a given time, usually 1 minute.

clear-based films have no dye in the base and have a low base fog and are particularly suited for ultrasound imaging.

clearing time the time taken in a fixer solution for the unexposed areas of the film to become transparent.

cleft lip a congenital defect in the lip; a fissure extending from the margin of the lip to the nostril; may be single or double, and is often associated with cleft palate.

cleft palate congenital failure of fusion between the right and left palatal processes. Often associated with cleft lip.

client quality the patient's view of how well the service or product provides what is expected by the patient.

clinical audit critical and systematic analysis of the quality of clinical care and treatment. It includes diagnostic procedures, treatment, resource use and outputs including quality of life.

clinical governance the framework within which all NHS organizations are accountable for their services, and are required to operate an active programme of continuous quality improvement within an overall, coherent framework of cost-effective service delivery.

clinical guidelines systematically developed statements that help the practitioner and patient in making decisions about care. *See also* **evidence-based practice**.

clinical target volume the total treatment field in relation to the tumour in radiotherapy.

clinical thermometer previously, glass and mercury thermometers of various types were used to take a patient's temperature. These have mostly been replaced by safer alternatives, such as electronic probes, for example, tympanic membrane thermometers, and single-use thermometers.

clinodactyly incurving of a finger, usually the fifth.

clitoris a small erectile organ situated at anterior junction of the labia minora. Involved in the female sexual response.

cloaca   the common intestinal and urogenital opening found in many vertebrates. In osteomyelitis, the opening through newly formed bone from a diseased area to enable pus to discharge.

clonal   derived from a single cell.

clonogenic cell   a cell that can proliferate into a colony of genetically identical cells.

clonus   a series of intermittent muscular contractions and relaxations.

closed fracture   a broken bone where the skin surface is intact.

closed manipulation   a method of manually realigning broken bones under general anaesthetic without the use of surgery.

clubbed fingers   a thickening and broadening of the bulbous fleshy portion of the fingers under the nails. The cause is not known but it occurs in people who have chronic heart and/or lung disease.

club foot   a congenital malformation, either unilateral or bilateral. *See also* **talipes**.

Clutton's joints   joints which show symmetrical swelling usually painless, the knees often being involved. Associated with congenital syphilis.

coagulation   the third of four overlapping processes involved in haemostasis. Coagulation (clotting) occurs through a series of complex reactions that use enzyme cascade amplification to start the formation of a fibrin clot to stop bleeding. There are two pathways/systems, intrinsic and extrinsic, which converge to follow a common final pathway. Coagulation starts when platelets break down, tissue is damaged and thromboplastins are released. Various factors are involved in coagulation: I, fibrinogen; II, prothrombin; III, tissue thromboplastin; IV, calcium ions; V, labile factor (proaccelerin); VII, stable factor (proconvertin); VIII, antihaemophilic factor (AHF); IX, Christmas factor; X, Stuart–Prower factor; XI, plasma thromboplastin antecedent; XII, Hageman factor; and XIII, fibrin-stabilizing factor. During the final common pathway, inactive prothrombin is converted to thrombin, the active enzyme. Thrombin converts soluble fibrinogen to insoluble fibrin, which forms a network of fibres in which blood cells are caught to form the clot. *See also* **haemostasis, platelet plug**.

coarctation   contraction, stricture, narrowing; applied to a vessel or canal. *coarctation of the aorta* congenital narrowing of the aorta, commonly affecting the area just after the origin of the left subclavian artery.

coating weight   the amount of phosphor per unit volume in a radiographic intensifying screen.

cobalt (Co)   an essential trace element, utilized as a constituent of vitamin B_{12} (cobalamins). Required for healthy red blood cell production and proper neurological function.

cobalt-60   a radioactive isotope of cobalt which is used as a source of radiation in teletherapy.

cobalt unit   a radiotherapy machine housing the isotope cobalt-60, the resultant radiation delivers the maximum dose below the skin surface and therefore reduces the likelihood of skin reactions.

cocaine   a powerful local anaesthetic obtained from the leaves of the coca plant. It is a controlled drug which is highly addictive and subject to considerable criminal misuse. Toxic, especially to the brain; may cause agitation, disorientation and convulsions. ***crack cocaine*** a highly potent and addictive form.

coccus   a spherical bacterium.

coccydynia   pain in the region of the coccyx.

coccygectomy   surgical removal of the coccyx.

coccyx   the last bone of the vertebral column. It is composed of four or five rudimentary vertebrae, cartilaginous at birth, ossification being completed at about the 30th year.

cochlea   a spiral canal resembling the interior of a snail shell, in the anterior part of the bony labyrinth of the ear.

Cockcroft–Walton generator   utilizes a number of rectifiers and capacitors, connected in series to produce a fully rectified voltage with less than 0.2% ripple. A single unit can cover the low-energy therapeutic X-ray range but for medium energy radiotherapy machines two units are used back to back. A voltage multiplier circuit using diodes and capacitors used in some X-ray generator systems.

code of practice   the guidelines setting out how healthcare professionals should fulfil their roles, duties, obligations and responsibilities, such as those produced by the statutory bodies whose functions are to regulate the registration and practice of healthcare professionals, for example, General Medical Council.

coeliac   relating to the abdominal cavity; applied to arteries and a nerve plexus.

coeliac disease (gluten-induced enteropathy)   due to intolerance to the protein gluten in wheat and rye. This results in subtotal villous atrophy of the mucosa of the small intestine and the malabsorption syndrome. Symptoms may become apparent at any age or patients may be asymptomatic. Treatment is with gluten-free diet.

coffee ground vomit   vomit containing blood, which in its partially digested state resembles coffee grounds. Indicative of slow upper gastrointestinal bleeding. *See also* **haematemesis**.

cognitive   the mental process of comprehension, judgement, memory and reasoning as opposed to emotional processes.

coherent scattering   when a photon interacts with an electron, is deflected from its path but does not lose energy. *See also* **elastic scattering**.

cohort   a group of people who have some common feature or characteristic, for example, year group at university.

cohort study   research that studies a population that shares a common feature, such as occupation.

coil   single or multiple loops of wire designed to produce (or transmit) a magnetic field when current flows through the wire or measure (or receive) an induced voltage in the loop caused by a changing magnetic field. *See also* **induction, transformer**.

coitus   insertion of the erect penis into the vagina; the act of sexual intercourse or copulation.

coitus interruptus   removal from the vagina of the penis before ejaculation of semen as a means of contraception. The method is considered unsatisfactory as it is not only unreliable but can lead to sexual disharmony.

cold spot   a term used in radionuclide imaging when a lower than expected quantity of radiation is detected.

cold water processor   an automatic film processor that only has a cold water supply and is more energy efficient than processors that use hot and cold water.

colectomy   excision of part or the whole of the colon.

colic   severe pain resulting from periodic spasm in an abdominal organ. *intestinal colic* abnormal peristaltic movement of an irritated gut. *renal colic* spasm of ureter due to the presence of a stone. *biliary colic* spasm of the biliary system due to the presence of a stone.

coliform   describes any of the enterobacteria (intestinal bacteria) such as *Escherichia coli*.

colitis   inflammation of the colon. May be acute or chronic, and may be accompanied by ulcerative lesions. *See also* **inflammatory bowel disease, ulcerative colitis**.

collagen   the main protein constituent of white fibrous tissue of skin, tendon, bone, cartilage and all connective tissue.

collagen diseases   there is inflammation of unknown aetiology affecting collagen and small blood vessels. They involve autoimmune responses and include dermatomyositis, polyarteritis nodosa, rheumatoid arthritis, scleroderma and systemic lupus erythematosus (SLE).

collapse   the 'falling in' of a hollow organ or vessel, for example, collapse of lung from change of air pressure inside or outside the organ. A vague term describing physical or nervous prostration.

collapsing pulse   also known as *Corrigan's pulse*. The water-hammer pulse of aortic regurgitation with high initial upthrust which quickly falls away.

collar bone   the clavicle.

collateral circulation   an alternative route provided for the blood by secondary blood vessels when a primary vessel is blocked.

collecting tubule   straight tube in the kidney medulla conveying urine to the renal pelvis.

Colles' fracture   a break at the lower end of the radius and ulna following a fall on the outstretched hand. The backward displacement of the radius produces the 'dinner fork' deformity. A common fracture in older women and associated with osteoporosis.

collimate   literally to make parallel. Restriction of the X-ray beam to a particular area. In CT this may be done pre patient or pre and post patient. ***pre-patient collimation*** restricts the incident beam to the required body area, determining the data set to be acquired. ***Post-patient collimation*** restricts scatter reaching the detectors: primarily on single slice units.

collimation   the restriction of the size of an X-ray beam to minimize radiation dosage.

collimator   a device for defining the size of the beam from an X-ray tube. ***primary collimator*** defines the maximum available beam size; the ***secondary collimators*** can be adjusted to restrict the field size to the treatment area in radiotherapy or the image size in diagnostic radiography. A device on a gamma camera designed to accurately project an image of radioactive distribution received from the patient on to the scintillator. *See also* **parallel-hole collimator, pin-hole collimator, converging collimator**.

collision   in computing a collision occurs if two computers access the network at the same time.

collodion   a solution forming a flexible film on the skin. Previously used as a protective dressing.

colloid   glue-like. A non-crystalline chemical; diffusible but not soluble in water; unable to pass through a semipermeable membrane. Some drugs can be prepared in their colloidal form.

colloid degeneration   that which results in the formation of gelatinous material, as in tumours.

colloid goitre   enlargement of the thyroid gland caused by the presence of viscid, iodine-containing colloid within the gland.

colloid solutions   ones containing large molecules used intravenously in the treatment of shock.

colon   the large bowel extending from the caecum to the rectum. Comprises the ascending, transverse, descending and sigmoid colon. *See also* **flexure, megacolon**.

colonic lavage   the washing out of the colon by using an enema, to empty the bowel prior to an examination or operation.

colonic washout   a method of clearing the bowel of faecal matter.

colonoscopy   the examination of the colon by the insertion of a fibreoptic instrument.

colony   a mass of bacteria resulting from the multiplication of one or more microorganisms. Containing many millions of individual micro-organisms it may be visible to the unaided eye; its physical features are often characteristic of the species.

colorectal   associated with the colon and the rectum.

colostomy   a surgically established fistula between the colon and the surface of the abdomen; to form either a temporary or permanent artificial anus (stoma) that discharges faeces.

colotomy   incision into the colon.

colour depth   the maximum number of colours a computer monitor is able to display and is determined by the bit depth, with 16 giving good colour and 24 giving true colour.

colour flow Doppler   the simultaneous ultrasound display of anatomical and flow information. Anatomy is shown as a grey scale image and blood flow in colour, for example, blood flowing towards the transducer is usually in red and away from the transducer is usually displayed in blue.

colour sensitizing   increasing the spectral sensitivity of the film by adding impurities to the film emulsion. *See also* **spectral sensitizing**.

colpocele   protrusion or prolapse of either the bladder or rectum so that it presses on the vaginal wall.

colpohysterectomy   removal of the uterus through the vagina. *See also* **hysterectomy**.

colpophotography   filming the cervix using a camera and colposcope.

colporrhaphy   surgical repair of the vagina. An *anterior colporrhaphy* repairs a protrusion of the bladder through the wall of the vagina (cystocele) and a *posterior colporrhaphy* repairs a protrusion of the rectum and posterior wall of the vagina into the vagina (rectocele).

colposcope   a binocular instrument used to obtain a high-power view of the cervix in cases of abnormal cervical smears. Used for diagnostic procedures and local treatments to the cervix.

colposcopy   the examination of the cervix using light and magnification.

coma   a state of unconsciousness from which the patient cannot be aroused, the severity can be assessed by corneal and pupillary reflexes and withdrawal responses to painful stimuli.

comet tail artefact   multiple reflections of ultrasound usually produced by small artefacts, usually in the gall bladder wall.

comminuted fracture   a break in a bone where the bone is fragmented.

Commission for Healthcare Audit and Inspection (CHAI) (Healthcare Commission)   a body with statutory powers to inspect and support the implementation of clinical governance arrangements in NHS Trusts. Their remit also includes targeted support when requested by organizations with a specific problem, and in more serious situations they may intervene by direction of the Secretary of State or at the request of Strategic Health Authorities, NHS Trusts or Primary Care Trusts. Also responsible for the second stage of the NHS Complaints procedure.

commissioning a complex process that aims to ensure that a specific population has an appropriate level of service provision. The stages include a needs assessment that is used to determine priorities, taking into account the overall national policy guidance from government. On completion of this process, an appropriate range of services are purchased from relevant providers. The final stage is evaluation.

commissioning tests checks made on new radiotherapy equipment to ensure that it is safe to treat patients; tests include radiation protection, leakage, accuracy of beam direction devices, beam modalities and output dose calibration.

committed dose the absorbed dose of radiation an individual receives as the result of the intake of radioactive material.

Committee on Safety of Medicines (CSM) in the UK the body that monitors drug safety and advises the licensing authority regarding the safety, efficacy and quality of medicines.

common variable immunodeficiency (CVID) one of the primary antibody deficiency syndromes, presenting in children or adulthood and associated with recurrent infections, autoimmunity, and an increased risk of malignancy.

communicable transmissible directly or indirectly from one person to another.

community care the care and support of individuals in community settings. Such care is delivered by health and social care professionals and unpaid carers such as family and neighbours. The community or primary care setting is increasingly important in the development and delivery of health services. *See also* **Primary Care Trust**.

comorbidity coexistence of two or more diseases.

compact bone the type of dense bone containing cylindrical structures called haversian systems which is found mainly in the shafts of long bones.

compact disk (CD) a 120-mm sheet of aluminium covered with a layer of acetate and with a polycarbonate backing. Used in computing to store data in digital form which can be read by a laser.

comparative study research study that compares two separate populations.

compartment syndrome swelling of the muscles in one of the limb compartments leading to ischaemia and necrosis of muscle tissue. Treatment is incision of the muscle fascia (fasciotomy).

compatibility suitability; congruity. The ability of a substance to mix with another without unfavourable results, for example, two medicines, blood plasma and cells.

complemental air the extra air that can be drawn into the lungs by deep inspiration.

complete abortion   a termination of pregnancy or a miscarriage when all the products of conception are expelled or removed.

complete miscarriage   the entire contents of the uterus are expelled.

complicated fracture   a break in bone continuity with associated injury of an organ or vessel.

complication   in medicine, an accident or second disease arising in the course of a primary disease; it can be fatal.

compound   a substance composed of two or more elements, chemically combined in a definitive proportion to form a new substance which displays new properties.

compound filters   beam-hardening filters made of tin, copper and aluminium used in radiotherapy. To be effective the filters must be fitted in the correct order, with those of the highest atom number nearest the target and the lowest nearest the patient.

compound (open) fracture   where part of the fracture is in contact with the external surface of the body.

compress   usually refers to a folded pad of lint, gauze or other material used to arrest haemorrhage or apply pressure, cold, heat, moisture or medication. Used to reduce swelling or pain, such as a cold compress to ease a headache.

compression   the state of being compressed. Pressing or squeezing together.

compression band   in radiography, an immobilization device which also displaces body tissue laterally and therefore enables a reduction in radiographic exposure factors and as a result radiation dose to the patient.

compression bandage/therapy   used in the management of venous leg ulcers to increase venous return and reduce venous hypertension. *compression stockings* are used to prevent venous leg ulcers occurring where there is venous insufficiency, or to reduce the risk of deep vein thrombosis following surgery or immobility.

compression fracture   usually of lumbar or dorsal region due to hyperflexion of spine; the anterior vertebral bodies are crushed together.

compressive force   a force applied along the length of a structure, causing the tissues to approximate one another. This force can be caused by muscular activity, weight bearing, gravity or external loading down the length of the bone. It is necessary for the development and growth of bone. If a large compressive force, which surpasses the stress limits of the structure, is applied, a fracture will occur.

Compton scattering   takes place when an X-ray photon collides with an electron and in doing so gives up some of its energy to the electron resulting in a decrease in the unit mass and an increase in the photon energy.

compulsive action   performed by an individual at the supposed instigation of another's dominant will, but against his own. ***impulsive action*** resulting from a sudden urge rather than the will.

computed radiography   the use of digital imaging in imaging departments. *See also* **digital imaging**.

computed tomography (CT)   computer-constructed imaging technique of a thin slice through the body, derived from X-ray absorption data collected during a circular scanning motion. Also known as ***computed axial tomography***.

computer algorithms   instructions within computer programs which translate the raw data into a usable form.

concentric   having a common centre or point.

concentric muscle work   the shortening of a muscle to pull its attachments closer together and produce movement at a joint. For example, the quadriceps muscles of the anterior thigh work concentrically to straighten the knee.

conchae   three bony projections that lie in the nasal cavity.

concomitant   several things occurring simultaneously such as chemotherapy and radiotherapy.

concretion   a deposit of hard material; a calculus.

concussion   a condition resulting from a blow to the head or the brain being shaken, characterized by headache, amnesia, memory loss and visual symptoms.

condensation   the process of becoming more compact, for example, the changing of a gas to a liquid.

conditioned reflex   a reaction acquired by practice or repetition.

conduction   the transmission of heat, light, or sound waves through suitable media; also the passage of electrical currents and nerve impulses through body tissues.

conduction band   an area containing electrons which are free of the nucleus of the atom and are therefore free to move around. They therefore take part in electrical conduction through the material.

conductive deafness   deafness due to interruption of the conduction of sound waves from the atmosphere to the inner ear.

conductor   a substance or medium which transmits heat, light, sound, electric current, etc. Material that allows the free flow of electrons. The degree of conductivity varies, some substances being good conductors, whereas others are non-conductors.

condylar joint   a synovial joint that allows flexion, extension and rotation, for example, the knee joint.

condyle   a rounded projection situated at the end of some bones, for example, tibia.

condyloma   a wart-like growth on the anus, vulva or glans penis, usually sexually transmitted.

cone   equipment slotted into the base of a light beam diaphragm to further collimate the emergent beam of radiation.

cones   photoreceptors in the retina, responsible for high-definition colour vision in good light. *See also* **rods**.

confidence interval   in statistics, a level, for example, 95%, that indicates the level of confidence that the test result, such as a mean, will occur within a specified range.

confidentiality   a legal and professional requirement to protect all confidential information concerning patients/clients obtained in the course of professional practice, and make disclosures only with consent, where required by specific legislation, or a court order, or where disclosure in the wider public interest is justified.

conformal therapy   radiotherapy techniques that try to ensure that the dosage given to the treatment area matches exactly the size and shape of the tumour while minimizing the dosage to healthy tissue. Employs the use of a multi-leaf collimator.

confounding factors   extraneous factors, apart from the variables already allowed for, that distort research findings.

confounding variable   one that affects the conditions of the independent variables unequally.

congenital   of abnormal conditions, present at birth, often genetically determined. Existing before or at birth, usually associated with a defect or disease, for example, developmental dysplasia of the hip (DDH) (previously known as congenital dislocation of the hip).

congenital deafness   present at birth, for example, caused by maternal rubella in early pregnancy. *sensorineural (perceptive) or nerve deafness* is due to a lesion in the inner ear, the auditory nerve or the auditory centres in the brain. *See also* **hearing impairment**.

congenital heart disease   developmental abnormalities in the anatomy of the heart, resulting postnatally in imperfect circulation of blood and often manifested by murmurs, cyanosis, breathlessness and sweating. *See also* **'blue baby'**.

congestion   hyperaemia. Passive congestion results from obstruction or slowing down of venous return, as in the lower limbs or the lungs.

congestive heart (cardiac) failure   a chronic inability of the heart to maintain an adequate output of blood from one or both ventricles, resulting in pulmonary congestion and overdistension of certain veins and organs with blood, and in an inadequate blood supply to the body tissues.

congruent   when describing a visual field defect implies the defect affects the same area of the field in both eyes.

conization   the removal of a cone-shaped sample of tissue.

conjugate   a measurement of the bony pelvis. ***diagonal conjugate*** the clinical measurement taken in pelvic assessment, from the lower border of the symphysis pubis to the sacral promontory = 111–126 mm. It is 18.5 mm greater than obstetrical conjugate, the available space for the fetal head, i.e. the distance from the sacral promontory to the posterior surface of the top of the symphysis pubis = 108–114 mm. ***true conjugate*** the distance from the sacral promontory to the summit of the symphysis pubis = 110.5 mm.

conjunctiva   the delicate transparent membrane which lines the inner surface of the eyelids (palpebral conjunctiva) and reflects over the eyeball (bulbar or ocular conjunctiva).

conjunctivitis   inflammation of the conjunctiva. Usually infective or allergic. Follicular and papillary types may indicate cause.

connective tissue   the diverse group of tissue that includes adipose, areolar, bone, cartilage, blood and blood-producing tissue, elastic, fibrous and reticular.

connective tissue massage   manipulations that stretch the superficial and deep connective tissue in order to stimulate the circulation.

Conradi–Hünermann syndrome   a skeletal dysplasia which is inherited as an autosomal dominant trait. Skeletal abnormalities are variable; they are present at birth. After the first few weeks, life expectancy is normal.

conscientious objection   a legal recognition that an individual is not bound to take part in some specific activities such as termination of pregnancy. It may also apply to other strongly held beliefs that are not acknowledged by law.

consciousness   a complex concept which implies that a person is consciously perceiving the environment through the five sensory organs, and responding to the perceptions. *See also* **anaesthesia**.

consent   patients are legally required to consent to treatment, surgery and any intervention that requires physical contact. Consent may be verbal, written, or implied, i.e. by non-verbal communication. However, where there are likely to be risks or disputes, written consent is advisable. It is the responsibility of the healthcare professional undertaking the procedure to provide a full explanation to the patient prior to treatment or surgery about what is involved and any additional measures that may be required and to obtain written consent. Previously this was the doctor concerned, but increasingly other healthcare professionals are undertaking treatments, for example, endoscopy by nurses. If the patient is a minor, or incapable of giving informed consent, the next-of-kin must sign the consent form.

consent form   a form signed prior to an invasive procedure to indicate that permission has been given for the procedure to take place.

conservative dentistry   the diagnosis, treatment and restoration of diseased or injured teeth.

conservative treatment   aims at preventing a condition from becoming worse without using radical measures. For example, the use of drug therapy rather than surgery.

consolidation   becoming solid, as, for instance, the state of the lung due to exudation and organization in lobar pneumonia.

constant potential (CP)   a constant voltage produced by smoothing a fully rectified voltage by using capacitors.

constipation   an implied chronic condition of infrequent and often difficult evacuation of faeces due to insufficient high-fibre food or fluid intake, immobility, or to sluggish or disordered action of the bowel musculature or nerve supply, or to habitual failure to empty the rectum. Other causes include pain on defecation, inability to respond to the urge to defecate, hypokalaemia, drugs such as iron preparations, pregnancy (hormonal), depression, colorectal cancer (alternating with diarrhoea) and some systemic diseases. *acute constipation* signifies obstruction or paralysis of the gut of sudden onset.

constituents of developer   developing agents, preservative, accelerator, restrainer, buffer, sequestering agent, solvent, hardening agent, wetting agent, anti-frothing agent, fungicide.

constituents of fixer   fixing agent, acid, buffer, preservative, hardener and solvent.

contact   direct or indirect exposure to infection. A person who has been so exposed.

contact lens   glass or plastic lens, worn under the eyelids in direct contact with conjunctiva (in place of spectacles) for therapeutic or cosmetic purposes.

contagious   capable of transmitting infection or of being transmitted.

containment isolation   the separation of a patient with any sort of infection to prevent the spread of infection to others. *See also* **protective isolation, source isolation**.

contiguous   touching, close. In CT scanning refers to slice reconstruction with no interslice spacing.

contingency fund   an amount of money included in the costings of a project that would be used for some unplanned or unpredictable expense.

continuity equation   used in ultrasound to assess the area of a heart valve using measurements of the velocity and mean pressure gradient of the blood flow through the valve and the width of the valve.

continuous ambulatory peritoneal dialysis (CAPD)   peritoneal dialysis carried out every day, by patients needing renal replacement therapy, at home.

continuous passive motion (CPM)   form of passive mobilization, used to help the recovery of cartilage after knee surgery.

continuous positive airways pressure (CPAP)   the application of gas at a constant positive pressure, to the airway of a spontaneously breathing patient, via an endotracheal tube or tightly fitting face mask. It reduces alveolar collapse at the end of expiration and reduces the work of breathing; used at night in patients with sleep apnoea.

continuous subcutaneous insulin infusion (CSII) the use of a pump to deliver insulin continuously, either with a fixed or variable basal rate, and with a facility for bolus dosing, to achieve almost physiological control of diabetes mellitus.

continuous wave Doppler when a fixed frequency ultrasound is transmitted continuously by one crystal and is received continuously by an adjacent crystal. Any motion within the beam will produce a measurable Doppler shift. It can measure very high flow velocities but has no range resolution.

continuous wave probe (CW probe) used in a Doppler scan where one half of the transducer head emits a continuous ultrasound beam and the other half continuously receives the reflected beam, for example, a pencil probe. *See also* **Doppler effect, Doppler scanner**.

contouring device an aid to radiotherapy planning. The device accurately records the patient outline to facilitate accurate dose distributions to be planned. *See also* **lead strip, adjustable template, rotation jig**.

contraceptive an agent used to prevent conception, for example, condom, spermicidal vaginal pessary or cream, rubber cervical cap, intrauterine device. *See also* **combined oral contraceptive, intrauterine device**.

contract draw together; shorten; decrease in size. Acquire by contagion or infection.

contracted pelvis one in which one or more diameters are smaller than normal; this may result in difficulties in childbirth.

contractile having the ability to shorten – usually following stimulation. A property of muscle tissue.

contraction shortening, for example, in muscle fibres.

contracture shortening of scar or muscle tissue, causing deformity. *See also* **Dupuytren's contracture**.

contraindication any factor or condition indicating that a certain type of treatment (usually used for that condition) should be discontinued or not used.

contralateral on the opposite side.

contrast the difference in density between two adjacent areas on a film, the higher the contrast the more black and white the film, the lower the contrast the more shades of grey. *See also* **gamma, subject contrast, film contrast, radiographic contrast, subjective contrast**.

contrast agent either positive substances (non-ionic iodine compounds or barium) or negative substances (air, water or carbon dioxide) which can be used to demonstrate organs, vessels or parts of the body more clearly during imaging investigations by changing the subject density.

contrecoup   injury or damage at a point opposite the impact, resulting from transmitted force. It can occur in an organ or part containing fluid, as the skull.

control group   in research, the group that is not exposed to the independent variable, such as a therapeutic intervention or experimental drug. *See also* **experimental group, variable**.

controlled area   an area where the dose rate exceeds a specific dose rate or an employee is likely to receive more than three tenths the relevant dose limit. Access is restricted to specific staff members and patients undergoing therapeutic or diagnostic procedures.

controlled-dose transdermal absorption of drugs   application of a drug patch to the skin: gradual absorption gives a constant level in the blood. Examples include hormone replacement, and nicotine for smoking cessation.

controlled drugs   preparations subject to regulatory control and include psychoactive drugs including narcotics, barbiturates, cocaine, morphine, hallucinogens, depressants and stimulants.

Control of Substances Hazardous to Health (COSHH)   regulations relating to obligatory risk assessment and action to be taken, such as during the use of certain anaesthetic agents.

contusion (bruise)   injury by a blow, when the skin is not broken.

convection   transfer of heat from the hotter to the colder part; the heated substance (gas or fluid), being less dense, tends to rise. The colder portion, flowing in to be heated, rises in its turn; thus convection currents are set in motion.

conventional fractionation   radiotherapy given once daily over a predetermined period of time.

converging collimator   gamma camera collimator where the piece of lead has holes which are shaped to focus the gamma rays on a single spot, the main use is in brain imaging.

conversion   in an intensifying screen is when energy is released from absorbed electrons in the form of light photons. In developer, when the chemical precipitates metallic silver from the silver salts in the film during processing. In the fixer when the unexposed, undeveloped silver halides are removed from the film to make the image stable.

convoluted tubule   coiled tube in the kidney cortex.

convolutions   folds, twists or coils as found in the intestine, renal tubules and the surface of the brain.

convulsion   uncontrolled, generalized movements which may be associated with a loss of consciousness.

Cooley's anaemia   thalassaemia.

coordination   moving in harmony. The body's ability to execute smooth, fluid, accurate and controlled movements.

copy film film used to produce exact copies of radiographs by direct contact printing.

coracobrachialis muscle a muscle of the upper arm.

cord a thread-like structure. *See also* **spermatic cord, spinal cord, umbilical cord, vocal cord**.

cordectomy surgical excision of a cord, usually reserved for a vocal cord.

cordotomy (chordotomy) division of the anterolateral nerves in the spinal cord to relieve intractable pain in the pelvis or lower limbs.

core central portion, usually applied to the slough in the centre of a boil.

core body temperature that in the organs of the central cavities of the body (cranium, thorax and abdomen).

cornea the outwardly convex transparent membrane forming part of the anterior outer coat of the eye. It is situated in front of the iris and pupil and merges backwards into the sclera.

corneal reflex a reaction of blinking when the cornea is touched.

corneoscleral associated with the cornea and sclera, as the circular junction of these structures.

coronal in dentistry relating to a crown.

coronal discharge when electrons are forcibly removed from their orbits to create an electric spark.

coronal plane an imaginary plane passing through the midline of the body dividing it into front and back halves. *See also* **frontal plane**.

coronary crown-like; encircling, as of a vessel or nerve.

coronary arteries those supplying the myocardium, the first pair to be given off by the aorta as it leaves the left ventricle. Spasm, narrowing or blockage of these vessels causes angina pectoris or myocardial infarction (heart attack). Diseased vessels may be cleared by balloon angioplasty, lasers or replaced with veins taken from the legs. *See also* **angioplasty**.

coronary care unit (CCU) high dependency area in a hospital specialized in the care of patients with heart problems, particularly after a heart attack.

coronary heart disease (CHD) also known as *ischaemic heart disease*. It includes angina pectoris and myocardial infarction. A deficient supply of oxygenated blood to the myocardium, causing central chest pain of varying intensity that may radiate to arms and jaws. The lumen of the blood vessels is usually narrowed by atheromatous plaques. If treatment with drug therapy is unsuccessful, percutaneous transluminal angioplasty, or surgery, may be considered. *See also* **angina pectoris, angioplasty, myocardial infarction**.

coronary sinus channel receiving most venous blood from the myocardium and opening into the right atrium.

coronary thrombosis occlusion of a coronary vessel by a thrombus. The area deprived of blood becomes necrotic and is called an infarct. *See also* **ischaemic heart disease, myocardial infarction**.

coronaviruses a group of RNA viruses responsible for acute respiratory infections such as the common cold.

coroner in England and Wales, an officer of the Crown, usually a solicitor, barrister or doctor, who presides over the Coroner's Court responsible for establishing the cause of death in cases where violence may be a possibility or suspected. Where doubts exist about the cause of death the doctor should consult the coroner and act on his or her advice. The coroner must be notified if a patient dies within 24 hours of admission to hospital. In addition all theatre/anaesthetic deaths must also be reported. Any death where the deceased has not been seen by a doctor recently requires that a coroner's postmortem is undertaken. In Scotland, reports about such deaths are submitted to the Procurator Fiscal but a postmortem is normally only ordered if foul play is suspected. The Scottish equivalent of the Coroner's Inquest is the Fatal Accident Enquiry, presided over by the Sheriff.

cor pulmonale heart disease resulting from disease of the lung (emphysema, silicosis, etc.) which strains the right ventricle.

corpus any mass of tissue which is easily distinguishable from its surroundings.

corpus callosum white matter joining the two cerebral hemispheres.

corpus luteum a yellow mass which forms in the ovary after ovulation. It secretes progesterone and persists to maintain pregnancy should it occur.

corpuscle outdated term for blood cells. *See also* **erythrocytes, leucocytes**.

correlation in statistics, associated with. *See also* **positive correlation, negative correlation**.

correlation coefficient (r) a value between $+1$ (perfect positive correlation) and -1 (perfect negative correlation). 0 equals no linear relationship.

cortex the outer layer of an organ or structure beneath its capsule or membrane such as the cerebral cortex or renal cortex.

corticosteroids hormones produced by the adrenal cortex. The word is also used for synthetic steroids such as prednisolone and dexamethasone.

cortisol hydrocortisone, one of the principal adrenal cortical steroids. It is essential to life. There is decreased secretion in Addison's disease and increased amounts in Cushing's disease and syndrome.

cortisone one of the hormones of the adrenal gland. It is converted into cortisol before use by the body. Used therapeutically as replacement in conditions that include Addison's disease. *cortisone suppression test* differentiates primary from secondary hypercalcaemia.

cosmesis the use of cosmetics or surgery for preserving or enhancing self-image.

cosmetic dentistry   the restoration or enhancement of dental aesthetics.

costal   associated with the ribs.

costal cartilages   those cartilages which attach the ribs to the sternum and each other.

cost–benefit analysis (CBA)   method of analysis used in the economic evaluation of healthcare interventions (programmes or procedures). Health outcomes are measured in monetary terms to enable comparisons between interventions from a variety of disciplines. There are problems with valuing life and health in monetary terms. So this method is not widely used.

cost centre   a department, for example physiotherapy or catering, for which a budget covering staff and other resources has been set.

cost effectiveness   analytical technique used in the economic evaluation of healthcare interventions (programmes and procedures). A *cost-effectiveness analysis* is used when the outcomes of the procedures are not necessarily the same, but can be measured in the same natural units. For example, the outcomes may be measured in death rates, healthy years of life gained, symptom-free days, or even blood pressures. The output of this type of analysis is 'cost per unit increase'. For example, cost of intervention against cost per life year gained. Health benefits are measured in natural units (for example, mortality rates, survival rates) or final clinical outcomes (for example, cost per life years gained, cost per days off sick reduced). Intermediate clinical outcomes are sometimes used (for example, number of cancers detected in a screening programme) but this is not valid if a clear association between cancer detected and survival or quality of life cannot be demonstrated.

cost minimization   analytic technique used in economic evaluation of healthcare interventions (programmes or procedures). A *cost-minimization analysis* is used when the outcomes or consequences of the procedures are the same. A prerequisite for such a study is that there is evidence (preferably from a randomized clinical trial) that the different procedures are equally effective. A cost minimization analysis therefore solely consists of the analyses of costs. Common examples include comparisons of home and hospital care for chronic and terminal conditions.

costochondral   associated with a rib and its cartilage.

costochondritis   inflammation of the costochondral cartilage.

costoclavicular   associated with the ribs and the clavicle.

costoclavicular syndrome   is a synonym for cervical rib syndrome.

cost utility   analytic technique used in economic evaluation of healthcare interventions (programmes or procedures). A *cost-utility analysis* is used when the outcomes cannot be measured in natural units, so a utility or value scale has to be employed. This may be because the important outcomes of the procedures are not directly comparable or they are multi-faceted, for example, a comparison of amputation against waiting for the treatment of a gangrenous foot – outcomes could be pain, mobility and/or survival. The commonly used utility scale is quality-adjusted life years (QALYs), which use survey tools such as the Nottingham Health Profile to allocate 'relative qualities' to different health states. However, different people value their health differently; therefore utility ratings are not unique. Research has provided 'average' utility. Cost utility analyses report results as 'costs per QALY (gained)'.

cot death *see* **sudden infant death syndrome**.

cotyledon one of the subdivisions of the uterine surface of the placenta.

cough explosive expulsion of air from the lungs. It may be volun-tary, or as protective reflex that expels a foreign body such as food or spu-tum. Cough may be a feature of numerous respiratory and cardiac conditions.

coulomb is equal to the charge carried by 6×10^{18} electrons or protons.

countertraction traction upon the proximal extremity of a fractured limb opposing the pull of the traction apparatus on the distal extremity.

count rate the number of gamma ray detections made by a gamma camera per minute.

coupling gel a gel put on a patient's skin during an ultrasound examination to exclude any air between the transducer and the skin surface to enable the transmission of ultrasound waves between the transducer and the patient.

covalent bond is when two atoms share electrons in such a way that each atom appears to share the number of electrons in an apparent closed shell.

Cowper's glands *see* **bulbourethral (Cowper's) glands**.

coxa the hip joint.

coxa valga an increase in the normal angle between neck and shaft of femur.

coxa vara a decrease in the normal angle plus torsion of the neck, for exam-ple, slipped femoral epiphysis.

coxalgia pain in the hip joint.

coxitis inflammation of the hip joint.

CP/M one of the most common 'universal' computer languages.

CPS (Characters Per Second) a measure of the speed of data output.

CPU (Central Processing Unit) the core of the computer.

cranial associated with the cranium, towards the head.

cranial cavity the brain box formed by the bones of the cranium.

craniofacia associated with the cranium and the face.

craniometry the science which deals with the measurement of skulls.

craniopharyngioma a congenital, benign tumour which develops between the brain and the pituitary gland.

cranioplasty operative repair of a skull defect.

craniosacral associated with the skull and sacrum. Applied to the outflow of the parasympathetic nervous system.

craniostenosis a condition in which the skull sutures fuse too early and the fontanelles close. It may cause increased intracranial pressure requiring surgery.

craniosynostosis premature fusion of cranial sutures resulting in abnormal skull shape and craniostenosis. Deformities depend on which sutures are affected.

craniotabes a thinning or wasting of the cranial bones occurring in infancy and usually due to rickets.

craniotomy a surgical opening of the skull in order to remove a growth, relieve pressure, evacuate blood clot or arrest haemorrhage.

cranium the part of the skull enclosing the brain. It is composed of eight bones: the occipital, two parietals, frontal, two temporals, sphenoid and ethmoid.

creatine a nitrogenous compound produced in the body.

creatine kinase (ATP: creatine phosphotransferase) occurs as three isoenzymes. It is found in brain tissue, skeletal muscle, blood and in myocardial tissue.

creatine kinase test increased levels of the myocardial isoenzyme in serum is indicative of acute myocardial infarction. ***phosphorylated creatine*** the important storage form of high-energy phosphate.

creatinine a waste product of protein (endogenous) and nucleic acid metabolism found in muscle and blood and excreted in normal urine. ***serum creatinine*** is raised in hyperthyroidism, muscle wasting disorders and in renal failure.

crepitus (crepitation) grinding noise or sensation within a joint, as in osteoarthritis. A feature of fracture in overuse injury. Crackling sound heard via stethoscope. Crackling sound elicited by pressure on tissue containing air (surgical emphysema).

crest a sharp ridge of bone.

cretinism obsolete term. *See also* **hypothyroidism**.

Creutzfeldt–Jakob disease (CJD) a progressive dementia transmissible through prion protein. ***new variant CJD*** mainly affecting young adults, is possibly linked with the prion causing bovine spongiform encephalopathy (BSE). CJD follows a rapid degenerative course often with spasmodic contraction of the muscles (myoclonus) and is usually fatal.

cribriform   perforated, like a sieve.

cribriform plate   that portion of the ethmoid bone allowing passage of fibres of olfactory nerve.

cricoid   ring-shaped. Applied to the cartilage forming the inferior posterior part of larynx.

cricoid pressure   a practical manoeuvre in which manual pressure is applied over the cricoid cartilage to occlude the oesophagus to prevent regurgitation and aspiration of gastric contents during induction of anaesthesia.

cricothyroidotomy (cricothyrotomy)   incision through the skin and cricothyroid membrane to secure a patent airway for emergency relief of upper airway obstruction. *See also* **tracheostomy**.

criminal law   the law that creates offences heard in the criminal courts such as theft.

criminal wrong   an act or omission that can be pursued in the criminal courts.

critical angle   when an incident beam of ultrasound strikes an interface at an angle equal to or greater than this angle, only reflection of the beam will occur.

critical appraisal   the process of making an objective judgement regarding a research study. Includes research design, methodology, analysis, interpretation of results and the applicability of the study findings to a particular area of health care.

Crohn's disease   a chronic recurrent granulomatous inflammation affecting any part of the bowel from mouth to anus. Inflammation may be discontinuous ('skip lesions') with normal bowel in between. May be complicated by fistulae and strictures. *See also* **inflammatory bowel disease**.

Crosby capsule   a special tube which is passed through the mouth to the small intestine. Allows biopsy of jejunal mucosa. Endoscopic biopsy is often used in preference to this time-consuming investigation.

cross infection   infection that a person receives from another person.

crossover effect   the amount of light transmitted to the opposite side of a film base expressed as a percentage.

crossover studies   a research study where the participants are exposed to both the experimental intervention and the placebo one after another.

croup   viral infection leading to laryngeal narrowing. The child has 'croupy', stridulous (noisy or harsh-sounding) breathing. Narrowing of the airway which gives rise to the typical attack with crowing inspiration may be the result of oedema or spasm, or both.

crown   the top part of a structure. ***artificial crown*** in dentistry, restoration used to cover the part of the tooth that projects above the gum line, usually made of metal, porcelain, or a combination of both. ***crown of a tooth*** that part of the tooth covered with enamel.

crown–rump length   a measurement, used in ultrasound imaging, of the length of the fetal head and body between the 6th and 14th week of pregnancy to assess the age of the fetus.

CRS (NHS Care Record Service)   provides computerized patient records and will be linked with PACS to provide full clinical information on patients.

cruciate   shaped like a cross such as the ligaments stabilizing the knee joint.

crus   a structure which is leg-like or root-like. Applied to various parts of the body, for example, crus of the diaphragm.

crutch palsy   paralysis of extensor muscles of wrist, fingers and thumb from repeated pressure of a crutch upon the radial nerve in the axilla.

cryoanalgesia   the relief of pain symptoms by blocking peripheral nerve conduction with extreme cold.

cryogenic   produced by low temperature. Also used to describe any means or apparatus involved in the production of low temperature.

cryoprobe   freezing probe which can be used to destroy tumours.

crystal defects   imperfections within a crystal which create areas of low energy called 'electron traps' and 'holes'. *See also* **point defects, line defects**.

cryosurgery   the use of intense, controlled cold to remove or destroy diseased tissue without harming the adjacent tissue.

cryotherapy   a method of freezing a tumour, the use of cold for the treatment of disease.

cryptogenic   of unknown or obscure cause.

cryptogenic fibrosing alveolitis   interstitial lung disease characterized by cellular infiltration and thickening of the alveolar walls. Pulmonary macrophages are implicated in fibrosis, and in recruiting other cell types such as neutrophils to the lung.

cryptorchism   a developmental defect whereby the testes do not descend into the scrotum; they are retained within the abdomen or inguinal canal.

crystalluria   excretion of crystals in the urine.

crystal violet (gentian violet)   a brilliant, violet-coloured, antiseptic aniline dye, used as 0.5% solution as a stain. It is only licensed for application to intact skin, the exception being marking the skin before surgery.

CT number   the number given to a pixel in a digital image to denote the calculated attenuation at that point of the image, expressed in Hounsfield Units.

CT scanner   computed tomography equipment now most commonly used to produce a volume of data which can provide multi planar sectional images of the patient using a beam of radiation that rotates continuously around

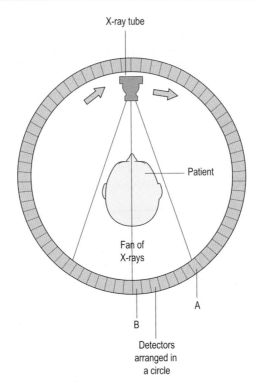

X-ray tube

Patient

Fan of
X-rays

A

B

Detectors
arranged in
a circle

Line diagram to show the main features of the scanning gantry of a CT scanner. The thick arrows show the direction of tube rotation. From Principles of radiological physics, 3rd edn, D T Graham, 1996, Churchill Livingstone, Edinburgh, with permission.

the patient as they move through the path of the beam. The image is produced by a computer which measures the attenuation of radiation in the body and reconstructs images on a monitor.

CT simulator   equipment for very accurate treatment planning prior to radiotherapy comprising of a CT scanner, laser positioning aids and a virtual simulation treatment planning computer.

cubital tunnel external compression syndrome   ulnar paralysis resulting from compression of the ulnar nerve within the cubital tunnel situated on the inner and posterior aspect of the elbow – sometimes referred to as the 'funny bone'.

cubital vein   situated in the arm.

cubitus   the forearm; elbow.

cuboid   shaped like a cube. One of the bones of the foot.

culdoscope   an endoscope used via the vaginal route.

culdoscopy   a form of peritoneoscopy or laparoscopy. Passage of a culdoscope through the posterior vaginal fornix, behind the uterus to enter the peritoneal cavity, for viewing same.

culture   the growth of microorganisms on artificial media under ideal conditions.

cumulative activity   total quantity of radiation produced over a period of time.

Cumulative Index to Nursing and Allied Health Literature (CINAHL)   computerized database of literature relevant to nursing and allied health.

cuneiform bones   three wedge-shaped bones in the foot, the medial, intermediate and lateral cuneiform bones.

curettage   the scraping of unhealthy tissue from a cavity. This may be treatment or may be done to establish a diagnosis after laboratory analysis of the scrapings.

curette   a spoon-shaped instrument or a metal loop which may have sharp and/or blunt edges for scraping out (curetting) cavities.

curie (Ci)   a measure of radioactivity, equal to 3.7×10^{10} nuclear disintegrations per second, now replaced by the Becquerel.

Curling's ulcer   acute peptic ulceration which occurs either in the stomach or duodenum as a response to the physiological stress of extensive burns or scalds.

cursor   a flashing marker on the computer screen which indicates where the next character is to be inserted.

curved array   in ultrasound, a set of elements mounted in a curved line to give a wide field of view, for example, obstetric scans.

Cushing's disease   a rare disorder, mainly of females, characterized principally by a cushingoid appearance, proximal myopathy, hyperglycaemia, hypertension and osteoporosis; due to excessive cortisol production by hyperplastic adrenal glands as a result of increased adrenocorticotrophin (ACTH) secretion by a tumour or hyperplasia of the anterior pituitary gland.

Cushing's reflex   a rise in blood pressure and a fall in pulse rate; occurs in cerebral space-occupying lesions.

Cushing's syndrome   clinically similar to *Cushing's disease* but including all causes: (a) adrenocortical hyperplasia, adenoma or carcinoma, which can be associated with excessive body hair and low levels of potassium due to excess of other adrenal steroids; (b) ectopic ACTH secretion by tumours, for example, small cell lung cancer, often associated with darkening of the skin; (c) iatrogenic due to treatment with glucocorticoids.

cusp   a projecting point, such as the edge of a tooth or the segment of a heart valve. The cardiac tricuspid valve has three, the mitral (bicuspid) valve two cusps.

cuticle   the epidermis or dead epidermis, as that which surrounds a nail.

cut-off sensitivity   the electromagnetic wavelength that a film emulsion is no longer sensitive to.

cyanosis   a bluish tinge to the skin due to a lack of oxygen, observed most frequently under the nails, lips and skin.

cycle   one complete waveform in alternating current, usually measured from zero to zero or from peak to peak.

cyclical vomiting   periodic attacks of vomiting in children, usually associated with ketosis and usually with no demonstrable pathological cause. Occurs mainly in highly strung children.

cyclotron   a device to accelerate charged particles or ions which then bombard a target in which nuclear reactions result in the production of radionuclides. These can then be used as a source of neutrons or protons for therapeutic radiopharmaceuticals.

cylindroma   a tumour of the endothelial element of apocrine tissue such as a sweat gland or a salivary gland. The supporting stroma is hyalinized.

cyst   a closed cavity or sac usually with an epithelial lining, enclosing fluid or semisolid matter.

cystadenoma   an innocent cystic new growth of glandular tissue. Liable to occur in the female breast.

cystectomy   usually refers to the removal of part or the whole of the urinary bladder. This necessitates urinary diversion.

cystic fibrosis (fibrocystic disease of the pancreas, mucoviscidosis)   the commonest genetically determined disease in Caucasian populations; there is abnormality of secretion of the exocrine glands. Thick mucus can block the intestinal glands and cause meconium ileus in a baby; later it can cause steatorrhoea and malabsorption. Thick mucus in the respiratory glands predisposes to repeated infections and bronchiectasis. Abnormality of the sweat glands increases the chloride content of sweat, which is a diagnostic tool.

cystinosis   a recessively inherited metabolic disorder in which crystalline cystine is deposited in the body. Cystine and other amino acids are excreted in the urine.

cystinuria   metabolic disorder in which cystine and other amino acids appear in the urine. A cause of renal stones.

cystitis   inflammation of the urinary bladder; the cause is usually bacterial. The condition may be acute or chronic, primary or secondary to stones, etc. More frequent in females, as the urethra is short.

cystocele   prolapse of the posterior wall of the urinary bladder into the anterior vaginal wall. *See also* **colporrhaphy**.

cystodiathermy   the application of a cauterizing electrical current to the walls of the urinary bladder through a cystoscope, or by open operation.

cystography   the radiographic examination of the urinary bladder following the introduction of a catheter via the urethra for the introduction of contrast agent.

cystolithiasis   the presence of a stone or stones in the urinary bladder.

cystometer   an apparatus for measuring the pressure under various conditions in the urinary bladder.

cystometrogram   a record of the changes in pressure within the urinary bladder under various conditions; used in the study of voiding disorders.

cystometry   the study of pressure changes within the urinary bladder.

cystoplasty   surgical repair or augmentation of the urinary bladder.

cystoprostourethrectomy   the surgical removal of the bladder and prostate with diversion of the ureters onto the abdominal wall.

cystoscope   an endoscope used to visualize the inner aspect of the bladder.

cystoscopy   use of a cystoscope to view the internal surface of the urinary bladder.

cystostomy (vesicostomy)   an operation whereby a fistulous opening is made into the urinary bladder via the abdominal wall. Usually the fistula can be allowed to heal when it is no longer needed.

cystotomy   incision into the urinary bladder via the abdominal wall.

cystourethritis   inflammation of the urinary bladder and urethra.

cystourethrogram   radiographic examination of the urinary bladder and urethra. *See also* **micturating cystourethrogram**.

cystourethroscopy   the examination of the urethra and urinary bladder under general anaesthetic using a cystoscope.

cytochrome   a series of proteins containing iron or copper. They have a similar structure to haemoglobin and are involved in mitochondrial oxidation–reduction reactions (electron transport chain) that produce ATP.

cytochrome P_{450}   liver enzyme important in the oxidation and clearance of lipid-soluble drugs.

cytodiagnosis   diagnosis by the microscopic study of cells.

cytogenetics   the scientific study of cells; particularly of chromosomes, genes and their behaviour. Chromosomes can be studied by culture techniques, using either tissue such as skin or lymphocytes, or fetal cells obtained by chorionic villus sampling or amniocentesis.

cytokines   proteins which act either on the cytokine-producing cell, or on other cells, via cell-surface receptors. The term is usually applied to proteins which act on immune cells (T cells, B cells, monocytes, etc.). Cytokines have many diverse effects on many different types of cell. Examples include interleukins (for example, IL-1, IL-2), tumour necrosis factor, interferon-alpha and interferon-gamma.

cytology   the study of isolated cells or those in tiny clusters.

cytoplasm (protoplasm)   the complex chemical compound constituting the main part of the living substance of the cell, other than the contents of the nucleus.

cytoreduction   the reduction of the size of a tumour using hormone or cytotoxic drugs.

cytotoxic   any substance which kills or inhibits the growth of cells.

cytotoxic drugs   drugs used mainly for the treatment of malignant diseases, but sometimes for other conditions. They work in different ways, but they all eventually cause cancer cell death by either disrupting DNA or causing programmed cell death. Some are cell cycle phase specific and others work at any point in the cell cycle. They also harm some normal cells and some have longer-term side-effects. There are five groups: (a) alkylating agents that disrupt DNA, for example, busulfan, cyclophosphamide; (b) antimetabolites that disrupt DNA by blocking enzymes required for its synthesis, for example, 5-fluorouracil; (c) antitumour antibiotics that disrupt DNA and the cell membrane, for example, bleomycin; (d) vinca alkaloids and other plant extracts that disrupt microtubules during cell division, for example, vincristine; (e) miscellaneous group that work in a variety of ways, for example, asparaginase. *See also* **chemotherapy**.

cytotoxins   antibodies which are toxic to cells.

D log E curve   applies to a particular film or film/screen combination and is the curve which results when the density is plotted against the log of relative exposure. *See also* **characteristic curve**.

dacryocystography   rarely used radiographic examination of the tear drainage apparatus following the introduction of a positive contrast agent. Superseded by CT and MRI.

dacty   a digit, finger or toe.

dactylitis   inflammation of finger or toe. The digit becomes swollen due to periostitis. Associated with congenital syphilis, tuberculosis, sarcoid.

dark adaptation   adjustments made by the eye in reduced light or darkness. The pupils dilate, cones function ceases, rhodopsin is formed and the rod activity increases. *See also* **light adaptation**.

data   items of information, usually collected for a specific purpose, for example to be used in the analysis of a problem.

data analysis   describes statistical analyses of data.

database   software designed to store information in a systematic way, and at the same time to allow easy retrieval and manipulation of all data.

data compression   in computing, the reduction in size of information to decrease transferred film size.

data processing   the storage, sorting and analysis of data, usually electronically with computers.

data protection   rules relating to information held about individuals, such as in Data Protection Act 1998. In computing only registered users can hold information about individuals on computer and all patients have a right under this act to see any records concerning themselves or their treatment.

data set   the data relating to a specific group such as a particular age group.

dating scan   an ultrasound scan taken between 11 and 14 weeks, using the crown–rump length to accurately age the fetus.

daughter radionuclide   a nucleus after it has decayed. *See also* **radioactive decay**.

day care centre   outpatient centres that provide company, psychological and nursing support.

day case surgery   the provision of surgery for out-patients who will return home the same day.

day hospital   a centre which patients attend daily. Recreational and occupational therapy and physiotherapy often provided. Greatest use is in the services for older people and those with mental health problems.

daylight systems   a system which enables the loading and unloading of radiographic film without the use of a darkroom. *See also* **dispersed daylight system, centralized daylight system**.

deafness   a partial or complete loss of hearing. *See also* **conductive deafness, congenital deafness**.

deamination   removal of an amino group (NH_2) from organic compounds such as excess amino acids.

debility   a condition of weakness with lack of muscle tone.

débridement   the removal of foreign matter and contaminated or devitalized tissue from or adjacent to a wound. *chemical/medical débridement* is accomplished by the external application of a substance to the wound, such as a specific wound dressing. *surgical débridement* is accomplished by using surgical instruments and aseptic technique.

debugging   the correction and, much more importantly, the finding of errors or bugs in a computer program.

decalcification   the removal of mineral salts, as from teeth in dental caries, bone in disorders of calcium metabolism.

deceleration time   used in cardiac ultrasound work to measure the function of a mitral valve, for example, a long mitral E wave deceleration time indicates diastolic dysfunction.

decibel (dB)   a unit of sound intensity (loudness).

decidua   the endometrial lining of the uterus thickened and altered for the reception of the fertilized ovum. It is shed at the end of pregnancy.

decidua basalis   that part which lies under the embedded ovum and forms the maternal part of the placenta.

decidua capsularis   that part which lies over the developing ovum.

decidua vera   the decidua lining the rest of the uterus.

deciduous   by convention refers to the teeth of the primary dentition.

deciduous teeth   temporary teeth in children, 20 in number and lettered abcde in each quadrant of the mouth.

decompression   removal of pressure or a compressing force.

decompression (of bladder)   in cases of chronic urinary retention, by continuous or intermittent drainage via catheter inserted per urethra.

decompression (of brain)   achieved by removing a circular area of the skull (trephining) in order to evacuate clot.

decompression illness   results from sudden reduction in atmospheric pressure, as experienced by divers on return to surface, aircrew ascending to great heights. Caused by bubbles of nitrogen which are released from solution in the blood; symptoms vary according to the site of these. The condition is largely preventable by proper and gradual decompression technique. Variously described as 'bends, chokes and creeps' depending on the symptomatology. Originally called caisson disease when identified as a hazard for divers. Later recognized as a complication of high altitude.

decontamination   the method of removing foreign material such as radioactive substances for the safety of the individual.

decubitus   the position of the person when lying down.

decubitus ulcer (pressure sore, bedsore)   a breakdown of the skin due to pressure or immobility, usual sites are buttocks, heels, elbows, shoulders.

decussation   intersection; crossing of nerve fibres at a point beyond their origin, as in the optic and pyramidal tracts.

deep vein thrombosis (DVT)   thrombus forming in a deep vein such as those in the legs or pelvis. It is associated with slowing of blood flow, abnormal or inappropriate clotting processes, or damage to veins. A thrombus may break off to form an embolus that travels in the venous circulation, through the heart to the lungs. *See also* **pulmonary embolus**.

defecation   voiding of faeces per anus.

defibrillation   the application of a direct current (DC) electric shock to arrest ventricular fibrillation of the heart and restore normal cardiac rhythm.

defibrillator   equipment for the application of a direct electric current to the heart to arrest ventricular fibrillation and restore normal cardiac rhythm.

deflection   when an ultrasound beam is refracted and therefore causes objects to appear to be in a different location from where they actually occur.

degaussing   a method of demagnetizing a cathode ray tube if the shadow mask becomes magnetized.

degeneration   deterioration in quality or function. Regression from more specialized to less specialized type of tissue.

deglutition   swallowing, a complex process that is partly voluntary, partly involuntary.

dehydration   loss or removal of fluid. In the body this condition arises when the fluid intake fails to replace fluid loss. This is liable to occur when there is bleeding, diarrhoea, excessive exudation from a raw area as in burns, excessive sweating, polyuria or vomiting, and usually upsets the body's electrolyte balance. If suitable fluid replacement cannot be achieved orally, then parenteral administration must be instituted.

delayed union   longer than expected healing of a fracture.

deliberate self-harm (DSH)   wilful non-fatal act(s) carried out in the knowledge that it was potentially harmful. Examples include self-poisoning (overdose), self-cutting and self-mutilation.

delirium   abnormal mental condition based on hallucinations or illusion. May occur in high fever, in mental health problems, or be toxic in origin.

delirium tremens   results from alcoholic intoxication and is represented by a picture of confusion, terror, restlessness and hallucinations.

Delphi technique   a research method where a consensus of expert opinion is obtained during a multiple-step process where the contributors are asked to rate a number of items, for example, research priorities, in order of importance.

deltoid   triangular.

deltoid muscle   muscle acting at the shoulder.

dementia (organic brain syndrome – OBS)   an irreversible organic brain disease causing disturbance of memory and personality, deterioration in personal care, impaired cognitive ability and disorientation. *See also* **presenile dementia, Creutzfeldt–Jakob disease**.

demographic indices   such as age distribution, birth and mortality rates, occupation and geographical distribution. They are used to obtain a profile of a given population, compare different areas and plan services.

demography   the study of population.

demyelination   destruction of the myelin sheaths surrounding nerve fibres. Can occur in the peripheral nerves (for example, Guillain–Barré syndrome), or in the central nervous system (for example, multiple sclerosis).

dendrite (dendron)   one of the branched filaments which are given off from the body of a nerve cell. That part of a neuron which transmits an impulse to the nerve cell.

dendritic cell   an antigen-presenting cell that presents a processed antigen to B and T lymphocytes bearing antigen-specific receptors. They are thought to be the cells important in determining the type of immune response generated against an antigen.

dendron   *see* **dendrite**.

Dennis Browne splints   splints used to correct congenital talipes equinovarus (club foot).

densitometer   an instrument for measuring the relative density of different steps on a film. *See also* **sensitometry**.

density   the amount of blackening on a radiographic or photographic film and is the log of the opacity.

dental   relating to teeth.

dental amalgam   a compound of a basal alloy of silver and tin with mercury, used for restoring teeth. *See also* **amalgam**.

dental attrition   non-carious, mechanical wearing of teeth, either through normal mastication or as a result of parafunctional habits, for example, bruxism.

dental caries   a microbial disease of the calcified tissues of the teeth, characterized by demineralization of the inorganic portion and destruction of their organic substance.

dental enamel   hard, acellular calcified tissue covering the crown of a tooth.

dental erosion   non-carious wearing away of the surfaces of the teeth due to chemical causes.

dental formulae   a method of identifying individual teeth: adult teeth are numbered and children's teeth have letters.

dental hygienist   dental auxiliary trained to scale and clean teeth, carry out certain preventive procedures and give oral hygiene instruction to the prescription of a dentist.

dental implant   artificial structure implanted surgically into the alveolar bone, usually made from titanium.

dental plaque   soft deposit of bacteria and cellular debris that rapidly forms on the surface of a tooth in the absence of oral hygiene.

dental pulp   tissue consisting of blood vessels, nerves and connective tissue that occupies the core of the crown and the root canal(s) of a tooth.

dental restoration   the process of replacing part or all of a tooth by artificial means; also the term given to the type of replacement used, for example, filling, crown, bridge.

dental scaling   the removal of calculus, using special instruments, from the surfaces of the teeth.

dental therapist   dental auxiliary who is trained to carry out certain dental operative procedures to the prescription of a dentist.

dentate   having natural teeth present.

dentine   calcified organic hard tissue forming the bulk of the crown and roots of teeth and surrounds the pulp cavity. *See also* **tooth**.

dentist   any person who practices dentistry, and is qualified and licensed to do so.

dentistry   profession concerned with the diagnosis, prevention and treatment of diseases of the teeth and their supporting tissues, including their restoration and replacement. *See also* **conservative dentistry, cosmetic dentistry, forensic dentistry, paediatric dentistry, preventative dentistry, prosthetic dentistry**.

dentition   the natural teeth collectively in an individual.

dento-alveolar abscess   localized collection of pus within the alveolar bone, of dental origin.

denture   a removable dental prosthesis. May be partial or full (replacing some, or all, of the teeth in either jaw respectively).

deoxygenation   the removal of oxygen.

deoxyribonucleic acid (DNA)   a double-strand nucleic acid molecule found in the chromosomes of all organisms (except some viruses). DNA (as genes) carries the coded instructions for passing on hereditary characteristics. DNA is a polymer formed from many nucleotides. These consist of the sugar deoxyribose, phosphate groups and four nitrogenous bases: adenine (A), guanine (G), thymine (T) and cytosine (C). Adenine and guanine are purine bases, and thymine and cytosine are pyrimidine bases. The nucleotide units are bound together to form a double helix with the adenine of one strand opposite the thymine of the other and the same for guanine and cytosine.

dependent variable   one that depends on the experimental conditions.

depolarization   in excitable cells the inside of the membrane becomes electrically positive with respect to the outside. Occurs during the transmission of a nerve impulse. *See also* **polarized**.

depressant   a drug that reduces functional activity of an organ.

depressed fracture   an indentation in the bone, usually occurs in the skull, when the bone is hit by a hard object or when a bone presses on an underlying organ such as the lungs.

depression   a hollow place or indentation. A downward or inward movement or displacement. Diminution of power or activity. An emotional disorder characterized by feelings of profound sadness, may be classified by severity (mild/moderate/severe), by the presence of somatic symptoms (anorexia, weight loss, impaired libido, sleep disturbance, etc.) and by the presence or absence of psychotic symptoms. Recognized cognitive symptoms include hopelessness, helplessness, guilt, low self-esteem and suicidal thoughts. The previous description of reactive versus endogenous depression is outdated and not thought to be relevant to treatment or prognosis.

deprivation indices   a set of census variables and weightings used to assess levels of deprivation within a specific community or population. They include: levels of unemployment, single-parent households, pensioners living alone and households without a car. *See also* **Jarman index**.

Derbyshire neck   goitre.

dermatitis   inflammation of the skin (by custom limited to an eczematous reaction). *See also* **eczema, atopic dermatitis, industrial dermatitis.**

dermatitis herpetiformis (hydroa)   an intensely itchy skin eruption of unknown cause, most commonly characterized by papules and vesicles, which remit and relapse. Associated with coeliac disease (gluten-induced enteropathy).

dermatofibroma   a small round, painless lump usually found on the extremities.

dermatologist   medically qualified individual who studies skin diseases and is skilled in their treatment. A skin specialist.

dermatology   the science which deals with the skin, its structure, functions, diseases and their treatment.

dermatomyositis   an autoimmune connective tissue disease mainly affecting the skin and muscles. Presents with a characteristic skin rash and muscle weakness. Can be associated with an underlying malignancy in more elderly people. *See also* **collagen**.

dermis   the true skin; the cutis vera; the layer below the epidermis.

dermoid   associated with or resembling skin.

dermoid cyst   a cyst which is congenital in origin and usually occurs in the ovary. It contains elements of hair, nails, skin, teeth, etc.

descriptive epidemiology   the retrospective analysis of the relationship between disease and suspected cause of the disease.

descriptive statistics   that which describes or summarizes the observations of a sample. *See also* **inferential statistics**.

desensitization   process of reducing subsequent immediate-type hypersensitivity reactions to venoms and other allergens by repeated injection of minute quantities of allergen in order to modulate the immune response away from the harmful allergic type reaction to a less pathological response. A behavioural therapy used for phobias where people are helped to overcome their irrational fear. There is a gradual introduction to the object or situation through imagining the object, looking at pictures or by eventually confronting the real thing.

desiccation   drying out. There can be desiccation of the nucleus pulposus, thus diminishing the cushioning effect of a healthy intervertebral disc.

designated area   an area where radiation is being used and therefore there are restrictions placed on who can be present in the area, areas are described as being controlled or supervised.

desloughing   the process of removing slough from a wound.

desquamation   shedding of the upper layers, usually of the skin either in flakes or powdery form.

detached retina   separation of the neurosensory retina from the pigment epithelium. May be caused by retinal tears or holes, fibrous traction on the retina, or by exudation of fluid under the neurosensory retina.

detained patient   a person with a mental disorder who has been detained under the relevant legislation such as the Mental Health Act.

detected quantum efficiency (DQE)   is the relationship between the density of useful quanta of light and the density of radiation quanta falling on the detector. Ideally this should be as near to 100% as possible.

detection acuity   the ability of an individual to see the presence of small objects.

detector   a device used to measure the amount of radiation transmitted through a patient. Modern CT units typically use solid state ceramic detectors. *See also* **scintillation detector**.

detergent   a cleansing agent, for example, cetrimide.

deterioration   progressive impairment of function: worsening of the patient's condition.

determinants of health   factors that may influence the health of an individual, or differences in health between individuals, apart from age, sex and constitution (physiological, genetic factors). These could be social and economic, environmental or psychological factors that increase the risk of ill health or disease (for example, heart disease, cancers, diabetes). These determinants, or indicators, are associated with better or worse health of populations as measured by mortality (standardized mortality ratios), valid measures of morbidity or self-reported health status (for example, health surveys, census, standardized illness ratios). For example, higher infant mortality may be associated with environmental factors, healthcare provision, social and community support, maternal deprivation and poverty. There may also be a cultural and behavioural perspective. *See also* **morbidity, mortality**.

deterministic effect   an effect that always occurs, with radiation dose it is an effect which occurs above a specific dose, skin reddening, hair loss, temporary depression of blood count, death. *See also* **stochastic effect**.

detoxication   the removal of the poisonous property of a substance.

detrusor   an expelling muscle such as that of the urinary bladder. ***detrusor instability*** failure to inhibit reflex detrusor contraction. *See also* **incontinence**.

developer   a chemical which reacts with exposed film and reduces exposed silver bromide crystals to black metallic silver by donating electrons to the crystals.

developing agent   the chemical which reduces exposed silver bromide crystals to metallic silver for example, a combination of phenidone and hydroquinone.

developmental dysplasia of the hip (DDH)   also known as ***congenital dislocation of the hip***. The term DDH is useful in describing the varying causes and severity of the condition. There is poor development of the acetabulum which allows the head of the femur to dislocate.

dextrocardia   transposition of the heart to the right side of the thorax.

diabetes   a disease characterized by the excretion of large quantities of urine, and therefore excessive thirst.

diabetes insipidus   a rare form of diabetes caused if the production of antidiuretic hormone decreases.

diabetes mellitus   a condition resulting from a deficiency in the amount of insulin produced by the pancreas.

diabetic   a person suffering from diabetes.

diabetic coma   a loss of consciousness in a patient with diabetes mellitus if the disease is undiagnosed or if insulin has been omitted.

diagnosis   the art or act of distinguishing one disease from another. ***differential diagnosis*** is the term used when making a correct decision between diseases presenting a similar clinical picture.

diagnostic   associated with diagnosis, evidence in diagnosis.

diagnostic ultrasonography   information is derived from echoes which occur when a controlled beam of sound energy crosses the boundary between adjacent tissues of differing physical properties.

dialyser (artificial kidney)   the machine used to remove waste products from the blood in the case of renal failure, the membrane used for dialysis.

dialysis   process by which solutes are removed from solution by diffusion across a porous membrane; requires the presence of a favourable solute gradient. *See also* **haemodialysis, peritoneal dialysis**.

diamagnetic   a substance that will slightly reduce the strength of the magnetic field in which it is placed, the magnetic field induced is opposed to that of the surrounding magnetic field and has negative magnetic susceptibility. *See also* **paramagnetic, superparamagnetic, ferromagnetic**.

diamagnetism   the influence of an applied magnetic field on the electrons orbiting the nuclei within the substance is rarely permanent. *See also* **paramagnetism, ferromagnetism**.

diapedesis   the passage of cells from within blood vessels through the vessel walls into the tissues.

diaphragm   the dome-shaped muscular partition between the thorax above and the abdomen below. Any partitioning membrane or septum. A cap which encircles the cervix to act as a barrier contraceptive, reliable when fitted correctly and used correctly with a spermicidal chemical.

diaphragmatic hernia   *see* **hiatus hernia**.

diaphysis   the shaft of a long bone.

diarrhoea   a change from the established bowel rhythm characterized by an increase in frequency and fluidity of the stools, may cause dehydration, hypokalaemia (low potassium levels in the blood), malabsorption of nutrients and perianal soreness. Causes include infection, food sensitivity, laxative misuse, drugs such as antibiotics, dietary change, anxiety, colorectal cancer (alternating with constipation) and some systemic diseases.

diarthrosis   a synovial, freely movable joint.

diastasis   a separation of bones without fracture.

diastema   a naturally occurring space between two teeth.

diastole   the relaxation filling period of the cardiac cycle. *See also* **systole**.

diastolic dysfunction   the inability of the left ventricle of the heart to spring back after it has opened.

diastolic notching   during an ultrasound procedure, a sudden and temporary dip towards the base line of the image display during the relaxation period of the cardiac cycle.

diathermy   the passage of a high-frequency electric current through the tissues causing heat to be produced. When both electrodes are large, the heat is diffused over a wide area according to the electrical resistance of the tissues. In this form it is widely used in the treatment of inflammation, especially when deeply seated (for example, sinusitis, pelvic cellulitis). When one electrode is very small the heat is concentrated in this area and becomes great enough to destroy tissue. In this form (***surgical diathermy***) it is used to stop bleeding at operation by coagulation of blood, or to cut through tissue.

dicephalous   two-headed.

dichroic fog   used to be seen when a film was manually processed and was caused by development continuing in the fixer, it appears as a pink stain if viewed by transmitted light and greenish blue when viewed by reflected light.

DICOM (Digital Imaging and COmmunications in Medicine)   a project to bring manufacturers together to agree standardization in computerized image transfer and communications so that clinical information can be communicated among all specialities.

dicrotic (associated with, or having)   a double beat, as indicated by a second expansion of the artery during diastole.

dicrotic notch   the second rise in the arterial tracing caused by the closure of the aortic valve (that between the left ventricle and the aorta). *See also* **anacrotic**.

dielectric   a substance that acts as an electrical insulator and can contain an electric field.

dielectric constant (K)   is the ratio of the capacitance of the capacitor with the dielectric to the capacitance with a vacuum between the plates of the capacitor.

dietetics   the interpretation and application of the scientific principles of nutrition to feeding in health and disease.

dietitian   one who applies the principles of nutrition to the feeding of an individual or a group of individuals. Dietitians are employed in a range of hospital and community settings, the food industry, by local authorities and by national and international agencies, for example, WHO.

differential blood count   the estimation of the relative proportions of the different leucocyte cells in the blood. The normal differential count is: polymorphonuclear 65–70%, lymphocytes 20–25%, monocytes 5%, eosinophils 0–3%, basophils 0–0.5%. In childhood the proportion of lymphocytes is higher.

differential diagnosis making a correct decision between diseases presenting a similar clinical picture. *See also* **diagnosis**.

differentiation the process during which cells and tissues expand the ability to perform specialized functions that distinguish them from other cell types. Cancer cells are graded by their degree of differentiation.

diffuse periostitis inflammation of the periosteum of long bones.

diffusion when water and other small molecules in tissue undergo random microscopic, parallel movement which can be measured by magnetic resonance techniques, for example, distinguishing cysts from solid tumours, strokes, and cerebrospinal fluid dynamic studies.

digestion the process by which food is changed so that it can be absorbed by the body.

digit a finger or toe.

digital literally to do with numbers, now refers to the electronic production of films and computer images. In computing, represents a quantity changing in steps which are discrete. *See also* **analogue**.

digital compression pressure applied by the fingers, usually to an artery to stop bleeding.

digital imaging system the production of a digital radiographic image by reading an imaging plate and then displaying an image on a computer screen (*digital radiography*) or reading the signal from a television camera attached to an image intensifier (*digital fluoroscopy*) (see figure on p. 124).

digitalis leaf of the common foxglove containing glycosides, such as digoxin.

digital radiography the production of a digital radiographic image by reading an imaging plate and then displaying an image on a computer screen.

digital scanner equipment used to produce a digital image from a conventional radiographic film by passing light through the image and recording the intensity of the light.

digital signal the measurement of a signal in terms of numbers rather than a continuously varying value producing higher-quality image transfer to computers and television monitors.

digital subtraction angiography a method of increasing the contrast between vessels containing radiographic contrast agent and the background. A digital radiograph with contrast agent is superimposed on a reversed digital image without contrast agent thus removing most of the background information.

digitally reconstructed radiograph the electronic capture, manipulation and storage of X-rays to form a two- or three-dimensional radiographic image. In

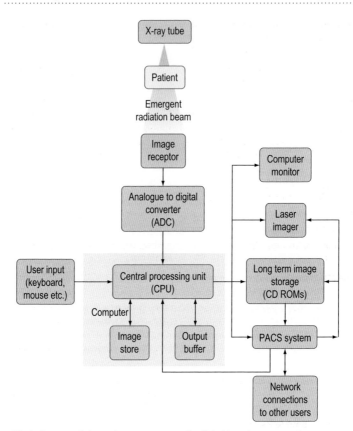

Block diagram of the major components of a digital imaging system. From Principles of radiological physics, 3rd edn, D T Graham, 1996, Churchill Livingstone, Edinburgh, with permission.

radiotherapy, computer reconstructions of radiographs from CT slices made to imitate the divergent X-ray beam.

digital verification   the use of either silicon diodes or ionization chambers placed in the exit beam during radiotherapy treatment to confirm the correct dose of radiation is being administered to the patient.

digital versatile disk (DVD)   a 120-mm sheet of aluminium covered with layer of acetate and an outer layer of metal and with a polycarbonate backing. Used in computing to store data in digital form which can be read by a laser.

digiti minimi quinti varus (congenital overlapping fifth toe) the smallest toe lies on the dorsum of the base of the fourth toe in a medially deviated position. It may be bilateral or unilateral.

dilatation stretching or enlargement. May occur physiologically, pathologically or be induced artificially.

dilatation and curettage (D and C) by custom refers to dilating the uterine cervix to obtain an endometrial sample by curettage. *See also* **hysteroscopy**.

dilatation and evacuation (D and E) dilatation of the cervix and evacuation of a fetus under anaesthetic for therapeutic termination of pregnancy or for the removal of a dead fetus in the second trimester of pregnancy.

dilution analysis when a known quantity of radioactive material is introduced into a space or cavity in a patient to enable the volume of the space to be calculated in radionuclide imaging.

diode a device containing an anode and a cathode in a vacuum and allows electrons to flow in one direction only, from the cathode to the anode.

dioxide oxide containing two atoms of oxygen in each molecule, for example, CO_2.

dipeptidases digestive enzymes that split dipeptides (paired amino acids) into individual amino acids.

2,3-diphosphoglycerate (2,3-DPG) substance present in red blood cells that decreases the affinity of haemoglobin for oxygen, thus allowing oxygen to be released to the tissues.

diplegia symmetrical paralysis of legs, usually associated with cerebral damage.

diploid (2n) describes a cell with a full set of paired chromosomes. In humans the diploid number is 46 chromosomes (44 autosomes and 2 sex chromosomes) arranged in 23 pairs in all cells except the gametes.

diplopia double vision.

direct cost a cost that can be directly attributed to the budget of a specific department, for example pharmacy costs in a given department.

direct current electricity the flow of electrons in only one direction.

direct exposure films films used without intensifying screens, for example, for intra-oral dental films.

disarticulation amputation at a joint.

discectomy surgical removal of a disc, usually an intervertebral disc.

discogenic arising in or produced by a disc, usually an intervertebral disc.

discography the introduction of a radiographic contrast agent into the nucleus of a spinal disc.

discrete distinct, separate, not merging. For example, used to describe some types of skin lesion.

discrete wedges   individual wedges produced with a limited range of angles, usually 15°, 30°, 45°, and 60° which are fitted to the light beam diaphragm during radiotherapy treatment.

disease   any deviation from or interruption of the normal structure and function of any part of the body. It is manifested by a characteristic set of signs and symptoms and in most instances the aetiology, pathology and prognosis is known.

disimpaction   separation of the broken ends of a bone that have been driven into each other during the impact which caused the fracture. Traction may then be applied to maintain the bone ends in good alignment and separate.

disinfectant   an agent that destroys or inhibits the growth of microorganisms, but not necessarily spore. The term is usually reserved for chemical germicides that are too corrosive or toxic to be applied to tissues, but which are suitable for application to inanimate objects.

disinfection   the removal or destruction of harmful microbes but not usually bacterial spores. It is commonly achieved by using heat or chemicals.

disinfestation   eradication of an infestation, especially of lice (delousing).

disk   a circular plastic disc coated with magnetic material used for storing computer data. Disks are usually high-speed devices.

dislocation   displacement of organs, or the articular surfaces of joints. The disruption of the joint is such that the articular surfaces no longer form a working joint. It may be congenital, spontaneous, traumatic or recurrent. Treatment may include reduction under anaesthetic.

disobliteration (rebore)   removal of that which blocks a vessel, most often intimal plaques in an artery, when it is called endarterectomy.

dispersed daylight system   a number of units of different sizes that are used to load films into cassettes and a cassette unloader that is fixed to an automatic film processor.

disposable items   articles that are used only once and then discarded thus reducing cross-infection.

dissecting aneurysm   a localized dilation of an artery, usually the aorta, when the outer and middle layers of the vessel wall are separated longitudinally. Rupture of the aneurysm may be fatal in less than 1 hour.

dissection   separation of tissues by cutting. When a group of lymph nodes are totally excised it is referred to as a block dissection of nodes: it is usually part of the treatment for cancer.

disseminated   widely spread or scattered.

disseminated intravascular coagulation (DIC)   an abnormal overstimulation of coagulation processes characterized by a rapid consumption of clotting factors which leads to microvascular thrombi and bleeding. It is associated with conditions leading to inadequate organ perfusion, such as hypo-volaemia and/or sepsis.

dissociation   separation of complex substances into their components. Ionization; when ionic compounds dissolve in water they dissociate or ionize into their ions.

distal   farthest from the head or source. *See also* **proximal**.

distribution server   in a PACS system a method of storing and sending images to an external user, the images can be encrypted to prevent unauthorized viewing.

diuresis   increased production/secretion of urine.

diuretics   substances that increase the secretion of urine by the kidney.

divers' paralysis   *see* **decompression illness**.

diverticulitis   inflammation of a diverticulum (a pouch or sac protruding from the wall of a tube or hollow organ).

diverticulosis   a condition in which there are many pouch-like hernias (diverticula) in the intestines. Colonic diverticula increase in frequency with age. May be asymptomatic, bleed, become infected or perforate.

diverticulum (diverticula)   a pouch or sac protruding from the wall of a tube or hollow organ. May be congenital or acquired.

dizygotic   relating to two zygotes. Describes non-identical twins that develop from two separate zygotes.

dolor   pain; usually used in the context of being one of the five classical signs and symptoms of inflammation – the others being calor, loss of function, rubor and tumor.

domain   an internet address.

domain name   used to locate an organization or individual on the internet.

dominant   describes a gene with the ability to override the expression of other recessive genes. ***dominant genes*** are expressed in both the homozygous state and the heterozygous state. Examples of dominant gene expression include: normal skin and hair pigmentation and Huntington's disease.

dominant hemisphere   on the opposite side of the brain to that of the preferred hand. The dominant hemisphere for language is the left in most right-handed people and about a third of left-handed people.

dongle   any device used to protect software from piracy.

dopa   a compound formed in an intermediate stage during the synthesis of catecholamines, for example, adrenaline (epinephrine), from tyrosine.

dopamine   a monoamine neurotransmitter. It functions in the central nervous system, especially the basal nuclei. Reduced levels are associated with Parkinson's disease. Used intravenously in some types of shock to increase cardiac output and blood flow to the kidneys.

dopants   impurities introduced into a crystal structure to control its characteristics. *See also* **activators, killers**.

doping   the addition of impurities to a substance, in extrinsic semiconductors impurities are added to the silicon or germanium to increase the electrical conductivity.

Doppler effect   when ultrasound echoes are reflected from a moving structure they are changed in frequency, the amount and direction depends on the velocity, the direction of the moving interface and the position of the observer. Moving towards an object produces an increase in the reflected frequencies and moving away from the object produces a decrease in frequency.

Doppler scanner   equipment used in ultrasound imaging to monitor a moving substance, for example, the flow of blood or the beating heart.

Doppler scanning   combines ultrasonography with pulse echo. Doppler ultrasound technique can be used to calculate cardiac output and stroke volume by measuring blood flow in the aorta via a probe passed into the oesophagus. Used to monitor haemodynamic status and response to treatment.

Doppler shift   a measurement obtained by subtracting the known frequency of the original transmitted ultrasonic waveform from the reflected waveform.

Doppler technique   can be used to measure the velocity of blood flow through a vessel to determine the degree of occlusion or stenosis.

dorsal   associated with the back, or the posterior part of an organ.

dorsal decubitus radiograph   patient is supine and the central ray passes through the body from side to side.

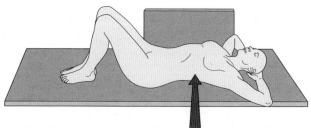

Dorsal decubitus. From Pocketbook of radiographic positioning, 2nd edn, Ruth Sutherland, 2003, Churchill Livingstone, Edinburgh, with permission.

dorsiflexion   bending backwards. In the case of the great toe – upwards.

dorsipalmar radiograph   a radiograph of the hand with the palm in contact with the cassette.

dorsiplantar   a radiograph of the foot with the sole in contact with the cassette.

dorsocentral   at the back and in the centre.

dorsolumbar   associated with the lumbar region of the back.

DOS (Disk Operating System)   the software which controls the computer disk drive.

dose build-up   each layer of tissue produces recoil electrons which in turn deposit their kinetic energy through several other layers of tissue. The energy in each layer will be determined by the number of electrons passing through the layer plus the absorbed kinetic energy.

dose-equivalent limits   the maximum dosage of radiation an individual can receive over a specific period of time in sieverts.

dose volume histogram   a graphical representation of dose distribution in a specific anatomical structure.

dosimeter, dosemeter   a device worn by personnel or placed within equipment to measure incident X-rays or gamma rays. ***thermoluminescent dosimeters***, using lithium fluoride powder impregnated into plastic discs, are used in personnel monitoring. Previously, photographic film in a special filter holder was used. *See also* **film badges, thermoluminescent dosimeters, solid state radiation detector, Geiger–Muller counter**.

dots per inch   a measure of image quality, the higher the number the better the image quality.

doubling time   time over which a tumour will double in size. A mark of tumour virulence and occasionally an indicator of chemoresponsiveness (faster doubling time often associated with high growth fraction and occasionally with higher chemoresponsiveness).

download   to transfer information from one computer to another.

Down's syndrome   a congenital condition in which there is learning disability and facial characteristics that include: oval tilted eyes, squint and a flattened occiput. The chromosome abnormality is of two types: (a) Primary trisomy, caused by abnormal division of chromosome 21 (at meiosis). This results in an extra chromosome instead of the normal pair: the infant has 47 chromosomes and is often born of an older mother. (b) Structural abnormality involving chromosome 21, with a total number of 46 chromosomes, one of which has an abnormal structure as the result of a special translocation. Such infants are usually born of younger mothers and there is a higher risk of recurrence in subsequent pregnancies.

drillers' disease (vibration syndrome)   caused by using vibrating machinery, resulting in cysts in the bones of the wrist and sometimes the hand.

drive wire   a wire used to hold a single radioactive source and cause it to oscillate over a prescribed length of a catheter.

drop attacks   periodic falling because of sudden loss of postural control of the lower limbs, without vertigo or loss of consciousness. Usually followed by sudden return of normal muscle tone, allowing the person to rise, if uninjured.

droplet infection   pathogen transmission in droplets of moisture such as during coughing or talking.

drug   the generic name for any substance used for the prevention, diagnosis and treatment of diagnosed disease and also for the relief of symptoms. *See also* **prescription only medicines, general sales list**.

drug dependence   a state arising from repeated administration of a drug on a periodic or continuous basis (WHO, 1964). Now a preferable term to drug addiction and drug habituation.

drug interaction   occurs when the action of one drug is affected by another drug, beverage or food taken previously or simultaneously.

drug misuse   term increasingly used to describe the illegal use of drugs. Substance misuse includes solvents and alcohol, as well as drugs.

drug reaction   an adverse reaction to a drug.

drug resistance   the increasing problem caused by the ability of some microorganisms to develop resistance to certain antibiotics, for example, vancomycin-resistant enterococci and methicillin-resistant *Staphylococcus aureus*.

drug tolerance   a situation where the therapeutic effects of a drug lessen over time, which necessitates the administration of a larger dose to achieve the same benefit.

drug trials   several levels of testing occurring during the development of new drugs. (a) *phase I trials* where small numbers of healthy volunteers (usually male) are given small doses and monitored for adverse reactions. Blood samples are tested to determine drug distribution and excretion. (b) *phase II trials* involve patients, and the new drug's efficacy is compared with existing treatments. (c) *phase III trials* involve large multiple centre studies carried out before the drug is approved and licensed for use by the appropriate bodies. *See also* **Committee on Safety of Medicines**. (d) *phase IV* trials take place after the drug has been approved for clinical use. Aim to monitor and report adverse and idiosyncratic reactions not seen earlier.

dry gangrene   death of part of the tissues of the body, occurs when the drainage of blood from the affected part is adequate; the tissues become shrunken and black.

dual dosemeter   two independent ionization chambers, that measure the integrated dose at the isocentre and feed signals to two independent dosimeters each capable of terminating a radiotherapy treatment exposure at a predetermined level. It provides a system of fail safe dose delivery control.

dual filament   two filaments in an X-ray tube to enable either broad or fine focus to be selected.

Dubowitz score   assesses gestational age.

Duchenne muscular dystrophy an X-linked recessive disorder affecting only boys. The disorder usually begins to show between 3 and 5 years and is characterized by progressive muscle weakness and loss of locomotor skills. Death usually occurs during the teens or early twenties from respiratory or cardiac failure.

duct a tube for carrying away the secretions from a gland.

ductless glands endocrine glands.

ductus arteriosus a fetal blood vessel connecting the left pulmonary artery to the aorta, to bypass the lungs in the fetus. At birth the duct closes, but if it remains open it is called persistent or patent ductus arteriosus, a congenital heart defect.

ductus venosus connection between the umbilical vein and inferior vena cava in the fetal circulation. Closes at birth.

Dukes' classification a staging system for colorecal tumours, A – confined to mucosa and submucosa; B – involvement of the musculature, C – metastatic involvement to regional lymph nodes; D – metastasized to distant organ tissues. It is based on the degree of tissue invasion and metastasis.

dulac technique positioning the patient so that the area of interest is in the centre of a sphere.

duodenal atresia closure of the duodenum, seen on ultrasound as a double bubble appearance of a fluid-filled, distended stomach and duodenal cap.

duodenal ulcer a peptic ulcer occurring in the duodenal mucosa. The majority are associated with the presence of the bacterium *Helicobacter pylori* in the stomach. Other factors include NSAIDs, smoking and genetic factors. Epigastric pain may occur some time after meals or during the night. The pain may be relieved by food, antacids and vomiting. The ulcer can bleed, leading to haematemesis and/or melaena, or it can perforate. Severe scarring following chronic ulceration may produce pyloric stenosis and gastric outlet obstruction. Management includes: (a) general measures; smoking cessation, avoiding foods that cause pain, avoiding aspirin and NSAIDs; (b) antibiotic drugs to eradicate *H. pylori*; (c) drugs to reduce gastric acid; H_2 receptor antagonists, for example, ranitidine, proton pump inhibitors, for example, omeprazole, antacids based on calcium, magnesium or aluminium salts; (d) rarely surgical treatment, for example, after perforation.

duodenitis inflammation of the duodenum.

duodenojejunal associated with the duodenum and jejunum.

duodenoscope a side-viewing flexible fibreoptic endoscope.

duodenostomy a surgically made fistula between the duodenum and another cavity, for example, cholecystoduodenostomy.

duodenum the fixed, curved, first portion of the small intestine, connecting the stomach above to the jejunum below.

duplex scan   a method of using real time imaging, colour and Doppler at the same time to demonstrate heart, blood vessels and in obstetrics.

duplicating film   film used to produce exact copies of radiographs by direct contact printing.

duplitized films   radiographic films in which the emulsion is coated on both sides of the base.

Dupuytren's contracture   painless, chronic flexion of the digits of the hand, especially the third and fourth, towards the palm. The aetiology is uncertain but some cases are associated with hepatic cirrhosis.

dura mater   the outer meningeal membrane. *See also* **falx cerebri, meninges, tentorium cerebelli**.

duty of care   the legal responsibility in the law of negligence that a person must take reasonable care to avoid causing harm.

DVD (Digital Versatile Disk)   a single- or double-sided disk used to record information from a computer using a laser to burn the surface of the disk.

DVI (Direct Video Interface)   a specialist computer connector for flat-panel computer monitors.

dwarf   person of stunted growth. May be due to growth hormone deficiency. Also occurs in untreated congenital hypothyroidism and juvenile hypothyroidism, achondroplasia and other conditions.

dwarfism   arrested growth and development as occurs in congenital hypothyroidism, and in some chronic diseases such as intestinal malabsorption, renal failure and rickets.

dwell time   the positioning of a radioactive source within a catheter for different intervals of time.

dye sensitizing   increasing the spectral sensitivity of the film by adding impurities to the film emulsion, because it is done by adding coloured dyes can be called *spectral sensitizing*.

dynamic CT   in early CT scanners when a number of scans were performed in rapid succession to demonstrate blood flow, now no longer used.

dynamic imaging   the monitoring of the change in radioactive uptake over time in radionuclide imaging.

dynamic incremental CT   in early CT scanners, when a number of dynamic CT scans were performed at different levels in the body, now no longer used.

dynamic range   in ultrasound imaging the difference between the maximum and minimum values in a set of data, that is how many degrees of black and white are found in the grey scale image.

dynamic wedge   a wedge angle produced by the rapid movement of the beam collimators, which does not affect the beam quality.

dysarthria a speech disorder that results from a problem in muscular control of the mechanisms of speech. It is caused by damage to either the central or the peripheral nervous system, or both. Loss of muscular control may involve incoordination and/or slowness and weakness. The problem may affect articulation, phonation, prosody, resonance and respiration.

dyschondroplasia a disorder of bone growth resulting in normal trunk, short arms and legs.

dysdiadochokinesia impairment of the ability to perform alternating movements, such as pronation and supination, in rapid, smooth and rhythmical succession; a sign of cerebellar disease but also seen in the so-called 'clumsy child' with minimal brain damage.

dysfunctional a body or a system which is unable to function normally.

dysgammaglobulinaemia impaired immunoglobulin production in terms of quantitative or qualitative humoral immunity. There are numerous primary and secondary causes including common variable immuno-deficiency, X-linked agammaglobulinaemia, X-linked hyper-IgM syndrome, myeloma and transient hypogammaglobulinaemia of infancy.

dysgenesis malformation during embryonic development.

dysgerminoma a rare ovarian tumour, benign or of low-grade malignancy. It originates from primitive/undifferentiated gonadal cells and occurs in young women.

dyskaryosis abnormality of nuclear chromatin, indicating a malignant or premalignant condition.

dyskeratosis abnormal keratin production by epithelial cells; may indicate malignancy.

dyskinesia (clumsy child syndrome) impairment of voluntary movement.

dysmaturity signs and symptoms of growth retardation at birth. *See also* **low birthweight**.

dysmelia limb malformation, including missing limbs or shortening of limbs.

dysmenorrhoea painful menstruation. It may be spasmodic or primary dysmenorrhoea, most often affecting young women once ovulation has become established, or congestive or secondary dysmenorrhoea usually affecting women in their late twenties and may be associated with pelvic pathology, such as fibroids or endometriosis.

dyspepsia indigestion.

dysphagia difficulty in swallowing. Dysphagia can occur in a variety of medical conditions including oesophageal cancer, cerebral palsy, motor neuron disease, cerebrovascular accident, dementia and head and neck cancer. The difficulty in swallowing may be experienced with fluids and/or solid food. The extent of difficulty can range from a mild to a very severe problem. Assessment and management of dysphagia is best conducted by a multidisciplinary team that may include a gastroenterologist, specialist nutrition nurse, dietitian, speech and language therapist. The composition of the team will be determined by the needs of the patient, the medical condition underlying the swallowing problem, whether surgery is indicated, the clinical setting and the aim of treatment (curative or palliative).

dysphasia   also sometimes known as ***aphasia***. Dysphasia is a disorder of language and has nothing to do with intelligence level or an intellectual disorder. It is most commonly associated with cerebrovascular accident affecting the left side of the brain, but can occur after a head injury or brain surgery. Dysphasia can affect the ability to understand language and also the use of language for expression. The presentation of dysphasia varies greatly and those affected·have very different skills and difficulties. It is important that detailed, individual consideration is given to their difficulties. The understanding of language includes understanding both what is said and what is written. Likewise, expression includes both verbal expression and written expression. Discrepancies between the level of understanding and expression of language are common. Most often, people with dysphasia have problems both in comprehension and in expression although the degree of impairment in each may vary. Assessment and treatment of dysphasia needs a detailed understanding and breakdown of language. Speech and language therapists can provide therapy to assist individuals and their carers to improve their communication. Dysphasia has a considerable impact on most areas of life such as relationships, work and leisure activities. Rehabilitation takes time and may last many months. People affected by dysphasia can become very withdrawn and isolated if they do not receive sufficient support. *See also* **aphasia**.

dysphonia   abnormality in the speaking voice such as hoarseness.

dysplasia   developmental abnormality of tissues and organs, often referring to a premalignant condition and graded according to severity.

dyspnoea   difficulty in, or laboured, breathing.

dyspraxia   lack of voluntary control over muscles, particularly the orofacial ones.

dysraphism   incomplete closure of a crease or ridge, for example of the neural tube.

dyssynergia   loss of fluency of movement; poor sequencing and timing of movements; loss of coordination of muscles that normally act in unison, particularly the abnormal state of muscle activity due to cerebellar disease.

dystaxia   difficulty in controlling voluntary movements.

dystonia   a movement disorder in which there is the abnormal posturing of a part of the body, examples of which are spasmodic torticollis and writer's cramp.

dystrophy   any abnormal condition caused by poor nutrition which usually results in muscle degeneration. *See also* **muscular dystrophy**.

dysuria   painful or difficult passing of urine.

E

ear the sensory organ concerned with hearing and balance. It has three parts, the outer (external), middle (tympanic cavity) and inner (internal) ear. The ***outer ear*** comprises the auricle (pinna) and the external auditory canal along which sound waves pass to vibrate the tympanic membrane which separates it from the middle ear. The ***middle ear*** cavity is air-filled and contains three tiny bones or ossicles: malleus, incus and stapes. The ossicles transmit the sound waves to the inner ear via the oval window. The middle ear communicates with the nasopharynx via the eustachian tube (pharyngotympanic tube). The fluid-filled ***inner ear*** comprises the cochlea (organ of hearing) and the semicircular canals which are concerned with balance. The cochlea and semicircular canals contain the nerve endings of the cochlear and vestibular branches of the vestibulocochlear or auditory nerve (eighth cranial). *See also* **cerumen, cochlea**.

eardrum the tympanic membrane at the end of the external auditory canal. The first auditory ossicle is attached to the inner surface.

eating disorders a term used to describe the range of conditions in which an individual's eating behaviour and nutrient intake is inappropriate for their needs. ***anorexia nervosa*** is characterized by distorted body image and a deliberate restriction of food intake, resulting in severe weight loss, malnutrition, endocrine disorders and electrolyte disturbances. ***bulimia nervosa*** – body weight is controlled by periods of restricted eating, purging and binge eating. Weight usually remains stable and within normal range. ***binge eating disorder*** – periods of binge eating without periods of food restriction or purging which result in the development of obesity. A complex mixture of social and psychological factors and life events predispose to and precipitate the development of eating disorders. Consequently they are best treated by a multidisciplinary team.

ecchondroma a benign tumour composed of cartilage which protrudes from the surface of the bone in which it arises.

ecchymosis bruise.

eccrine the most abundant type of sweat gland. *See also* **apocrine glands**.

echo the reflection of an ultrasound wave back to the transducer when the beam hits a surface at right angles.

echocardiography the use of ultrasound as a diagnostic tool for studying the structure and motion of the heart.

echoencephalography passage of ultrasound waves across the head. Can detect abscess, blood clot, injury or tumour within the brain.

echogenicity a characteristic of an ultrasound image, for example, benign masses are often homogeneous and malignant masses are often heterogeneous or fluid is black and solid areas appear white.

echo rephrasing the re-establishment of a magnetic resonance signal by either using a 180°radio frequency pulse or by gradient switching.

echo time (TE) the time between the centre of the excitation pulse and the peak of the echo.

echo train length the number of echoes that are individually phase encoded for a fast spin-echo sequence and corresponds to the number of lines of k-space measured per repetition time interval, they range from 3 to 128 depending on the type of pulse sequence. *See also* **k-space, repetition time**.

eclampsia occurrence of convulsions in a pregnant woman with signs of pre-eclampsia. A sudden convulsive attack.

ecmnesia impaired memory for recent events with normal memory of remote ones. Common in old age and in early cerebral deterioration.

ecological study a research study where a particular group of individuals rather than an individual, for example, schools, towns, etc., form the unit being observed.

economy describes spending or using as little as possible while still maintaining quality.

ectoderm the outer of the three primary germ layers of the early embryo. It gives rise to some epithelial and nervous tissues, for example, skin structures, inner ear, mammary glands, pituitary gland, the central nervous system, cranial, spinal and autonomic nerves, adrenal medulla and the lens and retina. *See also* **endoderm, mesoderm**.

ectogenesis (in vitro fertilization) the growth of the embryo outside the uterus.

ectopia malposition of an organ or structure, usually congenital.

ectopia vesicae an abnormally placed urinary bladder which protrudes through or opens on to the abdominal wall.

ectopic beat *see* **extrasystole**.

ectopic pregnancy (tubal pregnancy) pregnancy outside the womb (extra-uterine gestation), the uterine (fallopian) tube being the most common site.

ectrodactyly, ectrodactylia congenital absence of one or more fingers or toes or parts of them.

eczema an inflammatory skin reaction that may begin with erythema, then vesicles appear. These rupture, forming exudative areas that may crust. Scaling may occur. In chronic forms the skin becomes thickened. Some authorities limit the word 'eczema' to the cases with internal (endogenous) causes while those caused by external (exogenous) contact factors are called dermatitis. The skin of patients with eczema may be colonized or infected with *Staphylococcus aureus*. *See also* **dermatitis**.

eddy currents are induced electric currents in a transformer core and oppose the direction of the current in the windings of a transformer resulting in a power loss in the transformer, they can be reduced by laminating the core. In magnetic resonance imaging they are induced in the gradient coils or the structure of the magnet and degrade the image unless compensated for or eliminated.

edentulous without natural teeth.

editing altering a text or computer program.

effective current the value of current flowing for the same time that would produce the same electrical energy in a circuit as the equivalent alternating current.

effective dose a calculation to determine that amount of radiation received by a patient, for radiation protection purposes, which is weighted for each organ because different organs in the body show different sensitivity to radiation. The amount of a drug that can be expected to initiate a specific intensity of effect in people taking the drug.

effective half-life the time taken for the activity of a radionuclide in an organ to be reduced to half its original activity.

effective photon energy the energy of a homogeneous beam of photons having the same half value layer as the X-ray beam being evaluated.

effectiveness describes using resources to achieve the required outcomes.

effective voltage the value of voltage flowing for the same time that would produce the same electrical energy in a circuit as the equivalent alternating voltage.

effector a motor or secretory nerve ending in a muscle, gland or organ.

efferent carrying, conveying, conducting away from a centre. *See also* **afferent**.

efferent nerve one which conveys impulses outwards from the central nervous system to the muscles and glands. Also known as ***motor nerves***.

effervescent material used in radiotherapy to make an immobilizing device by placing the patient on an empty polythene bag, introducing the self hardening material and producing an impression of the patient's position, the impression can then be used during treatment to exactly replicate the patient position.

efficiency describes the use of minimum resources to achieve the maximum outcomes.

effusion extravasation of fluid into body tissues or cavities, such as a pleural effusion, or into joints where it causes swelling.

ejaculation   sudden emission of semen from the penis at the moment of male orgasm. ***retrograde ejaculation*** a situation where semen is discharged backwards into the bladder. It may follow prostate surgery or be associated with diabetic neuropathy.

elastic collisions   the mutual attraction of atoms, molecules etc. when the total energy is unchanged after the collision.

elastic scattering   when a photon interacts with an electron, is deflected from its path but does not lose energy. *See also* **coherent scattering**.

elbow joint   a synovial hinge joint formed by the humerus, radius and ulna.

elder abuse   physical, sexual, psychological, pharmacological or financial abuse of older people. May be by family, neighbours or carers.

electric circuit   the diagrammatic representation of electron flow through an electrical device.

Symbol and function of electric circuit elements[a]

Circuit element	Symbol	Function
Resistor		Inhibits flow of electrons
Battery		Provides electrical potential
Capacitor (condenser)		Momentarily stores electric charge
Ammeter		Measures electric current
Voltmeter		Measures electric potential
Switch		Turns circuit on or off by providing infinite resistance
Transformer		Increases or decreases voltage by fixed amount (AC only)
Rheostat		Variable resistor
Diode		Allows electrons to flow in only one direction

[a] From Radiologic science for technologists, 8th edn, 2005, S C Bushlong, Mosby, St Louis, with permission.

electric current   the rate of flow of electrons in a material. An electric current of one ampere flows at a point if a charge of one coulomb flows past the point per second.

electric field   the area surrounding an electrical charge, if an electric charge is placed inside the field a noticeable force will be exerted on it.

electrical potential   at a point is the measure of the work required to bring a unit positive charge from infinity to that point.

electric shock   shock caused when an electric current passes through the body, usually caused by accidental contact with an electric supply.

electrocardiogram (ECG)   a recording of the electrical activity of the heart muscle during the cardiac cycle made by an electrocardiograph. The normal heart produces a typical waveform, sinus rhythm, which consists of five deflection waves, known universally as PQRST. *See also* **ambulatory ECG, exercise (stress) ECG**.

electrocardiograph   an instrument that records the electrical activity of the heart from electrodes on the limbs and chest.

electrode   in medicine or therapy, a conductor in the form of a pad or plate, whereby electricity enters or leaves the body.

electroencephalogram (EEG)   a recording of the electrical activity of the brain, made by an electroencephalograph.

electroencephalograph   an instrument by which electrical impulses derived from the brain can be amplified and recorded, in a fashion similar to that of the electrocardiograph.

electrolysis   chemical decomposition by electricity, with ion movement shown by changes at the electrodes. Term used for the destruction of individual hairs (epilation), removal of moles, spider naevi, etc., using electricity.

electrolyte   a solution of a substance, such as sodium chloride, which dissociates into ions with an electrical charge (anions, cations). In medicine it describes the individual ion, for example, potassium and bicarbonate ions in the body. *electrolyte balance* the balance of relative amounts of electrolytes, for example, potassium, sodium, magnesium, calcium, chloride, bicarbonate (hydrogen carbonate) and phosphate in blood, other fluids and tissues. The balance between ions with a positive charge and those with a negative charge ensures overall electrical neutrality in the body. Many conditions and diseases cause *electrolyte imbalance*, which is often associated with loss of fluid and pH homeostasis.

electrolytic recovery   a method for recovering silver from radiographic fixer solution using a carbon anode and a stainless steel cathode, a direct current is passed between the two and the positively charged silver ions are attracted to the cathode where they are neutralized and form metallic silver, either a low or a high current density is used.

electromagnet   is formed when a piece of soft iron is placed inside a solenoid resulting in induced magnetism within the iron bar.

electromagnetic radiation   waves of energy that are caused by the acceleration of charged particles.

electromagnetic spectrum   the ordering of electromagnetic radiation into the various wavelengths and frequencies.

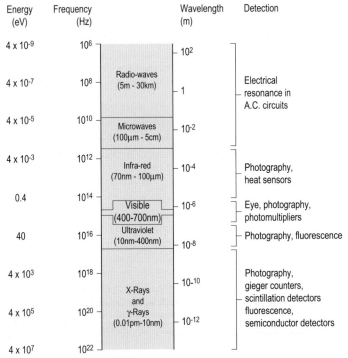

The electromagnetic spectrum (not drawn to scale). From Principles of radiological physics, 3rd edn, D T Graham, 1996, Churchill Livingstone, Edinburgh, with permission.

electromotive force (EMF)   measures the force needed for an electric current to flow between two points. A derived SI unit (International System of Units), the volt (V), is used.

electron   a negatively charged subatomic particle.

electron capture   the capture of an electron by the nucleus of an atom, the electron combines with a proton to form a neutron and a neutrino which is ejected from the nucleus.

electron gun   a piece of equipment that produces electrons by heating a spiral filament and then focussing them to form an electron beam.

electron microscopy   the use of a beam of electrons to visualize very small structures, such as virus particles.

electron shells   the orbits round the nucleus of an atom where the electrons are found in discrete levels, K is the nearest orbit to the nucleus and they are then labelled M, N, O, P etc.

electron transfer chain   a series of mitochondrial oxidation-reduction reactions that generate cellular energy as ATP.

electron trap   an area of low energy within a crystal which has the ability to catch and hold an electron for a period of time before it acquires the energy to escape.

electronic callipers   a method of measurement used to calculate the distance between two points identified during ultrasound imaging.

electronic collimation   used in PET cameras when an image is only recorded when two detectors simultaneously detect a photon of energy. *See also* **positron-emission tomography**.

electronic health record   a computerized summary of a patient's health record showing all their interactions with general practitioners and community healthcare workers.

electronic patient record   a computerized summary of all a patient's healthcare both in a primary and secondary care setting including written records, test results and medical images, for example, radiographs, scans, photographs, etc.

electronic portal imaging (EPI)   a method of capturing an image digitally in real time and the image is superimposed on the original radiotherapy simulation film or image to verify the accuracy of the field placement.

electrophoresis   a technique where charged particles are separated in a liquid medium by their characteristic speed and direction of migration in an electrical field. Used for measuring serum proteins.

element   a substance that cannot be broken down by chemical means into any other substance, each atom in the element contains a specific number of protons in the nucleus, a variable number of neutrons in the nucleus and a given number of electrons outside the nucleus. One of the constituents of a compound. The elements are the primary substances which in pure form, or in combinations as compounds, constitute all matter.

elevation   an upward movement such as the scapulae when the shoulders are lifted.

elimination   the passage of waste from the body – urine and faeces.

ellipsoid joint   a synovial joint that allows flexion, extension, abduction and adduction, for example, wrist joint.

eluting solution a liquid used to remove another substance by washing, used in a technetium generator where the eluting solution, saline, washes out the pertechnetate as sodium pertechnetate solution.

emaciation excessive leanness, or wasting of body tissue.

email an electronic mail system. Its current uses include sending imaging reports and pathology reports directly to GP surgeries from one computer to another via Healthlink. It may also be used by GPs for the direct referral of patients for examinations.

emasculation castration.

embolization the method of stopping, or drastically reducing the flow of blood in a vessel.

embolism obstruction of a blood vessel usually caused by a thrombus blood clot, but other causes include cancer cells, fat, amniotic fluid, gases, bacteria and parasites. Rarer emboli, such as fat, may follow long bone fractures, air may enter the circulation via a penetrating chest wound or during surgery, and amniotic fluid during labour. *arterial embolism*, originating from the left side of the heart or arterial disease, may travel to various sites including brain, bowel or limb; the effects dependent on the size of vessel affected and site, for example, gangrene of a limb or a portion of bowel. *See also* **cerebrovascular accident, deep vein thrombosis, pulmonary embolism**.

embolization therapeutic occlusion of a blood vessel using a foreign substance.

embolus solid body, for example a clot, or a gas bubble transported in the circulation. *See also* **embolism**.

embryo developmental stage starting 2 weeks after fertilization until the end of week 8 of gestation.

embryology study of embryonic development.

embryoma *see* **teratoma**.

embryopathy abnormality or disease of the embryo.

emesis vomiting.

emetic any agent used to produce vomiting.

emetogenic term that describes substances that cause vomiting or may do so, for example, cancer chemotherapy.

emission to send out. In physics all bodies emit electromagnetic radiation but a black body is the most efficient. In an intensifying screen when the light photons leave the screen and expose the film emulsion. An ejaculation or sending forth, especially an involuntary ejaculation of semen.

emphysema gaseous distension of the tissues. *See also* **crepitation, pulmonary emphysema, surgical emphysema**.

empirical based on observation rather than on scientific reasoning.

empyema pus in the pleural cavity.

emulsion   is the part of a radiographic film formed by light-sensitive salts for example silver halides in a gelatine binder, that records the radiographic image.

enamel   the outer layer covering the crown of a tooth.

encapsulation   enclosure within a capsule.

encephalitis   inflammation of the brain.

encephalocele   protrusion of brain substance through the skull. Often associated with hydrocephalus when the protrusion occurs at a suture line.

encephalography   a general term for techniques used to examine the brain. *See also* **echoencephalography, electroencephalography, pneumo-encephalography**.

encephalomalacia   softening of the brain.

encephalomyelitis   inflammation of the brain and spinal cord.

encephalomyelopathy   disease affecting both brain and spinal cord.

encephalon   the brain.

encephalopathy   any disease of the brain causing reduced levels of arousal and cognitive function.

enchondroma   a cartilaginous tumour.

encryption   a method of encoding computer data to prevent unauthorized people having access to the information.

endarteritis   inflammation of the intima or inner lining coat of an artery. *endarteritis obliterans* the new intimal connective tissue obliterates the lumen.

endemiology   the special study of endemic diseases.

endobronchial tube   plastic double-lumen tube introduced via the mouth into either of the two main bronchi in thoracic anaesthesia.

endocarditis   inflammation of the inner lining of the heart (endocardium) due to infection by microorganisms (bacteria, fungi or Rickettsia), or to rheumatic fever. There may be temporary or permanent damage to the heart valves.

endocardium   the smooth endothelium that lines the heart and covers the valves.

endocervical   associated with the inside of the cervix uteri.

endocrine   secreting internally. *See also* **exocrine**.

endocrine glands   the ductless glands that produce a hormone which passes directly into the blood or lymph. They include the hypothalamus, pineal body, pituitary, thyroid, parathyroids, adrenals, ovaries, testes and pancreas. Other structures also produce hormones, for example, placenta, gastrointestinal tract, kidneys and the heart.

endoderm   inner layer of the three primary germ layers of the early embryo. It gives rise to some epithelial tissue, for example, that of the pharynx, middle ear, respiratory tract, gastrointestinal tract and bladder. *See also* **ectoderm, mesoderm**.

endodontics   branch of dentistry concerned with the diagnosis and treatment of diseases of the dental pulp and periapical tissues.

endogenous   originating within the organism. *See also* **exogenous**.

endolymph   the fluid within the membranous labyrinth of the internal ear.

endometrial   associated with the endometrium. ***endometrial destruction*** transcervical destruction of the basal layer of the endometrium by transcervical resection, laser ablation or by using heat. Used in suitable cases as an alternative to hysterectomy in the treatment of menorrhagia.

endometrioma   a tumour of misplaced endometrium.

endometriosis   the presence of endometrium in abnormal sites, i.e. outside the uterus.

endometritis   inflammation of the endometrium.

endometrium   the specialized lining mucosa of the uterus.

endomyocardial   relating to the endocardium and myocardium.

endomysium   thin, inner connective tissue surrounding the muscle fibres.

endoneurium   the delicate, inner connective tissue surrounding the nerve fibres.

endorphins   a group of opioid-like neuropeptides. They are active in both central and peripheral nervous functions where they modulate pain interpretation and induce feelings of euphoria. *See also* **enkephalins**.

endoscope   an instrument for visualization of the interior of hollow tubular structures such as the urinary and gastrointestinal tracts, or body cavities, for example, joints. The older ones were rigid, tubular and made of metal. Those in general use are of the fibreoptic variety: light is transmitted by means of very fine glass fibres along a flexible tube. It permits examination, photography, biopsy and treatment of the cavities or organs of a relaxed (sedated) conscious person.

endoscopic retrograde cholangiopancreatography (ERCP)   introduction of an opaque contrast agent into the pancreatic and bile ducts via a catheter from an endoscope located in the duodenum.

endothelioid   resembling endothelium.

endothelioma   a tumour derived from endothelial cells.

endothelium   the lining membrane of serous cavities, heart, blood and lymph vessels.

endotracheal   within the trachea. ***endotracheal anaesthesia*** the administration of an anaesthetic through an endotracheal tube.

endotracheal tube   a plastic tube introduced via the nose or mouth into the trachea to maintain an airway during general anaesthesia and intermittent positive pressure ventilation.

enema the introduction of a liquid into the bowel via the rectum, to be returned or retained. The word is usually preceded by the name of the liquid used. It can be further designated according to the function of the fluid. The *evacuant enemas* are usually prepared commercially in small bulk as a disposable enema: the chemicals attract water into the bowel, promoting cleansing and peristaltic contractions of the lower bowel. The enemas to be retained are usually drugs, the most common being corticosteroids. *See also* **barium enema, laxatives**.

energy conservation techniques, including time management, problem solving and lifestyle planning, that enable an individual to make the best possible use of limited energy reserves. Commonly used in occupational therapy practice.

energy resolution the ability to distinguish between two different energy values. In a gamma camera, the width of the absorption peak at half the maximum count rate observed at the peak.

enhanced CT the use of a contrast agent to demonstrate more clearly vessels or organs of similar density to the surrounding tissue.

enkephalins (encephalins) neurotransmitters present in the central nervous system, pituitary gland and gastrointestinal tract. They have opioid-like analgesic effects. *See also* **endorphins**.

enophthalmos sunken position of an eyeball within its socket.

ensiform sword-shaped; xiphoid.

enteral within the gastrointestinal tract.

enteral diets those which are taken by mouth or through a nasogastric tube; low-residue enteral diets can be whole protein/polymeric, or amino acid/peptide.

enteral feeding method of providing nutrition when the gastrointestinal tract is functioning. Includes via nasogastric and nasoduodenal tubes or via gastrostomy or jejunostomy tubes. Enteral feeding can be administered by bolus, gravity or pump-controlled methods. *See also* **parenteral** feeding, **percutaneous endoscopic gastrostomy (PEG)**.

enteric relating to the small intestine.

enteric coating a coating applied to a pill that prevents drug release until it reaches the small intestine.

enteric fevers includes typhoid and paratyphoid fever.

enteritis inflammation of the intestine.

Enterobius vermicularis (threadworm) nematode which infests the small and large intestine.

enterocele prolapse of intestine. Can be into the upper third of vagina.

Enterococcus a genus of Gram-positive cocci commensal in the bowel, for example, *Enterococcus faecalis, E. faecium*. They cause urinary tract infection and wound infection and occasionally meningitis in neonates. It is increasingly common as a cause of hospital-acquired infection, and many strains are developing resistance to antibiotics.

enterokinase (enteropeptidase)   a proteolytic enzyme produced by duodenal mucosa. It converts inactive trypsinogen (pancreatic enzyme) into active trypsin.

enteron   the gut.

enteropeptidase   *see* **enterokinase**.

enterovesical   associated with the bowel and the bladder.

Entonox   proprietary name for a gaseous mixture of oxygen and nitrous oxide in equal measures that is inhaled by the patient to provide analgesia, for example, in obstetrics and intensive care.

entrance maze   a structure to prevent primary radiation and first scattered photons reaching the room door, used in radiotherapy treatment rooms so that lighter doors can be used and darkrooms so that people can enter while a film is being processed.

enucleation   removal of an organ or tumour in one piece. Removal of the eyeball due to malignant tumour, infection, trauma or control of pain in glaucoma.

Some colour codes[a]

Coloured indicator lights (e.g. on a control desk)	
RED:	Warning of danger requiring urgent action to terminate an unintended state of operation
YELLOW:	Requiring attention, caution (e.g. radiation on)
YELLOW (flashing):	Sources in transit (e.g. in remote afterloading equipment)
GREEN:	Ready for action
WHITE:	Equipment switched on but further operations required to bring it to the ready state
Coloured cables (single phase mains)	
BROWN:	Live
BLUE:	Neutral
GREEN/YELLOW:	Earth
Coloured cables (three phase mains)	
BROWN/BLUE/YELLOW:	Three live phases
GREEN/YELLOW:	Earth

[a] From Walter and Miller's textbook of radiotherapy, 6th edn, 2003, C K Bomford and I H Kunkler (eds), Churchill Livingstone, Edinburgh, with permission.

enuresis incontinence of urine, especially bed-wetting. **_nocturnal enuresis_** bed wetting during sleep.

environmental monitoring a mechanism for ensuring that the protective barriers in departments provide a safe working environment for all staff and the general public.

enzyme a protein that functions as a catalyst for specific biochemical reactions involving specific substrates. Many reactions in the body would proceed too slowly without an enzyme, for example, waste carbon dioxide would not be removed from the tissues without the enzyme carbonic anhydrase. Enzyme names often reflect their function, for example, dehydrogenases catalyse the removal of hydrogen in oxidation reactions.

eosinophil cells having an affinity for eosin. A type of polymorphonuclear leucocyte containing eosin-staining granules, it is associated with immune responses that involve allergies and immunoglobulin (IgE).

eosinophilia increased number of eosinophils in the blood.

ependymal cells a type of neuroglial cell that lines the fluid-filled cavities of the central nervous system (cerebral ventricles and the central canal of the spinal cord).

ependymoma a tumour arising from the lining cells of the ventricles, central canal of the spinal cord and the filum terminale.

epicardium the visceral layer of the pericardium.

epicondyle an eminence on some bones situated above the condyles, for example, femoral epicondyles.

epicondylitis inflammation of the muscles and tendons around the elbow. Can occur if the structures are subjected to excess or repetitive stress. It may affect the structures at the lateral (outer) or medial (inner) aspect of the elbow. **_lateral epicondylitis_** (tennis elbow) is associated with tennis, other racquet sports and weight training. **_medial epicondylitis_** (golfer's elbow) is primarily an overuse injury associated with golf and poor lifting techniques. *See also* **bursitis.**

epicritic describes cutaneous nerve fibres which are sensitive to fine variations of touch and vibration. Concerned with proprioception and two-point discrimination. *See also* **protopathic.**

epidemiology the scientific study of the distribution of diseases. It is concerned with the incidence, distribution and control of disease.

epidermis the outer avascular layer of the skin, the cuticle.

epididymis a small oblong body attached to the posterior surface of the testes. It consists of the seminiferous tubules which carry the spermatozoa from the testes to the deferent ducts (vas deferens).

epidural upon or external to the dura.

epidural anaesthesia local anaesthetic injected into the space external to the dura either by single injection or intermittently via a catheter, causing loss of sensation in an area determined by the site of the injection and volume of local anaesthetic used. ***epidural space*** the region through which spinal nerves leave the spinal cord. It can be approached at any level of the spine, but the administering of anaesthetic is commonly done at the lumbar level or through the sacral cornua for caudal epidural block.

epigastrium   the abdominal region lying directly over the stomach.

epiglottis   the thin leaf-shaped flap of cartilage behind the tongue which, during the act of swallowing, covers the opening leading into the larynx.

epilation   loss of hair.

epilepsy   conditions resulting from disordered electrical activity in the brain resulting in epileptic seizures or 'fits'. The seizure is caused by an abnormal electrical discharge that disturbs brain and results in a generalized or partial seizure, depending on the area of the brain involved. *See also* **grand mal, petit mal, Jacksonian epilepsy, status epilepticus**.

epileptic   a person with epilepsy.

epileptic aura   tingling in the hand or visual or auditory sensations that precede an attack of epilepsy. *See also* **aura**.

epimysium   outer fibrous coat surrounding an entire muscle.

epineurium   outer fibrous coat enclosing a nerve trunk.

epiphora   the continuous weeping of the eye, often due to blockage of the lacrimal apparatus.

epiphysis   the end of a growing bone. Separated from the shaft by the epiphyseal plate (cartilage) this is replaced with bone (ossification) when growth ceases.

episclera   loose connective tissue between the sclera and conjunctiva.

epistaxis   bleeding from the nose.

epithelialization   the growth of epithelium over a raw area; the final stage of healing.

epithelioma   a tumour arising from any epithelium.

epithelium   one of the four basic tissues. It lines cavities, covers the body and forms glands. It is classified according to the arrangement and shape of the cells it contains. It may be simple, single layer of squamous, cuboidal or columnar, or stratified with many layers, for example, stratified or transitional.

EPROM (Erasable Programmable Read Only Memory)   a memory store which can be programmed and then erased by UV light.

Epstein–Barr virus (EBV)   a herpesvirus, the causative agent of infectious mononucleosis. Also linked with the formation of some malignant tumours, including Burkitt's lymphoma and nasopharyngeal cancer.

epulis   a tumour growing on or from the gums.

equinus   a condition in which the toes point down and the person walks on tiptoe. *See also* **talipes**.

equity   fairness of distribution of resources such as health care. Access to resources is based on need and the ability to benefit. The ability of a health-care system to provide a comparable level of health care across the entire population. Covers the following dimensions: need for health care in the population (dependent on epidemiology of disease, determinants of health); availability, accessibility of healthcare resources; distribution of healthcare resources; use (utilization) of healthcare resources; geographic variation in need and healthcare utilization.

equivalent dose   a unit of dose that allows for the fact that different types of radiation will deposit different types of energy depending on the specific mass and charge.

equivalent square   a square which produces the same percentage scatter as an elongated or circular field, used to calculate depth dose in radiotherapy.

equivalent wavelength   the quality of a radiation beam by calculating Planck's constant times velocity over the maximum kilovoltage (Duane-Hunt's law).

erasable optical disks (Magneto-optical disks or MO disks)   read *and* write optical disks which combine magnetic and optical techniques.

Erb's palsy   paralysis involving the shoulder and arm muscles from a lesion of the fifth and sixth cervical nerve roots. The arm hangs loosely at the side with the forearm pronated ('waiter's tip position'). Most commonly a birth injury.

erectile   upright; capable of being elevated.

erectile dysfunction   an inability to achieve or maintain penile erection.

erectile tissue   vascular tissue, which, under stimulus, becomes rigid and erect from hyperaemia.

erection   the state accomplished when erectile tissue is hyperaemic.

erector   a muscle which achieves erection of a part. *erector spinae* muscle of the back.

eruption   the process by which a tooth emerges through the alveolar bone and gingiva.

erythema   redness or inflammation of the skin, can be as a result of mild sunburn or reaction to radiotherapy treatment.

erythroblast   a nucleated erythrocyte precursor found in the red bone marrow.

erythrocytes   non-nucleated red cells of the circulating blood. They carry oxygen and some carbon dioxide, and buffer pH changes in the blood.

erythrocyte sedimentation rate (ESR)   citrated blood is placed in a narrow tube. The red cells fall, leaving a column of clear supernatant serum, which is measured at the end of an hour and reported in millimetres. Inflammation and tissue destruction cause an elevation in the ESR.

erythrocytopenia   deficiency in the number of red blood cells.

erythroderma   abnormal redness of the skin, usually over a large area.

erythropoiesis   the production of red blood cells by the bone marrow. *See also* **erythropoietin, haemopoiesis**.

erythropoietin   a hormone secreted by some kidney cells in response to reduced oxygen content in the blood. It acts on the bone marrow, stimulating erythropoiesis. A recombinant human form is used therapeutically to treat anaemia associated with chronic renal failure and platinum-containing chemotherapy.

establishment   describes the planned staffing levels in a particular area. Usually described as the number of whole time equivalents (WTEs).

estradiol   *see* **oestradiol**.

estrogens   *see* **oestrogens**.

ethernet   a method of connecting a computer to a network to enable communication with other computers.

ethics   a code of moral principles derived from a system of values and beliefs. It is concerned with rights and obligations. ethics committees bodies that operate in academic institutions and NHS Trusts to consider proposals for research projects. The approval of the appropriate ethics committee is usually a prerequisite for obtaining a research grant.

ethmoid   a spongy bone forming the lateral walls of the nose and the upper portion of the bony nasal septum.

ethmoidal sinuses   numerous small, irregular-shaped cavities in the ethmoid bone.

ethnography   a study of individuals in their usual surroundings. Used in qualitative research by anthropologists to describe customs, culture and social life through observation, informal interviews, etc.

ethyl chloride   a volatile liquid used to test the onset of regional anaesthesia by reason of the intense cold sensation produced when applied to the skin.

ethylene oxide   a gas used to sterilize delicate equipment that would be damaged by high temperatures.

etoposide   a chemotherapeutic agent and mitotic inhibitor.

eustachian tube   *see* **pharyngotympanic tube**.

euthanasia   literally an 'easy death'. Inferring a painless death. Frequently interpreted as the act of causing a painless and planned death, such as relieving a person's extreme suffering from an incurable disease. Presently illegal in UK and opposed by many professional groups, it is practised in some European countries.

evacuant an agent which initiates an evacuation, such as of the bowel. *See also* **enema**, **laxatives**.

evacuation the act of emptying a cavity; generally refers to the discharge of faecal matter from the rectum. *See also* **manual evacuation**.

evacuation of retained products of conception (ERPC) emptying the uterus following an incomplete miscarriage.

even echo rephrasing in magnetic resonance imaging, the re-establishment of spin-echo coherence of moving spins on symmetric even echoes in multi-echo sequences as a result of sequential integration of signal phase shifts adding to zero.

evidence-based medicine (EBM) practice (EBP) describes the practice of medicine or delivery of healthcare interventions that are based on systematic analysis of information available in terms of effectiveness in relation to cost-effective health outcomes. The highest level of evidence (based on the robustness of the research methodology) is that gained from meta-analysis of randomized controlled trials (RCTs). Sometimes this level of evidence is not available and at the lowest level may be based on evidence from expert committee reports or opinions and/or clinical experience of respected practitioners.

evulsion forcible tearing away of a structure.

Ewing's tumour a malignant tumour that develops from bone marrow, usually in the long bones or the pelvis. Usually diagnosed in a child or young adult.

excision removal of a part by cutting.

excision biopsy the cutting out of a lesion and surrounding normal tissue for examination.

excitation the process of moving an electron in an atom into a higher orbit.

excrescence an abnormal protuberance or growth of the tissues.

excreta the waste material that is normally cleared from the body, particularly urine and faeces.

excretion the elimination of waste material from the body, and also the eliminated material.

excretion urography the radiographic investigation of the kidneys, ureters and bladder following the injection of a contrast agent.

exercise (stress) ECG performed during increasing levels of exertion, such as on a treadmill, to detect arrhythmias or ischaemic changes caused by physical stress. Frequently used for the diagnosis or prognosis of heart disease or to guide cardiac rehabilitation.

exfoliation the scaling off of tissues in layers. The shedding of the primary teeth.

ex gratia   as a matter of favour, for example, without admission of liability, of payment offered by a NHS Trust to a claimant.

exocrine   describes glands from which the secretion passes via a duct; secreting externally. *See also* **endocrine**.

exogenous   of external origin. *See also* **endogenous**.

exophytic   tendency to grow outwards, such as a tumour that grows into the lumen of a hollow organ rather than into the wall.

exostosis   an overgrowth of bone tissue forming a benign tumour.

expected date of delivery (EDD)   usually calculated as 280 days from the first day of the last normal menstrual period.

experimental epidemiology   the study of the effect of controlling the relevant suspected factors in the cause of a disease such as stopping cigarette smoking.

experimental group   a research term that describes the group exposed to the independent variable (the intervention or experimental agent such as a drug). *See also* **control group, variable**.

expiration   the process of breathing out air from the lungs.

expired air resuscitation   forced introduction or air into the lungs of someone who has stopped breathing, it may be administered mouth to mouth, mouth to nose or by using ventilating equipment.

exponential law   the decay or growth of a substance in which each step is half the value or double the value of the preceding step.

exposure   the measure at a particular point in a beam of X or γ rays and is the total charge of one sign over a small volume of air, unit coulombs per kilogram, now replaced by the kerma.

exposure factors   the settings used to produce the optimum radiographic image quality with the minimum radiation dose to the patient. The settings include the kilovoltage (kVp), milliamperes per second (mAs), source to image distance (SID), object to image distance (OID), source to object distance (SOD), the use of a secondary radiation grid, collimation and the type of film screen combination used. (See figure on p. 153.)

exposure rate   the measure of the intensity of a beam in unit time.

extended focus-to-skin distance techniques   radiotherapy treatment techniques where the focus to skin distance (FSD) is greater than 100 cm.

extension   traction upon a fractured or dislocated limb. The straightening of a flexed limb or part.

extensor   a muscle which on contraction extends or straightens a part.

external   outside.

external auditory meatus (auditory canal)   the canal between the pinna and eardrum.

Exposure factors. In selecting the exposure factors for an examination the radiographer is attempting to produce an image of optimum quality but at minimum radiation dose to the patient. Below is a summary of some of the factors which might be changed and their direct and indirect effect(s) on image quality and radiation dose to the patient[a]

Factor Increased ↑	Effect on the radiation beam leaving the tube	Direct effect on image quality	Indirect effect on image quality	Effect on radiation dose to the patient
mAs ↑	Quantity ↑	Image darker	May require larger focal spot to allow increased time	Dose ↑
kVp ↑	Quality ↑ Quantity ↑	Contrast ↓ Density ↑	Lower mAs	Less dose to area – gonad ↑
Collimation (tightened)	Smaller area no effect on quality/quantity	Improves contrast	Needs mAs ↑	Reduces dose ↓
SID	No effect	Alters magnification OID/SOD ratio	Requires mAs ↑	Slight reduction ↓
Use of secondary radiation grid	No effect	Contrast ↑	Requires mAs ↑	Dose ↑
Altering the speed class of the film/ screen combination	No effect	Increase photographic sharpness	Requires mAs ↑	Reduced ↓

[a] From Pocketbook of radiographic positioning, 2nd edn, 2003, Ruth Sutherland, Churchill Livingstone, Edinburgh, with permission.

external haemorrhage   bleeding when the skin surface is damaged.

external hydrocephalus   excess of cerebrospinal fluid mainly in the subarachnoid space.

external respiration   the exchange of gases between alveolar air and pulmonary capillary blood. Oxygen in the alveolar air moves into the blood, and carbon dioxide moves from the blood into the air in the lungs for excretion.

external rotation (lateral rotation)   a limb or body movement where there is rotation away from the vertical axis of the body.

extra-articular   outside a joint.

extracapsular   outside a capsule.

extracardiac   outside the heart.

extracellular   outside the cell membrane.

extracellular fluid (ECF)   fluid outside the cells such as plasma, interstitial fluid, lymph, gastrointestinal fluid and CSF. *See also* **intracellular**.

extracorporeal   outside the body.

extracorporeal circulation   blood is taken from the body, directed through a machine ('heart–lung' or 'artificial kidney') and returned to the general circulation. *See also* **cardiac bypass, cardiopulmonary bypass, extracorporeal membrane oxygenation (ECMO), haemodialysis**.

extracorporeal membrane oxygenation (ECMO)   a cardiopulmonary bypass device which uses a membrane oxygenator (artificial lung). Venous blood from the patient circulates through the device by a roller pump. A fresh flow of oxygen into the device passes through a semipermeable membrane that allows the diffusion of oxygen while simultaneously removing carbon dioxide and water. Once the blood is oxygenated it is returned to the patient through an artery or a vein.

extraction   the removal of a tooth.

extraction of lens   surgical removal of the lens from the eye. It may be extracapsular extraction, when the capsule is ruptured prior to delivery of the lens and preserved in part, or intracapsular extraction, when the lens and capsule are removed intact.

extradural   external to the dura mater.

extradural haematoma   a collection of blood external to the dura mater.

extrahepatic   outside the liver.

extrahepatic cholestasis   caused by a blockage to a large duct, for example, the common bile duct, by a gallstone or cancer of the pancreas.

extramural   outside the wall of a structure.

extraperitoneal   outside the peritoneum.

extrapleural   outside the pleura, i.e. between the parietal pleura and the chest wall.

extrapyramidal   outside the pyramidal tracts.

extrapyramidal effects/disturbances   include the tremor and rigidity seen in parkinsonism and the side-effects of drugs, such as phenothiazine neuroleptics (antipsychotic drugs), that may cause a parkinsonian-like syndrome.

extrapyramidal tracts   motor pathways that pass outside the internal capsule. They modify pyramidal tract motor functions and influence coarse voluntary movement and affect posture, coordination and balance.

extrarenal   outside the kidney.

extrasystole   premature beats (ectopic beats) in the pulse rhythm: the cardiac impulse is initiated by an abnormal focus.

extrathoracic   outside the thoracic cavity.

extrauterine   outside the uterus.

extrauterine pregnancy   *see* **ectopic pregnancy**.

extravasation   an escape of fluid from its normal enclosure into the surrounding tissues.

extravesical   outside the organ.

extrinsic   developing or having its origin from without; not internal. **extrinsic factor** vitamin B_{12}, essential for the maturation of erythrocytes and nerve function, cannot be synthesized in the body and must be supplied in the diet, hence it is called the *extrinsic factor*. Its absorption in the terminal ileum requires the presence of the intrinsic factor secreted by the stomach. *extrinsic sugars*, such as lactose in milk and sucrose as table sugar, that are not contained within cell walls.

extrinsic allergic alveolitis ('farmer's lung' or 'bird fancier's lung')   an inflammatory response in the lungs to the inhalation of organic dusts. The two main causes are microbial spores present in vegetable produce such as mouldy hay and animal proteins most commonly from pigeons and budgerigars. In an acute attack flu-like symptoms and breathlessness develop several hours after exposure; the symptoms generally subside spontaneously. If exposure continues a chronic condition with pulmonary fibrosis will develop.

exudate   the discharge of fluid or substances from cells or blood vessels onto the skin or organ surface.

eye   organ of vision. There are three layers, from outside in the sclera, the uvea, which forms the pigmented choroid, ciliary body and iris, and the inner light-sensitive retina containing photoreceptors (cones and rods) and pigment cells.

eye teeth   the canine teeth in the upper jaw.

F

. . . .

fabella   a sesamoid bone sometimes found posterior to the knee joint.

facet   a small, smooth, flat surface of a bone or a calculus.

facial   associated with the face.

facial hemiatrophy   a congenital condition, or a manifestation of sclero-derma in which the structures on one side of the face are shrunken.

facial nerve   seventh pair of cranial nerves. They supply the facial muscles, the salivary, lacrimal and nasal glands, and part of the tongue.

facial paralysis   paralysis of muscles supplied by the facial nerve.

facies   the appearance or the expression of the face. ***adenoid facies*** open mouthed, vacant expression due to deafness from enlarged pharyngeal tonsils (adenoids). ***Parkinson facies*** a mask-like appearance; saliva may trickle from the corners of the mouth.

facilitated diffusion   process whereby larger non-fat-soluble molecules such as glucose pass into the cell by using a protein carrier molecule. No energy is required but there must be a concentration gradient.

faecalith   a concretion formed in the bowel from faecal matter: it can cause obstruction and/or inflammation.

faecal softeners   *see* **laxatives**.

faeces   the waste material eliminated from the bowel, consisting mainly of indigestible cellulose, unabsorbed food, intestinal secretions, water, electrolytes and bacteria, etc.

failure to thrive   failure to develop and grow at the expected rate, ascertained by consistent measurement of height and weight plotted on a growth chart. It may result from an organic disorder or have non-organic causes, such as poor feeding, maternal deprivation or psychosocial problems. Careful investigation is required to establish the cause.

faint   a temporary loss of consciousness. *See also* **syncope**.

falciform   sickle-shaped.

fallopian tubes   *see* **uterine tubes**.

Fallot's tetralogy   a cyanotic congenital heart defect comprising a ventricular septal defect, narrowing of the right ventricular outflow tract (subvalvular pulmonary stenosis), right ventricular hypertrophy and malposition of the aorta overriding the ventricular septum. Amenable to corrective surgery.

false pelvis   the wide expanded part of the pelvis above the brim.

falx   a sickle-shaped structure.

falx cerebri   that portion of the dura mater separating the two cerebral hemispheres.

familial adenomatous polyposis   a dominantly inherited condition in which multiple polyps occur throughout the large bowel and which invariably leads to colon cancer. Polyps also occur in the stomach and duodenum.

Family Health Services (FHS)   community-based services provided by family doctors, dentists, opticians and pharmacists as independent contractors. They are not directly employed by the NHS, but have contractual arrangements to practise in the NHS.

farad (F)   a measure of capacitance, an electrical system has a capacitance of 1 farad if a charge of 1 coulomb held by the body results in a potential of 1 volt.

Faraday's laws of electromagnetic induction   (1) a change in the magnetic flux linked with a conductor induces an electromotive force in the conductor. (2) The size of the induced electromotive force is proportional to the rate of change of the magnetic flux linkage.

farmer's lung   *see* **extrinsic allergic alveolitis**.

fascia   a connective tissue sheath consisting of fibrous tissue and fat which unites the skin to the underlying tissues. It also surrounds and separates many of the muscles, and, in some cases, holds them together.

fasciculus   a little bundle, as of muscle or nerve.

fasciitis   an abnormal benign growth which develops in the subcutaneous oral tissue, usually in the cheek. Inflammation of the connective tissue.

Fatal Accident Enquiry   *see* **coroner**.

fatigue   weariness. Physiological term for diminishing muscle reaction to stimulus applied. In sports medicine the failure of muscle(s) to maintain force (or power output) during sustained or repeated contractions.

fatigue fracture   *see* **stress fracture**.

fatigue index (FI)   the decline in power divided by the time (in seconds) interval between maximum (peak) and minimum power, recorded during an anaerobic power exercise test.

fatty acid   hydrocarbon component of lipids. May be unsaturated (monounsaturated or polyunsaturated) or saturated depending on the number of double chemical bonds in their structure.

fatty degeneration   tissue degeneration that leads to the appearance of fatty droplets in the cytoplasm; found especially in disease of heart, liver and kidney.

fatty liver   accumulation of fat in the liver, an indication of diffuse liver disease or benign changes, demonstrated using grey scale ultrasound.

fat/water suppression   a method that suppresses signal within the imaging volume from either fat or water protons by applying a frequency selective, saturation, radio frequency pulse in magnetic resonance imaging.

fauces   the opening from the mouth into the pharynx, bounded above by the soft palate, below by the tongue. ***pillars of the fauces***, anterior and posterior, lie laterally and surround the palatine tonsil.

febrile   feverish; accompanied by fever. ***febrile convulsions*** occur in children who have an increased body temperature; they do not usually result in permanent brain damage. Most common between the ages of 6 months and 5 years. *See also* **convulsions**.

feedback   a homeostatic control mechanism. It is usually ***negative feedback*** where a physiological process is slowed or 'turned off' by an increasing amount of product, for example, temperature control. Much more rarely in ***positive feedback*** the process is speeded up by high levels of the product, for example, normal blood clotting. ***feedback treatment*** *See* **biofeedback**.

femoral   associated with the femur or thigh. Applied to the vein, artery, nerve and canal.

femoral arteriography   a contrast agent is injected via a catheter in the femoral artery to demonstrate the arterial circulation of the leg.

femoral hernia   protrusion through the femoral canal, alongside the femoral blood vessels as they pass into the thigh.

femoropopliteal   usually, referring to the femoral and popliteal vessels.

femur   the thigh bone, the longest and strongest bone in the body.

fenestra   a window-like opening.

fenestra ovalis   an oval opening between the middle and internal ear.

fenestra rotunda   a round opening which lies below the fenestra ovalis.

fenestration   a perforation, opening or pore, the glomerular capillaries of the nephron, which form part of the filtration membrane, are adapted for permeability and filtration by the presence of fenestrations. A surgical opening (or fenestra) in the inner ear to ease the deafness caused by otosclerosis.

ferritin   an iron–protein complex. A storage form of iron.

ferromagnetic   a substance that if placed in a magnetic field becomes magnetized and once the magnetic field is removed it retains its magnetism, for example iron, cobalt or nickel. *See also* **diamagnetic, paramagnetic, superparamagnetic**.

ferromagnetism   if an external magnetic force is applied to the material all the magnetic domains align in the same direction forming a strong magnet.

fetal age viability   defined as when a baby can survive outside the womb, that is, 24 weeks gestational age.

fetal alcohol syndrome (FAS)   stillbirth and fetal abnormality due to prenatal growth retardation caused by excessive maternal alcohol consumption during pregnancy.

fetal circulation   circulation adapted for intrauterine life. Extra shunts and vessels (ductus venosus, ductus arteriosus, foramen ovale and umbilical vein) allows blood to largely bypass the liver, gastrointestinal tract and lungs, as their functions are covered by maternal systems and the placenta.

fetus   the developmental stage from the eighth week of gestation until birth.

fetus papyraceus   a dead fetus, one of a twin which has become flattened and mummified.

fever (pyrexia)   an elevation of body temperature above normal. Designates some infectious conditions, for example, paratyphoid fever, scarlet fever, typhoid fever, etc.

fibre   a thread-like structure.

fibre distribution data interface (FDDI)   in computing a system similar to a token ring which uses fibreoptic cables to inform nodes when they can write to the network. *See also* **nodes**.

fibreoptics   light is transmitted through flexible glass fibres which enable the user to 'see round corners'. The technology utilized in endoscopic equipment.

fibril   a component filament of a fibre; a small fibre.

fibrillation   uncoordinated quivering contraction of muscle; referring usually to myocardial muscle. *See also* **atrial fibrillation, cardiac arrest, ventricular fibrillation**.

fibrin   the insoluble matrix on which a blood clot is formed. Produced from soluble fibrinogen by the action of thrombin.

fibrinogen   factor I of blood coagulation. A soluble plasma protein that is converted to fibrin by the action of thrombin.

fibroadenoma   a benign tumour containing fibrous and glandular tissue.

fibroblast (fibrocyte)   a blast cell that forms connective tissues. Involved during growth and tissue repair.

fibrocartilage   cartilage containing fibrous tissue.

fibrocaseous   a soft, cheesy mass infiltrated by fibrous tissue, formed by fibroblasts.

fibrocyst   a fibroma which has undergone cystic degeneration.

fibrocystic   associated with a fibrocyst.

fibrocystic disease   bone cysts which may be solitary or generalized. If generalized and accompanied by decalcification of bone, it is symptomatic of hyperparathyroidism.

fibrocystic disease of breast   the breast feels lumpy due to the presence of cysts, usually caused by hormone imbalance.

fibrocystic disease of pancreas   cystic fibrosis.

fibrocyte   *see* **fibroblast**.

fibroid   a fibromuscular benign tumour usually found in the uterus may be on a stalk (pedunculate) protruding from the uterus, in the wall of the uterus or in the endometrial cavity. The location of fibroids can be described as intramural (embedded in the wall of the uterus), subserous (protruding from the serosal surface into the peritoneal cavity), or submucous (protruding into the endometrial surface).

fibroma   a benign tumour composed of fibrous tissue.

fibromatosis   a gingival enlargement, believed to be hereditary, the tissue covers the surface of the adult teeth.

fibromuscular   associated with fibrous and muscle tissue.

fibromyalgia   a condition characterized by widespread pain and tender points. Many patients also complain of tiredness and of waking feeling unrefreshed.

fibromyoma   a benign tumour consisting of fibrous and muscle tissue.

fibroplasia   the production of fibrous tissue which is a normal part of healing.

fibrosarcoma   a form of sarcoma. A malignant tumour arising from fibrous tissue.

fibrosis   the formation of excessive fibrous tissues, for example, scar tissue, as a result of inflammation or pulmonary fibrosis caused by radiation, certain drugs and pneumoconiosis.

fibrositis   a lay term that denotes non-specific soft-tissue pain.

fibrous joint (synarthroses)   joints joined with fibrous tissue and have virtually no movement, for example, sutures.

fibrovascular   relating to fibrous tissue which is well supplied with blood vessels.

fibula   one of the longest and thinnest bones of the body, situated on the outer side of the leg and articulating at the upper end with the lateral condyle of the tibia and at the lower end with the lateral surface of the talus (astragalus) and tibia.

field defining wires   metal wires attached to the light beam diaphragm, which can be adjusted to outline the exact treatment area on the subsequent radiograph produced in the simulator.

field of view   the area of the scanned plane which may be included in the CT image.

field size   the size and shape of the X-ray beam. The maximum field of view of a gamma camera, usually between 25 and 50 cm.

filament   a thin, coiled, tungsten wire that when heated produces electrons in an X-ray tube.

filamented swab   a piece of gauze with a radiopaque strip. Used in theatre for internal swabbing as it can be traced radiographically if lost.

file   information stored on disk or cassette.

filiform   thread-like.

filiform papillae   small projections ending in several minute processes; found on the tongue.

film badge   a badge work by radiation workers which contains film, which when processed can be used to determine the amount of radiation received by that person.

film contrast   this is defined as the average gradient of the film. *See also* **characteristic curve**.

film entry system   the part of a radiographic film processor where the film enters the unit, it comprises of a pair of rollers and a microswitch which determines the length of time the film is between the rollers and can be linked to the replenisher system to ensure accurate replenishment.

film grain   formed by the coarse structure of the crystals in a radiographic film forming an overall density in the emulsion.

filter   a device designed to remove particles over a certain size or rays of specific wavelength while allowing others to pass through. Examples include intravenous fluid filters and optical filters.

filtrate   substance that passes through the filter.

filtration   the changes which occur in the X-ray beam when it passes through an object, it can reduce the amount of radiation and improve the quality of the beam by removing the low-energy photons. The process of straining through a filter under gravity, pressure or vacuum. Filtration under pressure occurs in the nephron of the kidney due to high-pressure blood in the afferent arteriole of the glomerulus.

filum   any filamentous or thread-like structure.

filum terminale   a strong, fine cord blending with the spinal cord above, and the periosteum of the sacral canal below.

fimbria   a fringe, for example, of the uterine tubes.

fine focus   the selection of a small filament to enable a small area of the anode to be bombarded with electrons and help reduce the unsharpness on the subsequent radiograph.

finger   a digit. *See also* **clubbed finger**.

firewall   either a programme or a dedicated computer used to protect a specific computer from external, unauthorized people accessing or changing information held on the computer.

firmware   software, but stored on a chip.

fission   occurs during radioactive decay when the nucleus of an atom elongates and breaks into two pieces.

fissure   a split or cleft. Can be moist or dry cracks in the epidermis or mucosa. They usually develop at 90° to the direction of the tension stress. Common sites include the anal mucosa and interdigitally for moist fissures, and the heel margins for dry fissures. ***palpebral fissure*** the opening between the eyelids.

fistula   an abnormal communication between two organs for example between bowel and bladder. May occur in conditions such as Crohn's disease, diverticulosis and cancer. *See also* **arteriovenous fistula**.

fits   *see* **convulsion**.

fixed costs   the costs incurred regardless of the level of activity, for example, related to the buildings and land, equipment maintenance.

fixer   a solution that converts and removes unexposed, undeveloped silver bromide into water-soluble silver complexes from the radiographic film during processing.

fixing agent   a chemical, ammonium thiosulphate, that converts unexposed, undeveloped silver bromide into water-soluble silver complexes that can be removed from the radiographic film by the solvent in the fixer solution.

flagellum   a fine, hair-like appendage capable of lashing movement. Characteristic of spermatozoa, certain bacteria and protozoa.

flail chest   unstable thoracic cage due to fracture. *See also* **paradoxical respiration**.

flap   a unit of skin and other subcutaneous tissues that maintains its own blood and nerve supply, used to repair defects in other parts of the body. Common in plastic surgery to treat burns and other injuries; skin flaps used to cover amputation stumps.

flat bone   the bones have a thin layer of cancellous bone enclosed by two layers of compact bone, they either protect underlying structures, for example, in the bones of the skull or are for muscle attachment, for example, the scapula.

flat foot   *see* **pes planus**.

flat pelvis   a pelvis in which the anteroposterior diameter of the brim is reduced.

flat screen monitor   a form of imaging monitor using a liquid crystal display to produce the image.

flattening filter   a metal filter, conical in section being thick at the centre and thinning towards the edges, used to reduce the intensity of the central beam and ensure that during radiotherapy the central 80% of the beam does not vary more than plus or minus 3% at maximum density.

flatulence   excessive gas in the gastric and intestinal tract.

flatus   gas in the gastrointestinal tract.

Fleming's left hand rule   the direction of force in a conductor placed in a magnetic field is at right angles to both the current and the magnetic field.

This can be predicted by holding the thumb, first and second fingers of the left hand at right angles to each other, thu*M*b = motion, *F*irst = force and se*C*ond = current.

Fleming's right hand rule   the direction of force in a conductor placed in a magnetic field is at right angles to both the electron flow and the magnetic field. This can be predicted by holding the thumb, first and second fingers of the right hand at right angles to each other, thu*M*b = motion, *F*irst = force and s*E*cond = electron flow.

flexible pes planus   is generally an asymptomatic abnormality of the foot in children but may become a semi-rigid condition in adulthood. It has been linked with excess laxity of the joint capsule and the ligaments supporting the arch, which allows it to collapse when weight is applied.

flexion   the act of bending by which the shafts of long bones forming a joint are brought towards each other.

flexor   a muscle which on contraction flexes or bends a part.

flexure   a bend, as in a tube-like structure, or a fold, as on the skin – it can be obliterated by extension or increased by flexion in the locomotor system. *See also* **left colic (splenic) flexure, right colic (hepatic) flexure, sigmoid flexure**.

flip angle   the angle through which the magnetization vector moves relative to the longitudinal axis of the static magnetic field as a result of the application of a radio frequency pulse in magnetic resonance imaging. The variation in flip angle is used in gradient-echo imaging to obtain various tissue weighted images. A 10–30° flip angle produces a T_2 weighted image and a 90° flip angle provides a T_1 weighted image. *See also* **T_1 relaxation time, T_2 relaxation time, gradient echo**.

flooding   a popular term to describe excessive bleeding from the uterus.

floppy baby syndrome   may be due to nervous system or muscle disorder as opposed to benign hypotonia (low muscle tone).

floppy disk   a flexible disk usually 3.5 inches in diameter.

floppy disk drive   an electronic device that allows information to either be written on to or removed from a floppy disk using a magnetic field.

flowchart   a diagrammatic representation of a computer program.

flowmeter   a measuring instrument for flowing gas or liquid.

flow-related enhancement   a process when the signal intensity of moving fluids can be increased compared with the signal from stationary tissue, when in-flowing, unsaturated, fully magnetized spins replace saturated spins within the imaging slice between successive radio frequency pulses in magnetic resonance imaging.

fluctuation   a wave-like motion felt on digital examination of a fluid-containing mass.

fluorescence　is when a material is irradiated and emits longer wavelength radiation, when the irradiation stops the light emission stops.

fluoride　an ion sometimes present in drinking water, toothpastes, tea, vegetables and sea food. It can be incorporated into the structure of bone and teeth, where it provides protection against dental caries but in gross excess it causes mottling of the teeth. As a public health preventive measure it can be added to a water supply in a strength of 1 part fluoride in a million parts of water (fluoridation).

Fluoro CT　equipment allowing the acquisition and immediate display of multiple CT images per second, is used in minimally invasive microtherapy procedures.

fluoroscopy　a real time radiographic examination of the human body, observed by means of an image intensifier and a television system.

fluorosis　results from an excessive intake of fluoride and results in a general increase in bone density and a mottled appearance to the teeth.

flux　the lines of force through a magnetic field.

focal epilepsy　an epileptic attack caused by a brain tumour, encephalitis or a head injury. Also known as *Jacksonian epilepsy*.

focal spot　the area of the anode bombarded by electrons; due to the angle of the anode the real focal spot is larger than the apparent focal spot.

focus　the point at which rays meet after reflection or refraction. The area of the anode that is bombarded by electrons.

focus groups　in research a method of obtaining data that involves interviewing people in small interacting groups.

focusing coils　produce magnetic fields to prevent divergence of the internal electron beam and therefore leakage of radiation from the equipment.

focusing cup　part of the cathode in an X-ray tube that helps direct the electrons to land on the target.

fold-over (aliasing, wrap around)　an artefact that occurs in magnetic resonance imaging due to the image encoding process. It occurs when the field of view is smaller than the area being imaged.

follicle　a small secreting sac. A simple tubular gland.

follicle stimulating hormone (FSH)　secreted by the anterior pituitary gland; it acts on the ovaries in the female, where it develops the oocyte-containing (Graafian) follicles; and to the testes in the male, where it stimulates spermatogenesis.

follicular carcinoma　a malignant tumour of the thyroid which spreads via the blood stream and metastasizes to bone and lung.

fomite　any article that has been in contact with infection and is capable of transmitting same.

fontanelle　a membranous space between the cranial bones. The diamond-shaped anterior fontanelle (bregma) is at the junction of the frontal and two parietal bones. It usually closes in the second year of life. The triangular posterior fontanelle (lambda) is at the junction of the occipital and two parietal bones. It closes within a few weeks of birth.

foot   that portion of the lower limb below the ankle.

foot drop   inability to dorsiflex foot due normally to damage of the nerve supply to the foot. Can be a complication of bedrest.

foramen   a hole or opening. Generally used with reference to bones.

foramen magnum   the opening in the occipital bone through which the spinal cord passes.

foramen ovale   a fetal cardiac interatrial communication which normally closes at birth. A foramen in the skull for the mandibular division of the trigeminal nerve.

forbidden energy gap   an area between the top energy level of the valence band and the bottom level of the conduction band, electrons can pass through the gap but cannot exist within the band.

force   the application of unit force to unit mass produces unit acceleration, unit Newton.

forced expiratory volume (FEV)   volume of air exhaled during a given time (usually the first second: FEV_1).

forced vital capacity (FVC)   the maximum gas volume that can be expelled from the lungs in a forced expiration.

forceps   a surgical instrument with two opposing blades used to grasp or compress tissues, swabs, needles and other surgical appliances.

forensic dentistry   the examination, interpretation and presentation of dentally related evidence in a legal context.

forensic medicine (medical jurisprudence, or 'legal medicine')   the application of medical science to questions of law.

foreskin   the prepuce or skin covering the glans penis.

formaldehyde   toxic gas used as a disinfectant. Dissolved in water (formalin), it is used mainly for disinfection and the preservation of histological specimens.

fornix   an arch; particularly referred to the vagina, i.e. the space between the vaginal wall and the cervix of the uterus.

FORTRAN   a programming language which is between BASIC and machine code in difficulty.

forward bias   is when a battery is connected across a PN junction the potential barrier is lowered to allow current to flow opp reverse bias.

fossa   a depression or furrow.

four-dimensional ultrasound   three-dimensional ultrasound with a real time, moving image.

fourchette   a membranous fold connecting the posterior ends of the labia minora.

Fourier analysis   the method of dividing an image into the various spatial frequency areas and expressing them in mathematical terms.

Fourier transform   used in electronic signal processing, a signal is analysed by taking a timed sample to identify its frequencies and their amplitudes and then to express them as a sum of frequencies multiplied by amplitude. This figure can then be electronically manipulated to improve the digital image.

fovea   a small depression or fossa; particularly the fovea centralis retinae, the site with many cones important for distinct colour vision.

fractional inspired oxygen concentration (FiO₂)   the concentration of oxygen in inspired gas, expressed as a fraction of 1 (for example, FiO₂ 0.6 equals 60% inspired oxygen concentration).

fractionation   in radiotherapy it is the process of administering smaller doses of radiation over a period of time, excluding weekends, to minimize tissue damage. *See also* **conventional fractionation, hyperfractionation, accelerated fractionation, accelerated hyperfractionation**.

fracture   loss in continuity of a bone as a result of injury or underlying pathology. *See also* **Bennett's fracture, closed fracture, Colles' fracture, comminuted fracture, complicated fracture, compression fracture, depressed fracture, incomplete fracture, impacted fracture, open (compound) fracture, pathological fracture, Pott's fracture, spontaneous fracture**.

fraenum   frenum.

fragilitas ossium   *see* **osteogenesis imperfecta**.

frame rate   the number of times an ultrasonic image is refreshed per second, a slow frame rate gives better resolution, a high frame rate better demonstrates movement.

free induction decay   a brief signal that occurs as the transverse magnetism decays towards zero following the application of a radio frequency pulse in magnetic resonance imaging.

Freiberg's infarction   death of bone tissue which most commonly occurs in the head of the second metatarsal bone.

Frenkel defect   the loss of an atom from a structure forming an interstitial ion or atom.

Frenkel's exercises   special repetitive exercises to improve muscle and joint sense.

frenulum   a small fold of mucous membrane that checks or limits the movement of an organ, for example, tongue, prepuce of the penis, frenulum linguae from the undersurface of the tongue to the floor of the mouth. Also called *frenum*.

frequency   the number of cycles of alternating current, measured in Hertz, that occur in 1 second. In statistics, the number of times a particular value occurs. Ultrasound is frequencies beyond 20 kiloHertz.

frequency distribution   the number of times (frequency) each value in a variable is observed.

friable   easily crumbled; readily pulverized.

Fricke dosimeter   a chemical dosimeter containing a solution of ferrous sulphate in sulphuric acid; when the chemical is irradiated ferric sulphate is produced. The quantity produced is assessed by measuring the optical density before and after irradiation.

frog plaster   conservative treatment of developmental dysplasia of the hip (congenital dislocation of the hip), whereby the dislocation is reduced by gentle manipulation and both hips are immobilized in plaster of Paris, both hips abducted to 80° and externally rotated.

front pointer   used in radiotherapy to indicate the central entry point of the radiation. *See also* **back pointer**.

frontal   associated with the front of a structure. The bone of the forehead.

frontal plane   a vertical plane running from head to foot. It divides the body into front and back parts and is at right angles to the median plane. Also called the *coronal plane*.

frontal sinus   cavity at the inner aspect of each orbital ridge on the frontal bone.

frozen shoulder   initial pain followed by stiffness, lasting several months. As pain subsides, exercises are intensified until full recovery is gained. Cause unknown.

fulcrum   the point at which two objects pivot.

Fulfield applicator   a secondary beam collimator with lead-lined sides which form a cone and a 3-mm thick Perspex end.

full-term   mature – when pregnancy has lasted 40 weeks.

fume cupboard   a cupboard with an external exhaust system to enable the handling of radioactive materials to prevent inhalation or ingestion of the dust or gaseous products.

fumigation   disinfection using the fumes of a vaporized disinfectant.

function   the ability to adapt consistently and competently to the demands of any normal situation in any normal environment. Describes the specific work done by a structure or organ in its normal state.

functional   relating to function. Of a disorder, of the function but not the structure of an organ. As a psychiatric term, describes a condition without primary organic disease.

functional incontinence   erratic and involuntary urinary incontinence in the absence of physical problems in bladder or nervous system. It may be due to immobility or cognitive defects.

fundus   the basal portion of a hollow structure; the part which is distal to the opening. In ophthalmology the inner surface of the eye as viewed through the pupil using an ophthalmoscope.

fungate   to grow rapidly and produce fungus-like growths, often occurs in the late stage of malignant tumours.

fungi   simple plants. Mycophyta, including mushrooms, yeasts, moulds and rusts, many of which cause superficial and systemic disease in humans, such as actinomycosis, aspergillosis, candidiasis and tinea.

fungicide   an agent that kills fungi. An addition to radiographic film emulsion, and developer to make them resistant to the growth of mould or bacteria.

fungiform   resembling a mushroom, like the fungiform papillae of the tongue.

funiculus   a cord-like structure.

funnel chest (pectus excavatum)   a congenital deformity in which the breast bone is depressed towards the spine.

fusiform   resembling a spindle.

fusiform aneurysm   localized dilatation of an artery in which the circumference of the vessel is dilated.

G

gag the reflex contraction of the pharyngeal muscles and elevation of the palate when the soft palate or posterior pharynx is stimulated. An instrument used to keep the mouth open.

gain (swept gain) the amount of sound received back by an ultrasonic transducer, increasing the gain visualizes the organs further away from the probe.

gain correction a factor used to compensate for the variation in electrical signal for an absorbed intensity of radiation between detector channels in CT scanning.

gait a manner or style of walking. *ataxic gait* an incoordinate or abnormal gait. *cerebellar gait* reeling, staggering, lurching. *scissors gait* one in which the legs cross each other in progressing. *spastic gait* stiff, shuffling, the legs being held together. *tabetic gait* the foot is raised high then brought down suddenly, the whole foot striking the ground.

Galeazzi fracture–dislocation fracture of the distal radius with dislocation of the radioulnar joint.

gallbladder a pear-shaped bag on the undersurface of the liver, it concentrates and stores bile.

gallows traction *see* **Bryant's 'gallows' traction**.

gallstones concentrations of cholesterol or other constituents of bile formed within the gallbladder or bile ducts; many small stones or one large stone may be formed.

galvanometer an instrument for measuring an electrical current.

gamete a female or male reproductive cell with the haploid (n) chromosome number; oocyte or spermatazoon.

gametogenesis production of gametes (oocytes and spermatozoa). *See also* **oogenesis, spermatogenesis.**

gamma the measure of the slope of a characteristic curve, the higher the gamma the higher the contrast on the radiographic film. *See also* **average gradient, sensitometry**.

gamma camera a large, stationery, scintillation counter, which records the activity over the whole field at the same time. Used to detect pathologies where the physiology of the structure is changed. The image is viewed on a cathode ray tube (see figure on p. 172).

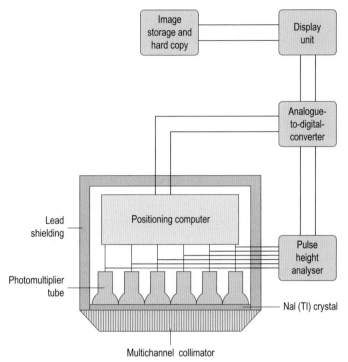

The main components of a gamma camera and its associated circuitry. From Principles of radiological physics, 3rd edn, D T Graham, 1996, Churchill Livingstone, Edinburgh, with permission.

gamma decay   the emission of gamma rays from a nucleus which has excess energy.

gamma encephalography   a small dose of isotope is given which is concentrated in many cerebral tumours, the pattern of radioactivity is then measured.

gamma knife   a method of treating tumours that are difficult to excise surgically by using multiple beams of radiation, focused at the tumour over a number of days.

gamma rays   short wavelength, penetrating rays of the electromagnetic spectrum produced by disintegration of the atomic nuclei of radioactive elements.

ganglion   a mass of nerve cell bodies in the peripheral nervous system such as those of the autonomic nervous system and those ganglia containing the cell bodies of sensory nerves. Localized cyst-like swelling near a tendon, sheath or joint. Sometimes occurs on the back of the wrist due to strain such as excessive use of a word processor. *See also* **gasserian ganglion**.

gangrene   death of part of the tissues of the body. Usually the results of inadequate blood supply, but occasionally due to direct injury (***traumatic gangrene***) or infection (e.g. ***gas gangrene***). Deficient blood supply may result from pressure on blood vessels (e.g. tourniquets, tight bandages and swelling of a limb); from obstruction within healthy vessels (e.g. arterial embolism, frostbite where the capillaries become blocked); from spasm of the vessel wall (e.g. ergot poisoning); or from thrombosis due to disease of the vessel wall (e.g. arteriosclerosis in arteries, phlebitis in veins). *See also* **dry gangrene, moist gangrene**.

gantry   a structure or support, in CT scanning a structure in which the X-ray tube, detectors and associated electronics are housed.

Gardner's syndrome   familial polyposis of the large bowel, with fibrous dysplasia of the skull, extra teeth, osteomas, fibroma and epidermal cysts.

gargoylism   congenital disorder of mucopolysaccharide metabolism with recessive or sex-linked inheritance. The polysaccharides chondroitin sulphate 'B' and heparitin sulphate are excreted in the urine. Characterized by skeletal abnormalities, coarse features, enlarged liver and spleen, learning disability.

gas   one of the three states of matter, the others being solid and liquid. A gas retains neither shape nor volume when released.

gas gangrene   a serious wound infection caused by anaerobic organisms of the genus *Clostridium*, especially *Clostridium perfringens* (*welchii*), a soil microbe often present in the intestine of humans and animals. *See also* **gangrene**.

gasserian ganglion   a mass of nerve cell bodies deeply situated within the skull, on the sensory root of the fifth cranial nerve. It is involved in trigeminal neuralgia.

gas transfer factor   measurement of the lung's ability to exchange gases. Particularly useful in the diagnosis and surveillance of interstitial lung diseases, sarcoidosis and emphysema.

gastrectomy   surgical removal of all or part of the stomach.

gastrin   a hormone secreted by the gastric mucosa on entry of food, which causes further gastric secretion.

gastritis   inflammation of the stomach.

gastrocnemius   the large two-headed muscle of the calf.

gastrocolic   associated with the stomach and the colon.

gastrocolic reflex   sensory stimulus when food enters the stomach, resulting in strong peristaltic waves in the colon.

gastroduodenal   associated with the stomach and the duodenum.

gastroenteritis   inflammation of the stomach and intestines.

gastrointestinal   associated with the stomach and intestine.

gastro-oesophageal   associated with the stomach and oesophagus.

gastro-oesophageal reflux   disease caused by passage of gastric contents into the oesophagus, typically causes heartburn, complications include ulceration, strictures and Barrett's oesophagus.

gastrophrenic   associated with the stomach and diaphragm.

gastroschisis   a portion of bowel appearing through a defect in the abdominal wall, near the umbilicus.

gastrulation   in early embryonic development the immense changes occurring as the blastocyst becomes the gastrula. The three primary germ layers are formed and cells move to their appointed locations in readiness for the start of structural development.

gate   a gate performs a single logical operation when subjected to a number of inputs. It is the basis of all computer operations.

Gauss   an electromagnetic unit of magnetic induction now replaced by the Tesla (1 Tesla=10 000 Gauss).

Geiger counter   a device for detecting and registering radioactivity.

Geiger–Muller counter   a device for measuring radiation dosage, it has a glass envelope containing argon, a positively charged central electrode and a negatively charged mesh cylinder.

Geiger–Muller tube   a radiation detector using an ionization chamber, used in personnel dosimetry and to detect the movement of gamma ray sources in brachytherapy.

gelatine   a complex compound used in the emulsion layer of a radiographic film to allow the absorption of water during chemical processing, keeping the silver halide grains in suspension, during manufacture to allow the grains to grow and bind the emulsion to the base of the film, it assists with forming and stabilizing the image during and after exposure to electromagnetic radiation.

gemellus muscles   muscles arising from the ischium.

general anaesthetic   a drug which causes unconsciousness by inhalation or injection of the drug.

General Medical Council (GMC)   the statutory body that regulates the practice of medicine in the UK. It oversees professional quality and continuing professional development standards for professional practice, discipline and conduct. It is responsible for the establishment and maintenance of a professional register for all doctors working in the UK, and has the power to remove individuals from the register in cases of professional misconduct, or in some cases to restrict practice or order specific training.

General Medical Services   the medical services provided by family doctors.

general sales list medicines   drugs that can be sold in shops and supermarkets under specific conditions.

genital   associated with the organs of reproduction.

genitalia   the external organs of reproduction.

genitocrural   associated with the genital area and the legs.

genitourinary   associated with the reproductive and urinary organs.

genitourinary medicine (GUM)   specialty concerned with the management of sexually transmitted infections and other medical conditions of the genital tract.

genu   the knee.

genu valgum (bow legs)   abnormal outward curving of the legs resulting in separation of the knees.

genu varum (knock knee)   abnormal incurving of the legs so that there is a gap between the feet when the knees are in contact.

geometric unsharpness   blurring of a radiographic image due to the size of the focal spot on the anode, and can be reduced by increasing the focus to film distance and the object film distance.

germicide   any agent capable of killing microorganisms (germs).

gestation sac volume   the volume of the sac which contains the fetus during pregnancy. Usually measured at 3 to 6 weeks using ultrasound.

ghosting   in ultrasound a mirror image which is produced when the gain is too high or when imaging objects with high acoustic reflections.

giant cell   an abnormally large tissue cell.

GIF (Graphics Interchange Format)   a compressed computer graphics file.

gigabyte   one billion (10^9) bytes, a measure of the size of a computer hard disk and denotes the quantity of information that can be stored on the system.

gigantism   abnormal overgrowth, especially in height, due to excess growth hormone in childhood prior to fusion of the epiphyses. Almost always due to a pituitary tumour.

gingiva   the keratinized oral mucosa immediately surrounding a tooth, i.e. the gum.

gingival sulcus   the pouch (invagination) made by the gingiva as it joins with the tooth surface.

gingivitis   inflammation of the gums caused by dental plaque.

girdle   usually a bony structure of oval shape such as the shoulder and pelvic girdles.

gland   an organ or structure capable of making an internal or external secretion. *See also* **endocrine, exocrine**.

glans   the bulbous termination of the clitoris and penis.

glass plasma display   the technology used for early flat screen computer monitors comprising of neon gas cells between two electrodes. When the electrodes are activated the gas glows therefore forming an image.

Gleason score (grade)   a method of grading prostate cancer based on the extent that tumour cells are arranged in recognizable glandular structures.

glenohumeral   associated with the glenoid cavity of scapula and the humerus.

glenoid   a cavity on the scapula into which the head of the humerus fits to form the shoulder joint.

glenoid labrum   fibrocartilagenous rim round the glenoid to deepen the cavity.

glia   *see* **neuroglia**.

gliding   one articular surface sliding smoothly over another.

glioblastoma multiforme   a malignant, rapidly growing tumour of the cerebrum or the spinal cord.

glioma   a malignant tumour composed of neuroglial cells affecting the brain and spinal cord, typically an astrocytoma or oligodendroglioma. *See also* **astrocyte, oligodendrocyte**.

gliomyoma   a tumour of nerve and muscle tissue.

globular grains   the type of grains found in some radiographic film emulsions and have the characteristic that the light-absorbing ability of the grain depends only on its volume, they are used in blue-sensitive or monochromatic systems.

globulins   a large group of proteins. Those in the plasma are classified as alpha and beta, which are concerned with substance transport, and gamma, which provides protection against infection. The gamma globulins comprise the immunoglobulins A, D, E, G and M.

globus pallidus   literally pale globe; a mass of motor grey matter situated deep within the cerebral hemispheres, lateral to the thalamus. Part of the basal nuclei.

glomerular filtration rate (GFR)   the volume of plasma filtered by the kidneys in 1 minute. It is usually about 120 mL per minute.

glomerulus   a coil of capillaries formed from a wide-bore afferent arteriole. It lies within the invaginated blind end of the renal tubule. Together with the renal tubule it forms a nephron. Part of the filtration membrane involved in the production of urine.

glossa   the tongue.

glossopharyngeal associated with the tongue and pharynx. The ninth pair of cranial nerves, they supply the tongue and pharynx.

glottis the opening between the abducted vocal folds in the larynx. It allows air to enter the respiratory tract and is involved in voice production.

glucagon hormone produced in the pancreatic islets of Langerhans. It causes the release of glucose from liver glycogen and thereby raises the blood glucose. Used by injection to reverse hypoglycaemia. *See also* **insulin**.

glucocorticoid any steroid hormone which promotes gluconeogenesis and which antagonizes the action of insulin. Occurring naturally in the adrenal cortex as cortisone and cortisol, and produced synthetically as, for example, prednisolone.

glucogenesis production of glucose.

gluconeogenesis the formation of glucose from non-carbohydrate sources, e.g. amino acids, lactate, etc.

glucuronic acid used in the liver for the conjugation of bile pigments.

glutathione a peptide needed for conjugation in the liver and for red cell integrity. Paracetamol overdose causes serious depletion.

gluteal associated with the buttocks.

gluteus muscles muscles of the buttock.

glycerol combines with fatty acids to form triglycerides (triacylglycerols) and phospholipids.

glycogen the main carbohydrate (polysaccharide) storage compound in animals. Many glucose molecules are linked together in a process called glycogenesis occurring in the liver and skeletal muscle. The conversion of liver glycogen back to glucose is called glycogenolysis.

glycogenesis glycogen formation from blood glucose.

glycogenolysis the breakdown of glycogen to glucose.

glycogen storage disease a recessively inherited metabolic disorder caused by various enzyme deficiencies. Glycogen accumulates in organs and tissues, e.g. liver. Hypoglycaemia occurs, and the body tends to use fat rather than glucose, leading to ketosis and acidosis.

glycolysis a metabolic pathway where glucose is broken down to form pyruvic acid and some energy (ATP).

glyconeogenesis *see* **gluconeogenesis**.

glycoproteins large group of proteins conjugated with a carbohydrate, e.g. collagen, mucins.

glycosuria the presence of sugar in the urine.

gnathalgia jaw pain.

gnathoplasty plastic surgery of the jaw or cheek.

goblet cells   mucus-secreting cells, shaped like a goblet, found in the mucosa lining the gastrointestinal and respiratory tracts.

goitre   an enlargement of the thyroid gland associated with a change of the level of thyroid function or a lack of iodine in the diet; may be smooth (simple) or nodular, and associated with normal or abnormal thyroid function; **hyperthyroid** with smooth enlargement in Graves' disease, or nodular enlargement in toxic multinodular goitre; **hypothyroid** with glandular enlargement in Hashimoto's disease.

gold (Au)   The radioactive isotope gold-198 is sometimes used in the treatment of some malignant diseases.

golfer's elbow   inflammation of the medial epicondyle of the humerus associated with playing golf.

Golgi tendon organ   specialized receptors in tendons that with skeletal muscle spindles monitor muscle stretching. Involved in proprioception.

Gompertzian growth curve   a mathematical model explaining the relationship between age and the expected time of death.

gomphoses   joints with minimal movement, for example, between the teeth and the jaw.

gonad   the female or male primary reproductive structure, ovary, testis.

gonadotrophic   having an affinity for, or influencing, the gonads.

gonadotrophin   gonad-stimulating hormone. *See also* **human chorionic gonadotrophin, luteinizing hormone**.

gonad protection   the use of lead rubber and/or collimation of the X-ray beam to reduce the radiation dosage to the reproductive system.

goose flesh   contraction of the tiny muscles attached to the hair follicles causing the hair to stand on end: it is a reaction to either cold or fear.

gouge   a chisel with a grooved blade for removing bone.

gout   a form of metabolic disorder in which blood levels of uric acid are raised (hyperuricaemia). Acute arthritis can result from inflammation in response to urate crystals in the joint. The big toe is characteristically involved and becomes acutely painful and swollen. Drugs that reduce uric acid levels can control the disease. If gout is untreated deposition of urate crystals can cause chronic arthritis, nodules (e.g. in the ear) and kidney damage. *See also* **pseudogout, tophus**.

Graafian follicle   a mature ovarian follicle. A minute vesicle in the ovarian stroma containing a single oocyte which is released when the vesicle ruptures at ovulation. After ovulation, the Graafian follicle forms the corpus luteum which, should fertilization occur, maintains the early pregnancy. In the absence of fertilization the corpus luteum only lasts for 12–14 days, after which it becomes the corpus albicans.

gracilis muscle   muscle of the leg.

gradient coils magnetic coils that are designed to alter the main magnetic field by a few percent. The magnetic field gradient is controlled by the electrical current passing through the coil. They are used in magnetic resonance imaging to localize a slice and spatially encode slice information.

gradient echo a basic pulse sequence that only uses magnetic field gradient reversal to re-phase the transverse magnetization and produce echoes of the magnetic resonance signal. This allows shorter repetition times and therefore faster scanning and flip angles of less than 90°. *See also* **flip angle**.

grading a classification of cancers based on histopathological characteristics. The level of malignancy of the tissue is determined by comparing the amount of cellular abnormality and the rate of cell division with normal cells in the same tissue. Low-grade cancer generally has slow tumour growth and spread, whereas high-grade cancer is aggressive with rapid spread. The grade of the disease is more important (for some types of cancer) than the stage as an indicator of prognosis and effective treatment. *See also* **differentiation, staging**.

grain technology the shape of the silver halide crystals in a radiographic film emulsion are referred to as grains and have two main formats, globular and tabular. *See also* **globular grains, tabular grains**.

graininess random density patterns visible on a radiographic film due to the grains in the film being distributed in both area and depth and can be 'clumped' together due to the manufacturing process.

Gram stain the method of staining microorganisms and therefore classifying them.

grand mal the commonest type of epileptic seizure with loss of consciousness and generalized convulsions.

granulocyte a cell containing granules in its cytoplasm. Describes the polymorphonuclear leucocytes, neutrophil, eosinophil and basophil.

granuloma a tumour formed of granulation tissue.

graph a diagrammatical representation of two or more groups of data.

graphics computerized 'drawing', known as CAD (computer-aided drawing). The ability of the computer to produce preprogrammed graphic characters. The mode the computer has to be placed in prior to drawing graphics.

graphics tablet a piece of equipment that can digitize drawing or graphs ready for input into the computer.

Graves' disease an autoimmune disorder characterized by hyperthyroidism, and exophthalmos.

Graves' ophthalmopathy a disease of the eye associated with Graves' disease.

gravid pregnant; carrying fertilized eggs or a fetus.

gravity   weight. *See also* **specific gravity**.

Grawitz's tumour   a renal cell adenocarcinoma.

gray (Gy)   the derived SI unit (International System of Units) for the absorbed dose of radiation. It has replaced the rad.

greater omentum   the fold which hangs from the lower border of the stomach and covers the front of the intestines.

greenstick fracture   a partial break in bone continuity occurring in young children when the bone appears bent.

Greinacher circuit   comprises of two rectifiers connected in series, and two capacitors connected in series to produce a fully rectified waveform with a ripple effect on the tube voltage but a constant tube current.

grey matter   unmyelinated nerve fibres and nerve cell bodies situated in the central nervous system. *See also* **white matter**.

grey scale   a method of showing the texture of tissue on an ultrasound display, the amplitude of each echo is represented by varying shades of grey, white outline from specular surfaces, mottled grey from various tissue areas and black from collections of fluid. The variation of shades of grey in which a CT image may be represented on screen.

grid   a device constructed of strips of high atomic number material (e.g. lead) which absorbs the scattered radiation and low atomic number material which allows the primary beam to pass through thus improving radiographic contrast of the image.

grid lattice   the number of lines of lead per centimetre in a secondary radiation grid.

grid ratio   the ratio of the height of the lead strips to the width of the spaces between them in a secondary radiation grid.

groin   the junction of the thigh with the abdomen.

grommet   ventilation tube inserted into the tympanic membrane. Frequently used in the treatment of glue ear in children.

groove   an uncovered passage.

gross tumour volume (GTV)   the total visible or palpable extent of a malignant growth.

grounded theory   research study where a hypothesis is elicited from the data gathered.

ground state   when the inner orbits of an atom are filled and therefore the atom is at its lowest energy state.

growth hormone (GH, somatotrophin)   hormone secreted by the anterior pituitary gland under the influence of two hypothalamic hormones, growth hormone releasing hormone, and growth hormone release inhibiting hormone (**somatostatin**). Growth hormone has widespread effects on body tissues and influences the metabolism of proteins, fats and carbohydrates. *See also* **acromegaly, dwarfism, gigantism**.

growth scan when 2 or 3 measurements are taken of the abdomen, head and femur of a fetus in the second and third trimester using ultrasound imaging. The weight of the fetus is calculated by using charts.

guidewire a device used to position an intravenous catheter, endotracheal tube, central venous line or gastric feeding tube.

gullet the oesophagus.

gumboil the opening on the gum of an abscess at the root of a tooth, dentoalveolar abscess.

Gurney Mott theory theory of latent image formation stating that electrons are trapped and then escape several times before another electron is trapped forming a stable two-atom silver speck called the latent sub-image centre, this attracts further electrons causing a build up of silver atoms which eventually destroys the crystal lattice and allows development to take place. *See also* **Mitchell theory**.

gut the intestines, large and small.

gut decontamination the use of non-absorbable antibiotics to prevent endogenous infection in patients having intestinal surgery or those who are immunocompromised because of drugs or neutropenia.

gynaecomastia enlargement of the male breast.

gyromagnetic ratio (γ) is a proportionality constant and is fixed for the nucleus, for example 42.6 MHz/Tesla for hydrogen.

gyrus a convoluted portion of cerebral cortex.

. . . .

habitual abortion   *see* **miscarriage**.

haem   the iron-containing pigment portion of haemoglobin.

haemangioma   a benign tumour formed by dilated blood vessels which may occur in any part of the body. When in the skin it is one form of birthmark, appearing as a red spot or a 'port wine stain'.

haemarthrosis   the presence of blood in a joint cavity.

haematemesis   the vomiting of blood, which may be bright red following recent bleeding – or 'coffee ground' appearance if it has been in the stomach for some time. The bleeding is usually from the upper gastrointestinal tract and causes include peptic ulcer, varices, neoplasms, drug erosions and coagulation defects.

haematin   a ferric-iron-containing derivative of haemoglobin.

haematinic   a substance required for the production of red blood cells.

haematocele   a swelling filled with blood.

haematogenous   originating or transported by the blood.

haematoma   a swelling composed of blood which can occur in any part of the body.

haematometra   an accumulation of blood (or menstrual fluid) in the uterus.

haematuria   blood in the urine; may be macroscopic, i.e. visible to the naked eye, microscopic when it is not.

haemoccult test   a test to detect minute quantities of blood in the faeces.

haemodialysis   a procedure in which impurities or wastes are removed from the blood. A method of renal replacement therapy used in patients in end-stage renal disease/failure (irreversible) or in acute renal failure (potentially reversible). The patient's blood is shunted from the body through a machine for diffusion and filtration and then returned to the patient's circulation. The procedure takes from 3–8 hours and may take place daily or two or three times a week.

haemodynamics   the study of blood circulation.

haemofiltration (CVVH)   form of renal replacement therapy (artificial kidney treatment), in which the patient's blood is passed through a filter allowing separation of an ultrafiltrate containing fluid and solutes. This is discarded and replaced with an isotonic solution. Usually continuous as in continuous veno-venous haemofiltration.

haemoglobin (Hb)   the red, respiratory pigment in the red blood cells. A molecule comprises four ferrous-iron-containing haem groups and four globin chains. It combines with oxygen and releases it to the tissues. Some carbon dioxide is carried by haemoglobin, which also acts to buffer pH changes. There is a special form of fetal haemoglobin (HbF) which has a high affinity for oxygen, and two major adult forms (HbA, HbA$_2$). HbF is replaced by adult forms during early childhood. *See also* **oxyhaemoglobin**.

haemoglobinopathy   usually hereditary abnormality of the haemoglobin molecule.

haemoglobinuria   haemoglobin in the urine.

haemolysin   an agent capable of causing disintegration of red blood cells.

haemolytic anaemia   a condition caused by the premature destruction of red blood cells, as with some drugs and toxins, autoimmune processes, or inherited red cell disorders.

haemolytic disease of the newborn (erythroblastosis fetalis)   a pathological condition in the newborn child due to Rhesus incompatibility between the child's blood and that of the mother. Red blood cell destruction occurs with anaemia, often jaundice and an excess of erythroblasts or primitive red blood cells in the circulating blood. Immunization of women at risk, using anti-D immunoglobulin, can prevent haemolytic disease of the newborn. Treatment of affected infants may include phototherapy, blood transfusion and exchange transfusion in severe cases.

haemoperitoneum   blood in the peritoneal cavity.

haemophilias   a group of conditions with inherited blood coagulation efects. In clinical practice the most commonly encountered defects are *aemophilia A* (factor VIII procoagulant deficiency) and *haemophilia B* or *Christmas disease* (factor IX procoagulant deficiency). Both of these conditions are X-linked recessive disorders resulting in an increased tendency to bleed, the severity of which depends on the amount of residual factor VIII or IX. Bleeding typically occurs into joints and muscles. *See also* **haemophilic arthropathy**.

haemophilic arthropathy   joint disease associated with haemophilia. The extent of joint damage has been 'staged' from radiological findings: (a) synovial thickening, (b) epiphyseal overgrowth, (c) minor joint changes and cyst formation, (d) definite joint changes with loss of joint space, (e) end-stage joint destruction and secondary changes leading to deformity.

haemopneumothorax   the presence of blood and air in the pleural cavity.

haemopoiesis (haematopoiesis)   the formation of blood. *See also* **erythropoiesis**.

haemoptysis the coughing up of blood which is bright red in colour and frothy. May be as a result of carcinoma of the bronchus, pulmonary tuberculosis, bronchiectasis.

haemorrhage loss of blood from a vessel. Usually refers to serious rapid blood loss. This may lead to hypovolaemic shock with tachycardia, hypotension, rapid breathing, pallor, sweating, oliguria, restlessness and changes in conscious level. Haemorrhage can be classified in several ways: (a) according to the vessel involved: arterial, venous or capillary; (b) timing: *primary haemorrhage* occurs at the time of injury or operation, *reactionary haemorrhage* occurs within 24 hours of injury or operation, *secondary haemorrhage* occurs within some days of injury or operation and usually associated with sepsis; (c) whether it is internal (concealed) or external (revealed).

haemorrhagic periostitis inflammation of the periosteum accompanied by bleeding between the periosteum and the bone.

haemorrhoids (piles) dilated veins around the anus. *external haemorrhoids* those outside the anal sphincter, covered with skin. *internal haemorrhoids* those inside the anal sphincter, covered with mucous membrane.

haemosiderin an iron–protein complex. A storage form of iron.

haemospermia blood in the semen.

haemostasis the process that controls bleeding from small vessels. Damage to the blood vessels starts a complex series of reactions between substances in the blood and others released from damaged platelets and tissue. There are four overlapping stages: vasoconstriction, platelet plug formation, coagulation and fibrinolysis. Also includes the measures used to stop bleeding during surgery or following injury.

haemothorax blood in the pleural cavity usually associated with chest injuries, for example fractured ribs.

halation the reflection back of light after it passes through a radiographic emulsion which may then re-expose the emulsion causing unsharpness on the film.

half-life amount of time taken for the radioactivity of a radioactive substance to decay by half the initial value. The half-life is a constant for each radioactive isotope, e.g. iodine-131 is 8 days. Or the time taken for the concentration of a drug in the plasma to fall by half the initial level. *biological half-life* time taken by the body to eliminate 50% of the dose of any substance by normal biological processes. *effective half-life* time taken for a combination of radioactive decay and biological processes to reduce radioactivity by 50%.

half-speed emulsion has half the speed of standard radiographic emulsions with an increase in image quality but also an increase in patient dosage. *See also* **standard contrast emulsion**.

half-value thickness the thickness of a substance that will transmit exactly one-half of the intensity of radiation falling on it.

hallucinations a false perception occurring without any true sensory stimulus.

hallucinogens   chemicals that cause hallucinations.

hallux   the great toe.

hallux rigidus   ankylosis of the metatarsophalangeal articulation due to osteoarthritis.

hallux valgus (hallux abducto-valgus, bunion)   a complex deformity of the medial column of the foot involving abduction and external rotation of the great toe and adduction and internal rotation of the first metatarsal (referenced to the midline of the body). Deformity exists when abduction of the hallux on the metatarsal is greater than 10 to 12°. Friction and pressure of shoes cause a bursa to develop. The prominent bone, with its bursa, is known as a bunion.

hallux varus   the great toe deviates toward the midline of the body and is commonly seen with metatarsus adductus.

halopelvic traction   a form of external fixation whereby traction can be applied to the spine between two fixed points. The device consists of three main parts (a) a halo, (b) a pelvic loop, and (c) four extension bars.

hamate   one of the eight carpal bones of the wrist.

hammer toe   a permanent hyperextension of the first phalanx and flexion of second and third phalanges.

hamstring muscles   flexor muscles of the posterior part of the thigh.

hamulus   a hook-like projection.

hand   that part of the upper limb below the wrist.

handshake   an electronic signal which indicates the end of the passage of data from the computer.

hard copy   the paper printout of the program or screen display.

hard rollers   part of the radiographic film transport system in an automatic processor made of paper wound round a stainless steel core and impregnated with epoxy resin.

hardener   an addition to the radiographic film emulsion to make it resistant to abrasions, an addition to the developer and the fixer to reduce mechanical damage and sticking of the films to the racks.

hard palate   the front part of the roof of the mouth formed by the two palatal bones.

hardware   the mechanical and electronic part of the equipment.

Harrington rod   a ridged, contoured, metal rod, surgically inserted, along with metal hooks, into the posterior aspect of the spine to treat scoliosis and other deformities.

Hashimoto's thyroiditis   a disease of the thyroid when the normal structures are replaced with lymphocytes and lymphoid germinal centres producing a goitre.

haustration   small pouches (sacculation), as of the colon.

haversian system   a cylindrical system found in compact bone. Comprises lamellae, lacunae, Volkmann's canals and canaliculi.

Hawthorne effect   a positive effect occurring from the introduction of change, of which people are less aware as time passes. Researchers doing observation research make allowances for this reaction to their presence by not including data from the first few days in the final data analysis.

head injury   injury resulting from a blow to the head causing haemorrhage or contusion. *See also* **extradural haematoma**.

healing   the natural process of cure or tissue repair. *See also* **wound healing**. In complementary or integrated medicine the term healing refers to a return to health; also the use of a therapy that may assist the healing process; a specific therapeutic form, such as spiritual healing and therapeutic touch.

healthcare systems   national or local organizations for providing medical/health care. The structure of the system has to accommodate progress in medical interventions, consumer demand and economic efficiency. Criteria for a successful system have been formulated: (a) adequacy and equity of access to care, (b) income protection (for patients), (c) macro-economic efficiency (national expenditure measured as a proportion of gross domestic product), (d) micro-economic efficiency (balance of services provided between improving health outcomes and satisfying consumer demand), (e) consumer choice and appropriate autonomy for care providers. There are four basic types of healthcare systems: socialized (UK NHS), social insurance (Canada, France), mandatory insurance (Germany), voluntary insurance (USA).

Health Development Agency   a statutory body set up to improve standards in public health. It is concerned with identifying the need for evidence and for commissioning research. Other roles include: standard setting, undertaking health promotion campaigns and distributing examples of good practice.

health gain   an attempt at measuring the benefit of health intervention on the population. For example, health gain from a cervical cytology screening programme may be measured as the reduction in deaths from cervical cancer; coronary heart disease prevention programme measured as a reduction in deaths from coronary heart disease in men under 65 years of age, or the number of deaths avoided over a specified period of time (e.g. 5 years).

Health Improvement Programme (HImP)   a focused action plan for improving health and healthcare provision at a local level. Involves a collaborative approach between Primary Care Trust(s), health professionals, local government, voluntary organizations and patient groups, etc.

health informatics   the process of using a computer to manage information.

health level 7   the international standard for textual communication of electronic data in and between any healthcare environment.

Healthlink a centralized, data communications network for healthcare professionals which enables authorized users to exchange documents and information cheaply and efficiently.

health promotion efforts to prevent ill health and promote positive health. Five key priority areas for action formulated by the World Health Organization (1986, 1998): (a) building healthy public policy, (b) creating supportive environments for health, (c) strengthening community action for health, (d) developing personal skills for health and (e) re-orientating health services (to focus on whole populations).

hearing impaired a loss or reduction of hearing.

heart the hollow muscular organ which pumps the blood around the pulmonary and general circulations. It is situated behind the sternum, lying obliquely within the mediastinum. It weighs approximately 300 g and is about the size of the person's fist. *heart block* partial or complete block to the passage of impulses through the conducting system of the atria and ventricles of the heart.

heart failure *see* **congestive heart failure**.

heart transplant surgical transplantation of a heart from a suitable donor.

heartburn retrosternal burning due to gastro-oesophageal reflux of acid.

heart–lung machine a machine that bypasses both the heart and lungs and may be used in cardiac surgery to oxygenate the blood.

heat exchanger a method of maintaining the temperature of solutions in an automatic film processor with a series of separate tubes through which water, developer or fixer flows; any waste heat from the developer is absorbed and passed to the water or heat from the water can be absorbed from the fixer.

Heberden's nodes small bony swelling at terminal (distal) interphalangeal joints occurring in osteoarthritis.

heel bruise (stone bruise) contusion to the subcutaneous fat pad located over the inferior aspect of the calcaneus.

heel spurs occur on the plantar surface of the calcaneus and are considered a variant of the normal point of attachment of the plantar fascia. They are insignificant when small, and may be well defined with smooth, regular cortical contours. However, when enlarged they cause pain on walking.

Heimlich manoeuvre a technique for removing foreign matter from the trachea of a choking person. Performed by holding the patient from behind and jerking the operator's clenched fist into the victim's epigastrium. Do not practice on volunteers.

helical CT *see* **spiral CT**.

helium–neon laser a laser which has helium-neon gas in the tube and produces red light.

helix   spiral. Outer ridge on the auricle (pinna) of the outer ear. Describes the structure of molecules such as DNA.

hemiatrophy   atrophy of one half or one side. *See also* **facial hemiatrophy**.

hemibody   half or on one side of the body.

hemiglossectomy   removal of approximately half the tongue.

hemiparesis   paralysis or weakness of one side of face or body.

hemiplegia   paralysis of one side of the body, usually resulting from a cerebrovascular accident on the opposite side.

hemiplegic   a patient paralysed down one side.

hepar   the liver.

hepatic   associated with the liver.

hepatic portal circulation   that of venous blood (collected from the intestine, pancreas, spleen and stomach) to the liver before return to the heart.

hepaticoenteric   associated with the liver and intestine.

hepatocellular   associated with or affecting liver cells.

hepatoma   primary carcinoma of the liver.

hepatomegaly   enlargement of the liver. It is palpable below the costal margin.

hepatosplenic   associated with the liver and spleen.

heredity   transmission from parents to children of genetic characteristics by means of the genetic material; the process by which this occurs, and the study of such processes.

hermaphrodite   individual possessing both ovarian and testicular tissue. Although they may approximate either to male or female type, they are usually sterile from imperfect development of their gonads.

hernia   the abnormal protrusion of an organ, or part of an organ, through an aperture in the surrounding structures: commonly the protrusion of an abdominal organ through a gap in the abdominal wall. *See also* **femoral hernia, hiatus hernia, incisional hernia, inguinal hernia, irreducible hernia, strangulated hernia, umbilical hernia**.

herpes simplex   a viral infection resulting in an inflammatory skin eruption.

hertz (Hz)   a SI unit (International System of Units) for wave frequency. One hertz equals one cycle per second.

heterogeneous   consisting of dissimilar elements or parts; unlike, not being uniform throughout. *See also* **homogeneous**.

heterosexual   of different sexes; often used to describe an individual who is sexually attracted to members of the opposite sex. *See also* **homosexual**.

heuristic   a 'trial and error' method of trying to solve a computer problem.

hexadecimal   a mathematical system which employs 16 digits from 0 to 9 plus A, B, C, D, E, F. For example, hexadecimal 24A is equal to decimal 570.

Comparison of decimal, hexadecimal and binary number systems 0–20[a]

Decimal	Hexadecimal	Binary
0	0	0
1	1	1
2	2	10
3	3	11
4	4	100
5	5	101
6	6	110
7	7	111
8	8	1000
9	9	1001
10	A	1010
11	B	1011
12	C	1100
13	D	1101
14	E	1110
15	F	1111
16	10	10000
17	11	10001
18	12	10010
19	13	10011
20	14	10100

[a]From Radiographic imaging, 3rd edn, 2002, Chris Gunn, Churchill Livingstone, Edinburgh, with permission.

hiatus   a space or opening.

hiatus hernia   movement of part of the stomach through the diaphragmatic hiatus into the chest. May be asymptomatic, cause gastro-oesophageal reflux or strangulate. *See also* **hernia**.

high-dependency unit (HDU)   an area within a hospital with augmented levels of staff and equipment in which patients can receive levels of observation monitoring, nursing and medical care between that available on a general ward and intensive care unit. Generally excludes those needing mechanical ventilation.

high-resolution CT   a method of using thinner slices in CT scanning in order to increase the image definition.

high spatial frequency algorithm   in CT scanning an algorithm used to provide high spatial resolution. Frequently used to demonstrate bone, or in high resolution chest studies. *See also* **algorithm**.

high-temperature chemistry   the chemistry used in automatic radiographic processing equipment that function in the range of 31–39°C at a pH of about 9.6, now superseded by low-temperature chemistry. *See also* **low-temperature chemistry**.

hilum   a depression on the surface of an organ where vessels, ducts, etc. enter and leave.

hinge angle   the angle between two radiotherapy beam axes at their point of intersection.

hinge joint   a synovial joint that allows only flexion and extension, for example, the elbow joint.

hip bone (innominate bone)   formed by the fusion of three separate bones, the ilium, ischium and pubis.

hip joint   a synovial ball and socket joint formed by the acetabulum of the pelvis and the head of femur.

Hirschsprung's disease   congenital intestinal absence of a ganglia (aganglionosis), leading to intractable constipation or even intestinal obstruction. There is marked hypertrophy and dilation of the colon (megacolon) above the aganglionic segment. Commoner in boys and children with Down's syndrome.

HIS (hospital information system)   a computerized system, the aim of which it to build a network of complementary centres, for example, hospitals, laboratories, primary care trusts and GP centres, etc. spread throughout Europe, to meet the social and healthcare needs in each area. The term can also be used to define the system used in an individual hospital or unit.

histamine   a compound found in all cells which is released in allergic, inflammatory reactions and causes dilation of capillaries, decrease in blood pressure, increase in secretions of gastric juice and a constriction of smooth muscle of the bronchi and uterus. *See also* **allergy, anaphylaxis, inflammation**.

histamine receptors   there are three types in the body, H_1 in the bronchial muscle, H_2 in the secreting cells in the stomach and H_3 in nerve tissue.

histamine test   test previously used to determine the maximal gastric secretion of hydrochloric acid.

histiocytes   macrophages or phagocytic tissue cells.

histiocytoma   benign tumour of histiocytes.

histogram   a graph displaying data in columns which are next to each other.

histology   microscopic study of tissues.

Hodgkin's disease   tumour of lymphoid tissue often originating in the mediastinum. Often occurs in young adults. A diagnostic feature is the presence of the large multinucleated Reed–Sternberg cells in the lymphatic system. The prognosis is related to the histological subtype and stage; cure rate is about 80%. Treatment may consist of radiotherapy and/or chemotherapy. *See also* **lymphoma**.

holes   the absence of an electron in the valence band, the 'hole' has a positive charge and therefore can attract electrons.

holistic   relating to the theory of holism. Describes health care that takes account of physical, psychological, emotional, social and spiritual aspects.

home-care team   nurses trained in palliative care who provide additional support in a patient's home.

homeostasis   autoregulatory processes whereby functions such as blood pressure, blood glucose and electrolytes are maintained within set parameters.

homogeneous   of the same type; of the same quality or consistency throughout.

homogenize   to make into the same consistency throughout.

homogenous   having a like nature; for example, a bone graft from another human being.

homolateral   on the same side.

hoop traction   fixed skin traction used for the treatment of fractures of the femoral shaft in children, and for the gradual abduction of the hip in children with developmental dysplasia of the hip.

horizontal plane   *see* **transverse plane**.

hormone   a specific chemical messenger produced by endocrine glands that is transported in the blood or lymph to regulate the functions of tissues and organs elsewhere in the body.

horseshoe kidney   an anatomical variation in which the inner lower border of each kidney is joined to give a horseshoe shape. Usually symptomless, but rarely interferes with drainage of urine into ureters.

hospice   specialist centres that care for the terminally ill.

hospital-acquired infection (HAI, nosocomial infection)   occurs in a patient who has been in hospital for at least 72 hours and did not have signs and symptoms of such infection on admission: 10–12% of hospital patients develop a HAI. Urinary tract infection is the most common type.

hospital sterilization and disinfection unit (HSDU)   central sterile supply units (CSSUs) that also provide disinfection of equipment.

host computer   the main computer in a system containing a number of computers.

hot spot   a term used for the high uptake of a radionuclide in part of the body and thus indicating the presence of a lesion.

Hough transform   a technique for electronically enhancing the edges of a feature in a digital image to improve its image quality.

Hounsfield unit   a standardized unit for reporting and displaying reconstructed CT values. Water is given a nominal value of 0, other structures are reproduced with values relative to water. A change in one Hounsfield unit corresponds to 0.1% of the attenuation coefficient difference between water (0 HU) and air (−1000 HU).

housemaid's knee   *see* **bursitis**.

HU   the measure of heat energy deposited in the anode by an exposure and is the product of the kilovoltage peak and the milliampere per second.

hub   a device for connecting computers together to form a network.

human chorionic gonadotrophin (HCG)   a hormone produced by the trophoblast cells and later the chorion. A tumour marker for testicular and choriocarcinoma.

human immunodeficiency virus (HIV)   currently designates the AIDS virus. There are two types: *HIV-1* (many strains), mainly responsible for HIV disease in Western Europe, North America and Central Africa, and *HIV-2*, causing similar disease mainly in West Africa.

human leucocyte antigen (HLA)   the major histocompatibility complexes, so called because they were first found on leucocytes.

human papilloma virus (HPV)   there are many types of HPV, including several that are associated with anogenital warts (particularly types 6 and 11), and a few types (particularly 16 and 18) that are associated with genital tract malignancy such as cervical carcinoma.

human T-cell lymphotropic viruses (HTLV)   two retroviruses; HTLV-1 and HTLV-2, both of which are linked with some forms of leukaemia.

humerus   the bone of the upper arm, between the elbow and shoulder joint.

humour   any fluid of the body. *See also* **aqueous, vitreous**.

Hurter and Driffield curve   an alternative name for the characteristic curve of a radiographic film.

Hutchinson's teeth   defect of the upper central incisors (second dentition) which is part of the appearance of congenital syphilis. The teeth are broader at the gum than at the cutting edge, with the latter showing an elliptical notch.

Huygens' principle　　when an ultrasound beam generated by a single source may be considered as the sum of the beams generated by a number of point sources.

hyaline　　like glass; transparent.

hyaline cartilage　　covers the ends of bones when forming a joint.

hyaline degeneration　　degeneration of connective tissue, especially that of blood vessels in which tissue becomes formless in appearance.

hyaloid　　resembling hyaline tissue.

hyaloid membrane　　the transparent capsule surrounding the vitreous humour of the eye.

hydatid cyst　　the cyst formed by larvae of a tapeworm, *Echinococcus granulosa*, found in dogs and other canines. The encysted stage normally occurs in sheep but can occur in humans after eating with soiled hands from contact with dogs or infected sheep. The cysts are commonest in the liver, but can affect the brain, lungs and bone.

hydatidiform　　associated with or resembling a hydatid cyst.

hydatidiform mole　　a condition of pregnancy when the chorionic villi of the placenta degenerate into a cluster of cysts which may become malignant. A ***complete hydatidiform*** mole shows abnormal proliferation of the trophoblast and the presence of hydropic placental villi with no fetal parts. An ***incomplete hydatidiform*** mole or partial mole has a chromosomally abnormal fetus (triploid chromosome complement). Malignant transformation to choriocarcinoma may occur, especially in pregnancies affected by a complete hydatidiform mole.

hydraemia　　a greater plasma volume than usual compared with cell volume of the blood; normally present in late pregnancy.

hydramnios　　an excess of amniotic fluid.

hydrarthrosis　　a collection of synovial fluid in a joint cavity.

hydrate　　combine with water.

hydrocele　　a swelling due to accumulation of serous fluid between the tunica vaginalis and tunica albuginea of the testis or in the spermatic cord.

hydrocephalus ('water on the brain')　　an excess of cerebrospinal fluid inside the skull due to a disruption in normal CSF circulation, or loss of brain tissue. *See also* **external hydrocephalus, internal hydrocephalus**.

hydrochloric acid　　acid formed from hydrogen and chlorine; secreted by the gastric oxyntic cells and present in gastric juice.

hydrocortisone　　*see* **cortisol**.

hydrogen (H)　　a colourless, odourless, combustible gas. ***hydrogen ion concentration*** (pH) a measure of the acidity or alkalinity of a solution, ranging from pH 0 to pH 14, 7 being approximately neutral; the lower numbers denote acidity, the higher ones denote alkalinity. ***hydrogen peroxide*** (H_2O_2)

a powerful oxidizing and deodorizing agent, used in suitable dilution in mouthwashes.

hydronephrosis an accumulation of urine in the pelvis of the kidney, if unrelieved may result in atrophy of the kidney due to the obstruction of the flow of urine from the kidney. The obstruction may be caused by an obstruction of the ureter by a tumour or stone, it may be congenital or caused by the constriction of the urethra by an enlarged prostate gland.

hydropneumopericardium the presence of air and fluid in the pericardial sac surrounding the heart. It may accompany pericardiocentesis.

hydropneumoperitoneum the presence of air and fluid and gas in the peritoneal cavity: it may accompany paracentesis of that cavity; it may accompany perforation of the gut; or it may be due to infection with gas-forming microorganisms.

hydropneumothorax pneumothorax further complicated by effusion of fluid into the pleural cavity.

hydroquinone a radiographic developer agent.

hydrosalpinx distension of a uterine tube with watery fluid.

hydrostatic pressure that exerted by a liquid on the walls of its container, such as blood on an artery.

hydrothorax the presence of fluid in the pleural cavity. Also known as a *pleural effusion*.

hydroureter dilation of the ureter and renal pelvis.

hydroxyapatite the calcium salts, carbonate, hydroxide and phosphate, that make bone extremely hard.

hydroxyl (OH^-) a monovalent ion, consisting of a hydrogen atom linked to an oxygen atom.

5-hydroxytryptamine (5-HT) a neurotransmitter. Also present in the gastrointestinal tract and platelets. Also known as *serotonin*.

hygiene the science dealing with the maintenance of health. *communal hygiene* embraces all measures taken to supply the community with pure food and water, good sanitation, housing, etc. *industrial hygiene* (occupational health) includes all measures taken to preserve the individual's health while he or she is at work. *mental hygiene* deals with the establishment of healthy mental attitudes and emotional reactions. *personal hygiene* includes all those measures taken by the individual to preserve his or her own health.

hygroma a cystic swelling containing watery fluid, usually situated in the neck and present at birth, sometimes interfering with birth.

hymen a perforated membrane across the vaginal entrance. *imperforate hymen* a congenital condition.

hyoid a U-shaped bone at the root of the tongue.

hyperacusis increased sensitivity to sound.

hyperbaric oxygen   term applied to gas at up to three times atmospheric pressure.

hyperbaric oxygen therapy   a form of treatment in which a patient is entirely enclosed in a pressure chamber breathing 100% oxygen at greater than one atmosphere pressure. Used for patients with carbon monoxide poisoning, decompression sickness, etc.

hypercalcaemia   excessive calcium in the blood usually resulting from bone resorption as occurs in hyperparathyroidism, metastatic tumours of bone, or Paget's disease. It results in anorexia, abdominal pain, muscle pain and weakness. It is accompanied by hypercalciuria and can lead to nephrolithiasis.

hypercalciuria   greatly increased excretion of calcium in the urine. Occurs in diseases which result in bone resorption. ***idiopathic hypercalciuria*** is the term used when there is no known metabolic cause. Hypercalciuria is of importance in the formation and development (pathogenesis) of kidney stones.

hypercholesterolaemia   excessive cholesterol in the blood. Predisposes to atheroma and gallstones. Also found in hypothyroidism (myxoedema).

hyperextension   overextension. Active or passive force which takes the joint into extension beyond its normal physiological range.

hyperflexion   excessive flexion.

hyperfractionation   the delivery of more than one dose of radiation a day over a period of time, the dose per fraction is lower compared with conventional fractionations resulting in an increase in the overall tumour dose.

hyperglycaemia   increased blood glucose, usually indicative of diabetes mellitus or impaired glucose tolerance, but sometimes due to pathological stress, e.g. myocardial infarction.

hyperglycaemic coma   occurs in diabetes if the disease is untreated or if insulin has been omitted.

hyperinsulinism   elevated circulating levels of insulin due to pancreatic tumour, insulinoma, or factitious administration of hypoglycaemic agents; resulting in hypoglycaemia, which may lead to episodic coma, confusion or even mental health disturbance.

hyperkeratosis   premalignant small warty nodules which may be due to sunlight, actinic or solar keratosis, tar or X-rays.

hyperkinesis   excessive movement.

hypermobility   excessive mobility. As in a joint that has an increase in the normal range of joint movement potentially leading to instability.

hypermotility   increased movement, as peristalsis.

hypernephroma (Grawitz tumour)   a malignant tumour of the kidney.

hyperostiosis   thickening of the skull vault.

hyperparathyroidism   overactivity of one or more parathyroid glands, usually due to parathyroid adenoma, and resulting in elevated serum calcium levels; rarely results in parathyroid bone disease, osteitis fibrosa cystica; may be primary, or secondary/tertiary usually in response to chronic renal failure. *See also* **hypercalcaemia, hypercalciuria, von Recklinghausen's disease**.

hyperpituitarism   *see* **acromegaly, Cushing's disease, gigantism, hyperprolactinaemia**.

hyperplasia   increase in the size of an organ due to an increase in the number of cells contained in the organ.

hyperprolactinaemia   elevation in circulating prolactin levels, sometimes due to stress; if pathological results in galactorrhoea, menstrual irregularity and subfertility; may be due to dopamine antagonists, such as metoclopramide or neuroleptic drugs, large, often non-functioning pituitary tumours, or prolactinomas.

hyperpyrexia   body temperature above 40–41°C.

hypertension   abnormally high blood pressure involving systolic and/or diastolic levels. There is no universal agreement on the upper limits of normal, especially with increasing age. Many cardiologists consider a resting systolic pressure of 140 mmHg and/or a resting diastolic pressure of 90 mmHg to be abnormal at age 20 years. Hypertension is considered to be a risk factor for the development of coronary heart disease. ***secondary hypertension*** may result from coarctation of the aorta, renal artery stenosis, renal disease, phaeochromocytoma, Cushing's disease/syndrome, Conn's syndrome, various drugs, such as oral contraceptives, NSAIDs, and the pre-eclampsia of pregnancy. *See also* **portal hypertension, pulmonary hypertension**.

hyperthermia   very high body temperature. *See also* **hyperpyrexia**.

hyperthyroidism (thyrotoxicosis)   condition due to excessive production of thyroid hormone (thyroxine, triiodothyronine), usually due to Graves' disease, but also multiple or solitary toxic nodules, and resulting classically in anxiety, tachycardia, sweating, increased appetite with weight loss, and a fine tremor of the outstretched hands; much commoner in women than men.

hypertrophy   increase in the size of tissues or structures, independent of natural growth. It may be congenital, compensatory, complementary or functional. *See also* **stenosis**.

hyperuricaemia   excess of uric acid in the blood.

hyperventilation   overbreathing. Increased respiratory rate; may occur during anxiety attacks, in salicylate poisoning or head injury, or passively as part of a technique of general anaesthesia in intensive care. Also associated with alkalosis and tetany.

hyperviscosity   an extremely viscous or thick fluid.

hyperviscosity syndrome   when the paraprotein level is raised and visual impairment, lethargy and coma therefore develop.

hypocalcaemia   decreased calcium level in the blood. Causes include: disturbed kidney function, excess calcium excretion, deficiency of vitamin D, alkalosis and hypoparathyroidism. Leads to tingling in the hands and feet, and stridor and convulsions in children.

hypochondria   unnecessary anxiety about one's health.

hypochondriac   associated with the regions of the upper abdomen beneath the lower ribs, associated with a person who is preoccupied with their health so that their state of mind itself becomes a disability.

hypochondriacal disorder   an excessive preoccupation with the possibility of having serious health problems associated with refusal to accept professional reassurance that there is no physical illness underlying the symptoms. Symptoms are often of a bodily nature or concerned with physical appearance.

hypochondrium   the upper lateral region (left and right) of the abdomen.

hypodermic   below the skin; subcutaneous.

hypofractionation   the practice of giving less than the conventional fractionations for a particular treatment, is used for treating tumours which have a higher capacity for repair such as melanomas.

hypogastrium   that area of the anterior abdomen which lies immediately below the umbilical.

hypoglossal   under the tongue.

hypoglossal nerve   the 12th pair of cranial nerves which innervate tongue movements.

hypoglycaemia   a condition when the blood sugar is less than normal.

hypoglycaemic   low blood sugar level.

hypoglycaemic coma   occurs in diabetes, the patient looses consciousness if they have an overdose of insulin or have not eaten at the appropriate time.

hypokalemia   lack of potassium in the blood.

hypomobility   decrease in the normal range of joint movement.

hypomotility   decreased movement, as of the gastrointestinal tract.

hypopharynx   that portion of the pharynx lying below and behind the larynx, correctly called the laryngopharynx.

hypophysis cerebri   *see* **pituitary gland**.

hypopituitarism   pituitary gland insufficiency, especially of the anterior lobe. Absence of gonadotrophins leads to failure of ovulation, uterine atrophy and amenorrhoea in women and loss of libido, pubic and axillary hair in both sexes. Lack of growth hormone in children results in short stature. Lack of adrenocorticotrophin (ACTH) and thyrotrophin (TSH) may result in lack of energy, pallor, fine dry skin, cold intolerance and sometimes hypoglycaemia. Usually due to tumour of or involving pituitary gland or hypothalamus but in other cases cause is unknown. Occasionally due to postpartum infarction of the pituitary gland.

hypotension   low blood pressure that is insufficient for adequate tissue perfusion and oxygenation; may be primary or secondary (e.g. reduced cardiac output, hypovolaemic shock, Addison's disease) or postural.

hypothalamus   literally, below the thalamus. It consists of an area of grey matter in the brain just above the pituitary gland. It has both endocrine and neural functions. The hypothalamus produces the hormones oxytocin and vasopressin (antidiuretic hormone); these are stored in the posterior pituitary prior to release. It is the major centre for the autonomic nervous system and controls physiological functions that include thirst and hunger, circadian rhythms and emotions such as anger.

hypothenar eminence   the eminence on the ulnar side of the palm below the little finger.

hypothermia   general lowering of body temperature, may occur when heat loss exceeds heat production. Occurs following shock or injury, often fatal if uncontrolled.

hypothesis   a declaration that can be tested by statistical (inferential) tests. It is a prediction based on the relationship between the dependent and independent variables.

hypothetico-deductive method   theories are examined and hypotheses for testing are derived in a deductive manner. The particular research study tests the hypotheses by data analysis that either supports or repudiates the original theory.

hypothyroidism   conditions caused by low circulating levels of one or both thyroid hormones (thyroxine, triiodothyronine). Much more common in women than men and may be: (a) associated with goitre, such as autoimmune thyroiditis, lack of iodine or as a drug side-effect, e.g. with lithium; (b) due to spontaneous atrophy; or (c) after surgical treatment for hyperthyroidism. Some individuals have a subclinical form and in others it may be transient. It results in decreased metabolic rate and may be characterized by some of the following: fatigue, bradycardia, angina, hypertension, aches and pains, carpal tunnel syndrome, low temperature and cold intolerance, weight gain, constipation, hair and skin changes (dry coarse skin), puffy face, anaemia, hoarseness, slow speech, menorrhagia and depression. Treatment is with replacement thyroxine. ***congenital hypothyroidism*** can be detected (by routine blood testing) soon after birth and treated successfully with thyroxine. Untreated, it leads to impaired mental and physical development. It is recognized by the presence of coarse facies and protruding tongue. The term cretinism was previously used.

hypovolaemic shock   shock caused by the loss of circulating blood volume as a result of dehydration, haemorrhage, vomiting, diarrhoea or severe burns. Used to be called medical shock.

hypoxaemia   an insufficient oxygen content in the blood.

hypoxia   diminished amount of oxygen in tissues.

hysterectomy   surgical removal of the uterus. ***abdominal hysterectomy*** effected via a lower abdominal incision. ***subtotal hysterectomy*** removal of the uterine body, leaving the cervix in the vaginal vault. ***total hysterectomy*** complete removal of the uterine body and cervix. ***vaginal hysterectomy*** carried out through the vagina.

hysteresis   is when a material is being magnetized the effect of magnetism lags behind the magnetizing force, the lag can be plotted to form a ***hysteresis loop***.

hysterosalpingectomy   excision of the uterus and uterine (fallopian) tubes.

hysterosalpingography   the radiographic investigation of the uterus and uterine tubes following the introduction of contrast agent via a cannula inserted into the cervix. *See also* **uterosalpingography**.

hysterosalpingostomy   anastomosis between a uterine (fallopian) tube and the uterus.

hysteroscopy   the passage of a small-diameter telescope through the cervix to visualize the uterine cavity. Also used for treatments such as transcervical resection of endometrium.

iatrogenic describes a secondary condition arising from treatment of a primary condition.

icon a pictorial representation on a computer screen.

identity bracelet a plastic band attached to either a patient's wrist or ankle when they are admitted to hospital, usually giving their name and patient number; it should not be removed until a patient leaves hospital.

idiopathic scoliosis characterized by a lateral curvature of the spine together with rotation and associated rib hump or flank recession. The treatment is by spinal brace or traction or internal fixation with accompanying spinal fusion. *See also* **halopelvic traction, Harrington rod, Milwaukee brace**.

IHE (Integrated Health Enterprise) a consultation exercise between manufacturers and health professionals to ensure that computerization of the healthcare system achieves what the users require.

ileal conduit a surgical procedure when the ureters are attached to the ileum, part of the ileum then forms a reservoir for urine which drains to the anterior abdominal wall through a fistula.

ileocaecal associated with the ileum and the caecum.

ileocolic associated with the ileum and the colon.

ileorectal associated with the ileum and the rectum.

ileostomy a surgically made fistula between the ileum and the anterior abdominal wall; a type of opening (stoma) discharging liquid faecal matter. Usually permanent when the whole of the large bowel has to be removed, for example, in severe ulcerative colitis.

ileostomy bags special plastic bags used to collect the liquid discharge from an ileostomy.

ileum the lower three-fifths of the small intestine, lying between the jejunum and the caecum. Concerned with the absorption of various nutrients such as vitamin B_{12}.

ileus intestinal obstruction. Usually restricted to paralytic as opposed to mechanical obstruction and characterized by abdominal distension, vomiting and the absence of pain.

iliac associated with the ilium. *iliac arteries* carry arterial blood to the pelvis and legs.

iliac crest   the highest point of the ilium.

iliac region/fossa   the abdominal region situated either side of the hypogastrium.

iliac veins   drain venous blood from the legs and pelvis.

iliococcygeal   associated with the ilium and coccyx.

iliofemoral   associated with the ilium and the femur.

iliopectineal   associated with the ilium and the pubis.

iliopectineal line   bony ridge on the internal surface of the ilium and pubic bones. It is the dividing line between the true and false pelvis.

iliopsoas   associated with the ilium and the loin.

ilium   the upper part of the innominate (hip) bone; it is a separate bone in the fetus.

Ilizarov frame   external fixation device used commonly in the management of fractures of the tibia.

image acquisition   the collection of data in order to produce a computed tomography or magnetic resonance image.

image acquisition time   the scanning time required to produce a set of images from a measurement sequence in magnetic resonance imaging. For a *two-dimensional sequence* it is the repetition time, times the number of signal excitations/averages times the number of phase encoded steps. For a *fast two-dimensional sequence* it is the two-dimensional sequence divided by the echo train length. For *three-dimensional volume sequence* it is the two-dimensional sequence multiplied by the number of partitions.

image annotation   the marking of information on a radiograph to denote the side of the body, the patient position and the exposure factors; digital systems allow preset terms, numbers and letters to be added alongside the patient image.

ImageChecker™   an aid to screening routine mammograms by automatically marking clusters of white areas and dense areas with radiating lines.

image format   the manner in which a computed tomography image is stored or displayed such as on screen, computer disk, magnetic tape or film.

image intensifier   a means of producing a real time image of a patient. The X-ray beam passes through the patient and onto the image intensifier which converts the image to light, this image is scanned and an electrical signal is sent to a television monitor where the image is viewed.

image manipulation   in CT scanning the ability to digitally alter the appearance of the acquired image to enhance depiction of the required anatomy.

image quality   the ratio of signal over noise.

image reconstruction   the process of producing an image from computer data or a set of unprocessed measurements.

image segmentation   in digital imaging, dividing an image into its various parts or taking the image from the background to increase the definition of the object.

imaging plate   a re-usable plate coated with barium phosphate that, when exposed to radiation excites the electrons, and then, when scanned by a helium-neon laser, produces an image which can be recorded.

imaging techniques   diagnostic techniques used to investigate the condition and functioning of organs and structures. They include radiographic examination, radionuclide scans, ultrasonography, computed tomography, magnetic resonance and positron emission tomography.

imbalance   want of balance. Term refers commonly to the upset of acid–base relationship and the electrolytes in body fluids.

immersion foot   *see* **trench foot**.

immobilization device   a method of reducing movement during radiotherapy treatment or diagnostic imaging.

immobilize   to keep from moving, splints or plaster of Paris bandages are used to prevent realigned broken bones from becoming displaced.

immune   protected against infection by specific or non-specific mechanisms of the immune system. Altered reactivity against an antigen, caused by previous exposure to that antigen.

immune response   the response of the immune system to a perceived threat, either from non-self antigens, or from self antigens during a pathological immune response. This may be against microorganisms, malignant cells, and damaged or healthy tissues.

immunity   an intrinsic or acquired state of immune responsiveness to an antigen. *active immunity* is acquired, naturally during an infection or artificially by immunization. It involves the production of antibodies and specific T cells in response to exposure to an antigenic stimulus. The primary response to exposure is followed by a lag phase of 2–3 weeks before enough antibodies are produced, but the secondary response following a subsequent exposure is more intense and has a much reduced lag phase because the memory cells are able to produce antibodies very quickly. This type of immunity tends to be of long duration. *cell-mediated immunity* T-lymphocyte-dependent responses which cause graft rejection, immunity to some infectious agents and tumour rejection. *humoral immunity* from immunoglobulins produced by plasma cells derived from B lymphocytes. Immunity can be innate (from inherited qualities), or it can be acquired, actively or passively, naturally or artificially. *passive immunity* is acquired, naturally when maternal antibody passes to the fetus via the placenta or in colostrum and breast milk, or artificially by administering immunoglobulins (usually human in origin). This type of immunity tends to be short-lived because the immune response is not stimulated to produce specific antibodies.

immunization   a process by which resistance to an infectious disease is induced or increased.

immunocompromised patients (immunosuppressed patients)   patients with defective immune responses, which can be inherited or acquired. Often produced by treatment with drugs or irradiation. Also occurs in some patients with cancer and other diseases affecting the lymphoid system. Depending on the immune defect, different patterns of infection result. Patients with cellular defects are likely to develop infections with opportunistic organisms such as *Candida*, *Pneumocystis carinii* and *Cryptococcus neoformans*. Patients with antibody defects are more liable to infections with encapsulated bacteria such as pneumococcus.

immunocytochemistry   staining cells with specific antibodies for diagnostic purposes.

immunodeficiency   the state of having defective immune responses, leading to increased susceptibility to infectious diseases.

immunoglobulins (Igs) (antibodies)   high-molecular-weight glycoproteins produced by plasma cells (derived from B lymphocytes) in response to specific antigens. The basic structure of immunoglobulins is Y-shaped, consisting of two identical heavy chains, each linked to two identical light chains. Immunoglobulins are found in the blood and other body fluids where they form part of body defences. Immunoglobulins function in a variety of ways, but all involve combining with the antigen to form an immune complex. There are five classes of immunoglobulins, IgG, IgA, IgD, IgM and IgE, each with different characteristics, functions and locations.

immunohistochemistry   staining tissue with specific antibodies for diagnostic purposes.

immunological response   *see* **immunity**.

immunology   the study of the immune system of lymphocytes, inflammatory cells and associated cells and proteins, which affect an individual's response to antigens.

immunosuppression   the administration of agents to significantly interfere with the ability of the immune system to respond to antigenic stimulation by inhibiting cellular and humerol immunity. May be deliberate such as before bone marrow transplants to prevent rejection by the host or incidental such as following chemotherapy for the treatment of cancer.

immunosuppressive   that which reduces immunological responsiveness. Describes an agent such as a drug that suppresses immune system function.

immunotherapy   the use of knowledge about immunity to prevent and treat disease. Can be used to mean desensitization therapy against specific allergens, for example, insect venom, or can refer to therapeutics which use agonists or antagonists based on immune system components, for example, treatment based on biological modifiers such as interleukin-2.

impacted   firmly wedged, abnormal immobility, for example, faeces in the rectum; a fetus in the pelvis; a tooth in its socket or a calculus in a duct.

impacted fracture   a break in bone continuity when the ends of the bone overlap, the most common site is just above the wrist joint.

impedance   the general opposition of flow of electric current measured in ohms. In ultrasound a measure of the tissue's resistance to distortion by ultrasound and depends on the tissue density and the velocity of the sound.

imperforate   lacking a normal opening.

imperforate anus   a congenital absence of an opening into the rectum.

imperforate hymen   a fold of mucous membrane at the vaginal entrance which has no natural outlet for the menstrual fluid.

implant   any drug, structure or substance inserted surgically into the human body, for example, implants of progestogens for contraception, or implants used in plastic surgery. Those used to augment tissue contour may be of two types: *alloplastic* synthetic foreign body implants such as those used in breast reconstruction, or *autologous implants* tissue obtained from the same patient. *dental implant* artificial structure implanted surgically into the alveolar bone, usually made from titanium.

implantation   the insertion of living cells or solid materials into the tissues, for example, accidental implantation of tumour cells in a wound; implantation of radioactive material or solid drugs; implantation of the fertilized ovum into the endometrium.

incidence rate   the total number of new cases, of a specific disease, occurring in a given period of time among a given number of people.

incident beam   the beam of radiation striking an object.

incident light   the light travelling from the light source.

incipient   initial, beginning, in its early stages.

incision   in surgery, a cut into soft tissue, the act of cutting.

incisional hernia   protrusion through the site of a previous abdominal incision.

incisor tooth   an anterior tooth with a cutting edge and single root, placed first and second from the midline in both primary and secondary dentition.

incompetence   inadequacy to perform a natural function, for example, mitral valve regurgitation.

incomplete abortion   a termination of pregnancy or a miscarriage when the products of conception are not fully expelled or removed. *See also* **miscarriage**.

incomplete fracture   the bone is only cracked or fissured, called greenstick fracture when it occurs in children.

incomplete miscarriage   part of the fetus or placenta is retained in the uterus. *See also* **evacuation of retained products of conception**.

incontinence   inability to control the evacuation of urine or faeces. *See also* **functional incontinence, neurogenic incontinence, stress incontinence**.

incubator   an apparatus with controlled temperature and oxygen concentration used for preterm or sick babies. A low-temperature oven in which bacteria are cultured.

incus anvil-shaped bone of the middle ear. *See also* **malleus, stapes**.

independent variable the variable conditions of an experimental situation, e.g. control or experimental.

indicator a substance used to make visible the completion of a chemical reaction or the achievement of a certain pH.

indicator lamps situated on a control panel to give the status of equipment, for example, if the door of the treatment room is closed, or outside the room to indicate treatment is in progress.

indigenous of a disease, etc., native to a certain locality or country.

indigestion (dyspepsia) a feeling of gastric discomfort, including fullness and gaseous distension, which is not necessarily a manifestation of disease.

indirect cost a cost that cannot be attributed to any one department and its budget. It is shared between various budgets, for example, the cost of heating a building.

indolent slow growing, reluctant to heal.

induction the production of an electromotive force in a conductor when it is moving relative to a magnetic field of changing intensity. The act of bringing on or causing to occur, as applied to anaesthesia and labour.

induration the hardening of tissue, as in hyperaemia, infiltration by tumour, etc.

industrial dermatitis a term used in the National Insurance (Industrial Injuries) Act to cover occupational skin conditions.

industrial disease (occupational disease) a disease contracted by reason of occupational exposure to an industrial agent known to be hazardous, for example, dust, fumes, chemicals, irradiation, etc., the notification of, safety precautions against and compensation for which are controlled by law.

inelastic collisions the mutual attraction of atoms, molecules, etc. when either the energy from one particle is given to the other or only kinetic, excitation or ionization energy is transferred after the collision.

inevitable abortion miscarriage.

inevitable miscarriage loss of the pregnancy cannot be prevented.

in extremis at the point of death.

infant a child of less than 1 year old.

infarct area of tissue affected when the end artery supplying it is occluded by atheroma, thrombosis or embolism, for example, in myocardium or lung.

infarction irreversible premature tissue death. Necrosis (death) of a section of tissue because the blood supply has been cut off. *See also* **myocardial infarction, pulmonary infarction**.

infection the successful invasion, establishment and growth of micro-organisms in body tissues. It may be acute or chronic. *See also* **autoinfection, cross infection, hospital-acquired infection, opportunistic infection**.

infectious disease a disease caused by a specific, pathogenic microorganism and capable of transmission to another individual by direct or indirect contact.

infective infectious. Disease transmissible from one host to another.

inferential statistics also known as inductive statistics. That which uses the observations of a sample to make a prediction about other samples, i.e. makes generalizations from the sample. *See also* **descriptive statistics**.

inferior lower; beneath.

inferosuperior radiograph a radiograph taken from below to above.

infestation the presence of animal parasites.

infibulation circumcision.

infiltration the entry into cells, tissues or organs of abnormal substances or cells, for example, cancer cells, fat. Penetration of the surrounding tissues; the oozing or leaking of fluid into the tissues.

infiltration anaesthesia analgesia produced by infiltrating the tissues with a local anaesthetic.

inflammation local defence mechanism initiated by tissue injury. The injury may be caused by trauma, microorganisms, extremes of temperature and pH, UV radiation, or ionizing radiation. It is characterized by heat, redness, swelling, pain and loss of function. See also **calor, dolor, rubor, tumor**.

inflammatory bowel disease (IBD) a condition of unknown (idiopathic) intestinal inflammation. Mainly ulcerative colitis and Crohn's disease. Also lymphocytic and collagenous colitis.

inflammatory response a reaction of the immune system to protect the body against harmful substances or physical agents.

influenza (flu) a viral infection of the respiratory tract.

informatics information management and technology (IM&T). Information is needed to ensure the effective running of any organization. Data are pieces of material which, when compiled effectively, form information. Information is managed in a number of different ways but increasingly it is managed using technological means (*information technology, **IT***). Non-technological means may be more appropriate for the target group/recipient. For example, telephone calls and notice boards are ways in which information might be managed.

informed choice in order to make decisions about their own care and management clients/patients need information from healthcare professionals. This means the provision of accurate, appropriate information about the person's condition, and about the treatment options available. Healthcare professionals may disagree with the patient/client's decisions, but the latter takes precedence where an adult patient is deemed to be mentally competent.

informed consent in the UK consent forms must include a signed declaration by the doctor or other healthcare professional that he/she has explained the nature and purpose of the operation or treatment to the patient in non-technical terms. Any questions that the patient may have after signing the form should be referred to the doctor or other health professional who is to carry out the treatment. *See also* **consent**.

infundibulum any funnel-shaped passage, for example, the ends of the uterine tubes.

infusion fluid flowing into the body either intravenously or subcutaneously over a long period of time, an aqueous solution containing the active principle of a drug.

infusion cholangiography the radiographic investigation of the biliary tract following the infusion of a radiographic contrast agent into the median cubital vein.

ingestion taking food or drugs into the stomach. The means by which a phagocytic cell takes in material such as microorganisms.

inguinal associated with the groin.

inguinal canal a tubular opening through the lower part of the anterior abdominal wall, parallel to and a little above the inguinal (Poupart's) ligament. In the male it contains spermatic cord; in the female the uterine round ligaments.

inguinal hernia protrusion through the inguinal canal in the male. *See also* **hernia**.

inhalation the breathing in of air, or other vapour, etc. A medicinal substance which is inhaled, such as an inhalation anaesthetic or in the aerosols used for asthma treatment.

inherent innate; inborn.

inherent filtration the filtration of the beam which is outside the operator control for example, the target material, the glass envelope and the X-ray window of the X-ray tube.

inherent wedge a microprocessor controlled wedge used to attenuate part of the beam in radiotherapy treatment.

inhomogeneities variations within a patient due to the different densities of bone, tissue and organs.

inhomogenicity the slight variation in uniformity of the static magnetic field in parts per million as a fractional deviation from the average value of the field.

initialize at the beginning of computation all variables are given specific values in the program.

injection the act of introducing a fluid (under pressure) into the tissues, a vessel, cavity or hollow organ, air can be injected into a cavity, the substance injected. *See also* **pneumothorax**.

inkjet printer a printer which sprays streams of quick-drying ink through very fine jets, building up the characters or images in very fine dots to produce an image on paper. Often a separate cartridge is used for each of the main ink colours, black, red, green and yellow.

inlay in dentistry, a restoration made from cast gold or porcelain to fit a prepared cavity, into which it is then cemented.

innervation the nerve supply to a part.

innocent benign; not malignant.

innominate unnamed. *See also* **hip bone**.

inquest in England and Wales, a legal enquiry by a coroner into the cause of sudden or unexpected death.

insecticide an agent which kills insects.

insensible without sensation or consciousness. Too tiny or gradual to be noticed.

insensible perspiration the water lost by evaporation through the skin surface other than by sweating. It is significantly increased in inflamed skin.

insert the part of an X-ray tube which contains the anode, and cathode in a vacuum.

insertion the act of setting or placing in, the attachment of a muscle to the bone it moves.

in situ in the normal position, undisturbed.

insomnia sleeplessness.

inspiration inhalation; breathing in.

instep the arch of the foot on the dorsal surface.

instillation insertion of drops into a cavity, for example, conjunctival sac.

insufflation the blowing of air along a tube (pharyngotympanic, uterine) to establish patency. The blowing of powder into a body cavity.

insulator a substance which has a high resistance to the flow of electricity or heat.

insulin a polypeptide hormone produced by the beta cells of the pancreas. Insulin secretion is regulated by the blood glucose level and it opposes the action of glucagon. It has an effect on the metabolism of carbohydrate, protein and fat by stimulating the transport of glucose into cells. An absolute or relative lack of insulin results in hyperglycaemia, a high blood glucose with decreased utilization of carbohydrate and increased breakdown of fat and protein; a condition known as diabetes mellitus. Three types of insulin are available commercially: ***bovine insulin***, ***porcine insulin*** and ***human insulin***, produced using recombinant techniques. Insulin is produced in U100 strength, i.e. 100 units per mL, a standardization replacing the previous 20, 40 and 80 unit strengths.

insulin coma   when a diabetic patient loses consciousness due to either an overdose of insulin or fails to eat at the appropriate time.

insulin-dependent diabetes mellitus (IDDM)   *see* **diabetes mellitus** type 1.

insulinoma   pancreatic islet beta cell adenoma.

integral dose   the sum total of dose to all elements of irradiated tissue and represents the total absorbed energy.

integument   a covering, especially the skin.

intelligent peripheral   a keypad linked to a computer that can act as a computer in its own right.

intensifying factor   the ratio of the radiation exposure required to produce a density of 1.0 on a radiographic film without screens compared to the exposure required to produce a density of 1.0 with screens and using the same film.

intensity   the total energy of a beam of electromagnetic radiation per second at a given point. In ultrasound the intensity of the ultrasound beam is the energy flow rate per unit area in watts per square centimetre.

intensity-modulated radiotherapy (IMRT)   the use of a computer system to optimize the beam shape and profile to the target tissues by using multileaf, moving collimators and therefore maximizing the radiation delivery technique by evaluating millions of possible beam arrangements to create a clinically accurate treatment plan.

intensive therapy unit (ITU) (intensive care unit)   an area within a hospital with augmented levels of staff and equipment in which highly specialized monitoring, resuscitation and therapeutic techniques are used to support critically ill patients with actual or impending organ failure, particularly those needing artificial ventilation.

interaction cross section   the size of the area of the patient that lies in the field of the X-ray beam.

interarticular   between joints.

interatrial   between the two atria of the heart.

intercellular   between cells.

intercostal   between the ribs.

interface   the connection from the computer to other hardware, allowing free communication between the two.

interferons (IFNs)   protein mediators that enhance cellular resistance to viruses. They are involved in the modulation of the immune response. Interferon has caused regression of some cancers and is used in the management of some types of multiple sclerosis.

interlacing   the construction of an image when an electron beam scans a tube phosphor, first the odd lines are scanned and then the even lines.

interleukins (IL)   large group of signalling molecules (cytokines). They are non-specific immune chemicals produced by various cells, such as macrophages. Interleukins are also involved with the regulation of haematopoiesis.

interlobar   between the lobes.

interlobular   between the lobules.

interlock   a safety device, for example, to protect the X-ray unit from over-heating, to prevent exposure if the room door is open.

internal   inside.

internal conversion   the transfer of energy from the nucleus of a heavy atom to an electron in the K shell.

internal ear   that part of the ear which comprises the vestibule, semicircular canals and the cochlea.

internal haemorrhage   bleeding inside the body, often with no external signs.

internal hydrocephalus   excess of cerebrospinal fluid mainly in the ventricles of the brain. A valve (e.g. Spitz–Holter type) is used to drain excess CSF and return it to the bloodstream.

internal respiration (tissue respiration)   the reverse of external respiration, involving gaseous exchange between the cells and blood. Oxygen moves from the blood, via the tissue fluid, to the cells, and waste cellular carbon dioxide moves into the blood for onward transport to the lungs. *See also* **respiration**.

internal (medial) rotation   a limb or body movement where there is rotation towards the vertical axis of the body.

internal secretions   those produced by the endocrine glands; hormones.

internal version   *see* **version**.

Internet   a network of computers, accessible to anyone throughout the world who has access to a computer and modem, giving access to the World Wide Web and email.

interosseous   between bones.

interphalangeal   between the phalanges.

interpretive approach   a research approach that incorporates the meaning and significance individuals attach to situations and behaviour. May be used in social science research.

interprofessional   intense teamwork among practitioners from different healthcare professions focused on a common problem-solving purpose and requiring recognition of the core expertise and core knowledge of each profession and blending of common core skills to enable the team to act as an integrated whole.

interprofessional education (IPE)   shared (or common) learning of common (or generic) core skills among students and qualified practitioners of different healthcare professions that fosters respect for each other's core knowledge and expertise, capitalizes on professional differences, and cultivates integrated teamwork to solve patients' problems.

interpupillary line   line joining the centre of the two orbits and is perpendicular to the median sagittal plane. *See also* **median sagittal plane**.

interserosal   between serous membrane, as in the pleural, peritoneal and pericardial cavities.

intersexuality   the possession of both male and female characteristics.

interspinous   between spinous processes, especially those of the vertebrae.

interstices   spaces.

interstitial   the space between cells; distributed through the connective structures or the space between organs.

interstitial cell stimulating hormone (ICSH, luteinizing hormone)   a hormone released from the anterior lobe of the pituitary gland; causes production of testosterone in the male.

interstitial fluid (tissue fluid)   the extracellular fluid situated in the spaces around cells.

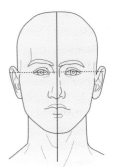

Interpupillary line. From Pocket book of radiographic positioning, 2nd edn, Ruth Sutherland, 2003, Churchill Livingstone, Edinburgh, with permission.

interstitial lamellae   plates of bone filling the spaces between haversian systems.

interstitial lung disease   a wide range of respiratory disorders characterized by inflammation and eventually, fibrosis of the connective tissue of the lungs.

interstitial therapy   brachytherapy where the sources are implanted directly into the affected tissue.

intertrochanteric   between trochanters such as those on the proximal femur.

interval cancer   one that is discovered in the time interval between screening episodes, such as breast cancer detected between mammography examinations.

interval data   measurement data with a numerical value, for example, temperature, that has an arbitrary zero. The intervals between successive values are the same, for example, a 1 degree increase from 38 to 39 is exactly the same as one from 39 to 40. *See also* **ratio data**.

interval status   when the numbers are ordinal and the steps between each number are of equal size.

interventricular   between ventricles, as those of the brain or heart.

intervertebral   between the vertebrae, as discs and foramina. *See also* **nucleus, prolapse**.

intestinal obstruction   a blockage that stops the contents of the intestine passing into the lumen of the bowel.

intestine   a part of the alimentary canal (extending from the stomach to the anus). Consists of the small and large intestine (bowel).

intima   the internal coat of a blood vessel.

intra-abdominal   inside the abdomen.

intra-amniotic   within or into the amniotic fluid.

intra-aortic   within the aorta. ***intra-aortic balloon pump*** (IABP) device used to increase cardiac output in ventricular failure or shock.

intra-arterial   within an artery.

intra-articular   within a joint.

intrabronchial   within a bronchus.

intracanalicular   within a canaliculus.

intracapillary   within a capillary.

intracapsular   within a capsule, for example, that of the lens or a joint. *See also* **extracapsular**.

intracardiac   within the heart.

intracaval   within the vena cava.

intracavitary therapy   brachytherapy where the sources are arranged in a suitable applicator to irradiate the walls of a body cavity from the inside.

intracellular   within cells. ***intracellular fluid*** (ICF) that fluid inside the cells. *See also* **extracellular**.

intracerebral   within the cerebrum, such as a haemorrhage.

intracranial   within the skull.

intracranial pressure (ICP)   the pressure inside the cranial cavity. It is maintained at a normal level by brain tissue, intracellular and extracellular fluid, cerebrospinal fluid and blood. A change in any of these compartments can increase the pressure, for example, after head injury. *See also* **raised intracranial pressure**.

intradural   inside the dura mater.

intragastric   within the stomach.

intragluteal   within the gluteal muscle of the buttock.

intrahepatic   within the liver.

intrahepatic cholestasis   caused by blockage of the small bile ducts within the liver, such as in hepatitis or cirrhosis.

intralobular   within the lobule, for example, vessels draining a hepatic lobule.

intraluminal   within the lumen of a hollow tube-like structure.

intralymphatic   within a lymphatic node or vessel.

intramedullary   within the bone marrow.

intramural   within the wall of a hollow tube or organ.

intramuscular   within muscle tissue.

intranasal   within the nasal cavity.

intranet   a small network of computers, for example, within a Hospital Trust to allow limited access and enable the sharing of confidential files within the organization.

intraocular   within the globe of the eye.

intraoperative probe   a very small footprint, high-frequency ultrasound probe which is inserted into blood vessels to visualize their anatomy, for example, in cardiac work.

intraoperative radiotherapy   radiotherapy that takes place during an operative procedure.

intraoral   within the mouth.

intraoral radiograph   a radiograph of a tooth when the film is placed inside the mouth. *See also* **periapical film**.

intraorbital   within the orbit.

intraosseous   inside a bone. The intraosseous route has been developed as a way of giving fluids when rapid establishment of systemic access is vital and venous access is impossible. It provides an alternative route for the administration of drugs and fluids until venous access can be achieved.

intraperitoneal   within the peritoneal cavity.

intrapharyngeal   within the pharynx.

intraplacental   within the placenta.

intrapleural   within the pleural cavity.

intrapulmonary   within the lungs, as intrapulmonary pressure.

intraspinal   within the spinal canal.

intrasplenic   within the spleen.

intrasynovial   within a synovial membrane or cavity.

intrathecal   within the meninges; into the subarachnoid space. A route used for the administration of certain drugs, such as antibiotic drugs for meningitis.

intrathoracic   within the cavity of the thorax, such as pressures.

intratracheal   within the trachea.

intrauterine   within the uterus.

intrauterine contraceptive device (IUCD, IUD)   a device which is inserted in the cavity of the uterus to prevent conception. Its exact mode of action is not known.

intrauterine fetal death   death of a fetus weighing at least 500 grams or after 24 weeks gestational age.

intrauterine growth restriction (IUGR) the impairment of fetal growth rate commonly arising due to placental insufficiency.

intrauterine transfusion of the fetus endangered by Rhesus inco-mpatibility. Red cells are transfused directly into the abdominal cavity of the fetus, on one or more occasions. This enables the induction of labour to be postponed until a time more favourable to fetal welfare.

intravaginal within the vagina.

intravascular within the blood vessels.

intravenous (IV) within or into a vein.

intravenous infusion (IVI) commonly referred to as a '*drip*': the closed administration of fluids from a containing vessel into a vein for such purposes as hydrating the body, correcting electrolyte imbalance or introducing nutrients.

intravenous injection the introduction of drugs, including anaesthetics, into a vein.

intravenous urography (IVU) demonstration of the urinary tract following an intravenous injection of a contrast agent.

intraventricular within a ventricle, especially a cerebral ventricle.

intrinsic detector efficiency the ability of a detector to produce a signal for each quanta of radiation falling on it.

introitus any opening in the body; an entrance to a cavity, particularly the vagina.

intubation placing of a tube into a hollow organ. *tracheal intubation* is used during anaesthesia. *duodenal intubation* a double tube is passed as far as the pyloric antrum under fluoroscopy, the inner tube is then passed along to the duodenojejunal flexure.

intussusception a condition in which one part of the bowel telescopes into another, causing severe colic and intestinal obstruction. It occurs most commonly in infants around the time of weaning.

intussusceptum the invaginated portion of an intussusception.

intussuscipiens the receiving portion of an intussusception

invagination the act or condition of being ensheathed; a pushing inward, forming a pouch.

invasion the entry of bacteria into the body or the spread of cancer cells.

inverse square law the intensity of radiation from a small isotropic source is inversely proportional to the square of the distance from the source, used in radiography for calculating the dose rate and exposure factors when changing the focus film distance.

inverse piezo-electric effect when an electric current is applied to a material it expands and contracts producing an ultrasound pulse.

inverse treatment planning   computer software to determine optimal isodose contours and maximum tumour dose for a given radiotherapy treatment, used in intensity modulated radiotherapy.

inversion   turning inside out, as inversion of the uterus.

inversion recovery   in magnetic resonance imaging it is the basic pulse sequence which inverts the magnetization and measures the time taken for the nuclei to return to equilibrium. The rate of recovery depends on the relaxation rate (T_1).

inversion time (TI)   in magnetic resonance imaging it is the time after the middle of a 180° radio frequency inverting pulse and the inversion recovery sequence to the middle of the 90° read pulse, and monitors the amount of longitudinal magnetization.

in vitro   in glass, as in a test tube.

in vitro fertilization (IVF)   human oocytes are fertilized by spermatozoa in test tubes in laboratories that are specialized in this technique.

in vivo   in living tissue.

involucrum   a sheath of new bone, which forms around necrosed bone, in conditions such as osteomyelitis. *See also* **cloaca**.

involuntary   independent of the will, as muscle of the thoracic and abdominal organs.

iodine (I)   an element required for the formation of thyroid hormones (T_3, T_4). *oral iodine* may be prescribed preoperatively for patients with hyperthyroidism to control the release of thyroid hormones and reduce vascularity of the gland. *radioactive isotopes of iodine*, for example, ^{131}I, are used in the diagnosis and treatment of thyroidconditions, such as cancer. Iodine is bactericidal and is used as *povidone iodine* for skin disinfection prior to invasive procedures. It is used within several proprietary wound dressings.

iodine seeds   a source of iodine^{125} used to treat the pituitary by permanently implanting the seeds and as surface applicators to treat the cornea.

ion   when an atom either loses or gains an electron it forms an ion. *See also* **anion, cation**.

ion channel   water-filled channels in the cell membrane that allow certain ions to pass through as in the transmission of nerve impulses. Some drugs act at the level of the ion channels.

ion-exchange resins   substances administered orally to reduce the level of specific ions (calcium and potassium) in the body such as in renal failure.

ionic bond   when one or more electrons move from one atom to another and then form ions which are attracted to each other as they have an opposite charge, after the electron exchange the shells in each ion appear to be intact.

ionization   the process of removing an electron from an atom, thus forming a positive ion.

ionization chamber   a device, containing air for measuring the potential dosage of a beam of radiation by collecting charge on an electrode, ***thimble ionization chamber*** a modification to enable the device to be used practically, it is smaller in size and uses an air equivalent medium in the capsule. Used in radiotherapy planning to record the output of the X-ray tube.

ionizing radiation   form of radiation that destabilizes an atom, forming an ion. Examples include gamma rays, X-rays and particle radiation. It has the ability to cause tissue damage. *See also* **radiation**.

ions   when an atom either loses or gains an electron it forms an ion.

IP address (Internet Protocol Address)   a unique number given to any computer when it is connected to the internet, it is formed by four blocks of three numbers, the highest being 255.

ipsilateral   affecting the same side of the body.

iridium (^{192}Ir)   a radioactive element used in brachytherapy to treat cancers in anus, tongue, breast as implanted wires or hair pins. Can also be used as a Selectron source.

iridium wire   a source of Iridium^{192} used in manual afterloading systems and is purchased by specifying the activity per unit length required.

iris   the circular pigmented structure forming the anterior one-sixth of the middle coat of the eyeball. It is perforated in the centre by an opening, the pupil. Contraction of its muscle fibres regulates the amount of light entering the eye. ***iris bombe*** bulging forward of the iris due to pressure of the aqueous behind, when posterior synechiae are present around the pupil.

iron (Fe)   a metallic element needed in the body as a constituent of haemoglobin and several enzymes.

irradiated volume   in radiotherapy, the quantity of tissue that receives a radiation dose that is considered to be significant in relation to normal tissue tolerance.

irradiation   exposure to any form of radiant energy such as heat light or X-rays. The lateral scattering of light in the emulsion layer of a radiographic film causing unsharpness.

irreducible hernia   when the contents of the sac cannot be returned to the appropriate cavity, without surgical intervention.

irregular bones   cancellous bones surrounded by a thin layer of compact bone and irregular in shape, for example the vertebrae, facial bones.

irritable   capable of being excited to activity; easily stimulated.

irritable bowel syndrome (IBS)   functional intestinal symptoms not explained by organic bowel disease. Symptoms include abdominal pain, bloating and change in bowel habit (alternating constipation and diarrhoea).

irritant   describes any agent which causes irritation.

ischaemia   deficient blood supply to any part of the body. *See also* **angina**.

ischaemic heart disease (IHD)   *see* **coronary heart disease**.

ischiorectal   associated with the ischium and the rectum, as an ischiorectal abscess which occurs between these two structures.

ischium   the lower part of the innominate bone of the pelvis; the bone on which the body rests when sitting.

ISDN (Integrated Services Digital Network)   a set of standards for the transfer of digital information over a telephone wire and other media.

islets of Langerhans   collections of special cells scattered throughout the pancreas, mainly concerned with endocrine function. The pancreatic islets contain four types of hormone-secreting cells: alpha cells, which secrete glucagon; beta cells, which secrete insulin; the delta cells, which secrete several substances, including somatostatin or growth hormone inhibiting hormone (GHIH); and others that produce regulatory pancreatic polypeptide.

isobar   any nucleus that has the same atomic mass number as another nucleus but with different atomic numbers. A line joining points of equal pressure.

isocentre   the point in space at which the central beams from each beam angle intersect. In CT this is the point of greatest accuracy of the reconstructed image, hence its importance when positioning a patient on the table prior to scanning. In radiotherapy, the point where the axis of rotation of the diaphragm, the horizontal axis of rotation of the gantry and the vertical axis of rotation of the couch intersect.

isocentric gantry   a C-shaped structure that connects the X-ray tube to the image intensifier so that the central beam from the X-ray tube is always aligned to the centre of the image intensifier.

isocentric reference mark   a point marked onto the patient to enable accuracy of repositioning, for example, in radiotherapy.

isodose chart   a number of isodose lines to represent the output from a specific source of radiotherapy equipment.

isodose contour   a line on an isodose chart that plots doses of equal value.

isodose curve   the graphical representation of the distribution of radiation dose within a uniform area.

isodose distribution   lines plotting the radiation dose received by the patient throughout the radiotherapy treatment area.

isodose lines   the lines that plot the areas of a patient that receive a radiation dose of equal value.

isodose surface   the graphical representation of the area of skin surface receiving a radiation dose.

isoelectric point   the pH value in which a substance or system is electrically neutral. In a film emulsion it determines some characteristics of the emulsion: the minimum solubility, viscosity, conductivity and swelling and determines how easily products are removed from the emulsion.

isolated limb perfusion   a method of introducing cytotoxic drugs into an isolated arterial supply by administering a tourniquet to the limb, under general anaesthetic.

isolation   separation of a patient from others for a number of reasons. *See also* **containment isolation, protective isolation, source isolation**.

isolator   apparatus ranging from what is virtually a large plastic bag in which a patient can be nursed to that in which surgery can be performed. It aims to prevent pathogenic microorganisms either gaining entry or leaving the enclosed space.

isometric transition   is the move from an excited state of a nucleus to a stable state.

isotonic   equal tension; applied to any solution which has the same osmotic pressure as the fluid with which it is being compared. *isotonic saline* (normal saline, physiological saline), 0.9% solution of sodium chloride in water.

isotope of an element   any nucleus which contains the same number of protons as the element but has a different mass number.

isotopes   two or more forms of the same element having identical chemical properties and the same atomic number but different mass numbers. Those isotopes with radioactive properties are used in medicine for research, diagnosis and treatment of disease.

isotropic   to emit radiation in all directions.

ISP (Internet Service Provider)   a company that enables access to the internet.

isthmus   a narrowed part of an organ or tissue such as that connecting the two lobes of the thyroid gland.

iteration   to repeatedly execute an instruction in a computer program.

iterative reconstruction algorithm   a mathematical method of image reconstruction which involves continually updating and adjusting the image as data are acquired. Back projection methods are more commonly used today.

J

Jacksonian epilepsy (focal epilepsy)   an epileptic attack caused by a brain tumour, encephalitis or a head injury, symptoms include limb twitching.

jargon   technical or specialized language that is understood only by a particular group, for example health professionals. Often used to describe the use of obscure and pretentious language, together with a roundabout way of expression.

Jarman index   system for weighting general practice populations according to social conditions. A composite index of social factors that general practitioners considered important in increasing workload and pressure on services. These factors were identified through a survey of one in ten general practitioners in the UK in 1981. An underprivileged area (UPA) score was then constructed based on the level of each variable in each area, weighted by the weighting assigned from the national general practitioner survey. Eight variables were used: (a) elderly living alone, (b) children aged under five years, (c) unskilled, (d) unemployed (as % economically active), (e) lone-parent families, (f) overcrowded accommodation (>1 person/room), (g) mobility (moved house within 1 year), (h) ethnic origin (new Commonwealth and Pakistan). Information on the variables were derived from the census.

jaundice   a condition characterized by a raised bilirubin level in the blood (hyperbilirubinaemia). Minor degrees are only detectable using tests. Major degrees are visible in the yellow discoloration of skin, sclerae and mucosae. Jaundice without the excretion of bilirubin in the urine is termed *acholuric*. Jaundice may be classified as follows: (a) *haemolytic or prehepatic jaundice* where excessive breakdown of erythrocytes releases bilirubin into the blood, such as in haemolytic anaemia. *See also* **haemolysis, haemolytic disease of the newborn**. (b) *hepatocellular jaundice* arises when liver cell function is impaired, such as with hepatitis or cirrhosis. (c) *obstructive* or *cholestatic jaundice* where the flow of bile is obstructed either within the liver (intrahepatic) or in the larger ducts of the biliary tract (extrahepatic). Causes include: cirrhosis, tumours, parasites and gallstones. *See also* **cholestasis**.

java   a programming language that works on all computer systems.

jaw-bone   describes either the upper jaw (maxilla) or lower jaw (mandible).

jejunum   that part of the small intestine between the duodenum and the ileum.

jig   a device for immobilizing patients during radiotherapy treatment.

joint the articulation of two or more bones (arthrosis). There are three main classes: (a) *fibrous* (*synarthroses*), e.g. the sutures of the skull; (b) *cartilaginous* (*amphiarthroses*), e.g. between the manubrium and the body of the sternum; and (c) *synovial* or freely movable (*diarthroses*), e.g. shoulder or hip. *See also* **Charcot's joint**.

joint cavity the space between the articular surfaces of bones. In the most common, synovial cavity, the ends of the bone are covered with articular hyaline cartilage and synovial fluid fills the space.

joule (J) the SI unit for measuring energy, work and quantity of heat. The unit (J) is the energy used when 1 kg (kilogram) is moved 1 m (metre) in the direction of the force of 1 N (newton). The *kilojoule* (kJ = 10^3 J) and the *megajoule* (MJ = 106 J) are used by nutritionists for measuring large amounts of energy.

JPEG (Joint Picture Experts Group) a compressed, computer graphics file used to store images on a computer.

jugular pertaining to the throat. *jugular veins* two veins passing down either side of the neck.

jukebox an electromechanical device for handling large numbers of optical computer disks to enable the rapid retrieval of archived data.

juvenile chronic arthritis (JCA) now more commonly termed *juvenile idiopathic arthritis*.

juvenile idiopathic arthritis (juvenile chronic arthritis) chronic inflammatory arthritis in children (previously termed *Still's disease*) features such as fever, rash and anaemia may be early signs of the disease.

juvenile osteochondritis a condition of the epiphyses or centres of ossification. It may be due to a poor blood supply causing the 'death of bone'.

juxtaglomerular close to the glomerulus. *juxtaglomerular apparatus (JGA)* cells in the distal tubule and the afferent arteriole of the nephron. They monitor changes in pressure and sodium levels in the blood, and initiate the release of renin. *See also* **macula densa**.

juxtapose to place side by side.

K-space the space that is filled with information and undergoes Fourier transformation to form a magnetic resonance image. By manipulating the K-space, faster sequences can be implemented.

Kaposi's sarcoma neoplasm characterized by new blood vessel growth producing red, purple or brown lesions, often on the skin, may metastasize to the lymph nodes and viscera. Originally common in Africa but now often seen in immunocompromised individuals, for example, those with acquired immunodeficiency syndrome (AIDS).

karyorrhexis disintegration of nuclear chromatin.

Keller's operation for hallux valgus or rigidus. Removal of the proximal half of the proximal phalanx, plus any bone growths (osteophytes) and bony outgrowths (exostoses) on the metatarsal head. The toe is fixed in the corrected position; after healing a pseudarthrosis results.

keloid an overgrowth of collagenous scar tissue at the site of a skin injury.

Kelvin the unit of thermodynamic temperature.

keratin a fibrous protein found in nails and the outer part of the skin and horns, etc.

keratitis inflammation of the cornea.

keratoacanthoma a benign, rapidly growing, flesh-coloured nodule on the skin with a central plug of keratin. The tumour is most common on the face, back of the hands and the arms.

kerma kinetic energy released per unit mass of an absorber, unit joules per kilogram or grays.

ketonaemia ketone bodies in the blood.

ketones organic compounds (e.g. ketosteroids) containing a keto group. *ketone bodies* include acetone, acetoacetate (acetoacetic acid) and β-hydroxybutyric acid produced normally during fat oxidation. Can be used as fuel but excess production leads to ketoacidosis. This may occur when blood glucose level is high, but unavailable for metabolism, as in poorly controlled diabetes mellitus.

ketonuria ketone bodies in the urine.

ketosteroids steroid hormones that contain a ketone group. The 17-ketosteroids are excreted normally in urine and are present in excess in overactivity of the adrenal glands and the gonads.

keV   the energy given to an electron when passing through a potential difference of 1 kilovolt in a vacuum.

keyboard   a microprocessor with a range of keys which when depressed send an electrical code to a computer which then displays the appropriate image on a monitor or carries out an appropriate action.

kidney   paired retroperitoneal organs situated on the upper posterior abdominal wall in the lumbar region. Help to maintain stability by producing urine to excrete waste such as urea, control water and electrolyte balance and blood pH. They also secrete renin and renal erythropoietic factor (REF) and are involved in vitamin D metabolism.

kidney failure   inability of the kidneys to maintain normal function. *See also* **renal failure**.

kidney function tests   a series of tests that include: routine urine testing, urine concentration/dilution tests, serum urea and electrolytes, serum creatinine and renal clearance to estimate glomerular filtration rate (GFR).

kidney machine (artificial kidney)   the machine used to remove waste products from the blood in the case of renal failure. *See also* **dialyser**.

kidney transplant   surgical transplantation of a kidney from a previously tested suitable live donor or a donor who has recently died. Kidneys may also be transplanted from the renal bed to other sites in the same individual in cases of ureteric disease or trauma.

killers   impurities added to the intensifying screen crystal to control after-glow.

kilogram (kg)   one of the seven base units of the International System of Units (SI). A measurement of mass.

kilojoule (kJ)   a unit equal to 1000 joules. It is used to measure large amounts of energy. It replaces the kilocalorie (kcal) which is still commonly used. *See also* **calorie**.

kilovoltage treatment unit   radiotherapy units operating in the region of either 50–150 kV for the treatment of external, superficial lesions or 150–300 kV for treatment of metastatic bone lesions and some primary bone lesions.

kinase   an enzyme activator that converts a zymogen to its active form. Enzymes that catalyse the transfer of a high-energy group of a donor, usually adenosine triphosphate (ATP), to some acceptor, usually named after the acceptor (e.g. fructokinase).

kinetic   relating to or producing motion.

kinetic energy   the energy which a body possesses by virtue of its motion, unit joule.

Kirschner wire   a wire drilled into a bone to apply skeletal traction. A hand or electric drill is used, a stirrup is attached and the wire is rendered taut by means of a special wire-tightener.

Klumpke's paralysis   paralysis and atrophy of forearm and hand muscles, sometimes caused by birth injury.

klystron   a microwave device which amplifies the power of radiofrequency radiation. When used with a radiofrequency driver it acts as the radiofrequency power source in some linear accelerators.

knee   the synovial condylar joint formed by the lower end of the femur and the tibial condyles and the patella with the patellar articular surface of the femur.

knee jerk   a reflex contraction of the relaxed quadriceps muscle caused by a tap on the patellar tendon: usually performed with the lower femur supported behind, the knee bent and the leg limp. Persistent variation from normal usually signifies organic nervous disorder.

knuckles   the dorsal aspect of any of the joints between the phalanges and the metacarpal bones, or between the phalanges of the hand.

Köhler's disease   osteochondritis of the navicular bone. Confined to children of 3–5 years.

Korotkoff sounds   the sounds audible when recording non-invasive arterial blood pressure with a sphygmomanometer and stethoscope. The phases are: (1) a sharp thud – systolic pressure, (2) a swishing sound, (3) a soft thud, (4) a soft blowing that becomes muffled, (5) silence. Opinion is divided as to whether phase 4 or 5 should represent diastolic pressure.

Krebs cycle (citric acid cycle, tricarboxylic acid cycle)   the final common pathway for the oxidation of fuel molecules: glucose, fatty acids, glycerol and amino acids. These enter the cycle as acetyl coenzyme A (CoA) and are oxidized to produce energy ATP (adenosine triphosphate), carbon dioxide and water.

Krukenberg tumour   a secondary (metastatic) malignant tumour of the ovary, usually spread from primary stomach (gastric) cancer.

Küntscher nail   used for intramedullary fixation of fractured long bones, especially the femur. The nail has a 'clover-leaf' cross-section.

kV_p   the maximum kilovoltage applied across an X-ray tube in a forward direction during an exposure.

kypholordosis   coexistence of kyphosis and lordosis.

kyphoscoliosis   coexistence of kyphosis and scoliosis. May prevent proper lung expansion and respiratory problems.

kyphosis   as in **Pott's disease**, an excessive backward curvature of the dorsal spine. Commonly associated with osteoporosis.

L

labia (lips) ***labia majora*** two large lip-like folds of skin extending from the mons veneris to form the vulva. ***labia minora*** two smaller folds lying within the labia majora.

labial (buccal) adjacent to the lips or cheeks.

labioglossolaryngeal relating to the lips, tongue and larynx.

labyrinth the cavities of the internal ear including the cochlea and semicircular canals. ***bony labyrinth*** that part which is directly hollowed out of the temporal bone. ***membranous labyrinth*** the membrane lining the bony labyrinth.

labyrinthectomy surgical removal of part or the whole of the membranous labyrinth of the internal ear. Sometimes carried out for Ménière's disease.

labyrinthitis inflammation of the internal ear.

laceration a wound with torn and ragged edges.

lacrimal, (lachrymal, lacrymal) associated with tears.

lacrimal bone a tiny bone at the inner side of the orbital cavity.

lacrimal duct connects lacrimal gland to upper conjunctival sac.

lacrimal gland situated above the upper, outer canthus of the eye.

lacrimonasal associated with the lacrimal and nasal bones and ducts.

lactacid (lactic) anaerobic system a series of chemical reactions occurring within the cells where a very small amount of adenosine triphosphate (ATP) for energy use is produced from glucose, without oxygen. The end product being lactic acid.

lactacid oxygen debt component the amount of oxygen required to remove lactic acid from muscle tissue and blood during the process of recovery from intense exercise.

lactase (β-galactosidase) digestive enzyme present in the small intestine mucosa. It catalyses the hydrolysis of lactose to glucose and galactose.

lactation secretion of milk, the period during which an infant receives nourishment from breast milk.

lacteals the commencing lymphatic ducts in the intestinal villi; they absorb digested fats and convey them to the cisterna chyli.

lactiferous conveying or secreting milk.

lactose deficiency the management depends on severity and may involve the exclusion or restriction of lactose-containing foods.

lacuna a space between cells; usually used in the description of bone.

lamella a thin plate-like scale or partition. A ring of bone round a haversian system. A gelatine-coated disc containing a drug; it is inserted under the eyelid.

lamina a thin plate or layer, usually of bone.

lamina dura a layer of bone forming the outer layer of the socket in which a tooth lies.

lamination layering, soft iron sheets with insulation between each sheet found in a transformer core to reduce eddy currents.

laminectomy removal of vertebral laminae – to expose the spinal cord nerve roots and meninges. Most often performed in the lumbar region, for removal of degenerated intervertebral disc.

LAN (Local Area Network) a number of computers connected together, for example in a hospital.

laparoscopic cholecystectomy removal of the gallbladder using minimally invasive surgical techniques. *See also* **laparoscopy**.

laparoscopy (peritoneoscopy) endoscopic examination of the internal organs by the transperitoneal route. A laparoscope is introduced through the abdominal wall after induction of a pneumoperitoneum. A variety of surgical procedures are performed in this way, including biopsy, cyst aspiration, division of adhesions, tubal ligation, assisted conception techniques, appendicectomy and cholecystectomy.

laparotomy incision of the abdominal wall. Usually reserved for exploratory operation.

Larmor equation ($\omega = \gamma B_0$) the proportional relationship between the precessional angular frequency of a nuclear magnetic moment (ω in Hertz) and the main magnetic field (B_0 in Tesla). The gyromagnetic constant (γ) is a proportionality constant and is fixed for the nucleus, for example, 42.6 MHz/Tesla for hydrogen.

Larsen syndrome multiple joint dislocations.

laryngeal associated with the larynx.

laryngeal mask airway with inflatable cuff placed via the mouth into the oropharynx to maintain the airway during general anaesthesia.

laryngeal mirror mirror for inspecting the oral cavity and larynx.

laryngectomy surgical removal of the larynx.

laryngitis inflammation of the larynx.

laryngopharynx the lower portion of the pharynx.

laryngoscope instrument for visualization of the larynx, for diagnostic or therapeutic purposes or to facilitate the insertion of an endotracheal tube into the larynx under direct vision.

laryngoscopy   direct or indirect visual examination of the interior of the larynx.

laryngostenosis   narrowing of the glottic aperture.

laryngotomy   surgical opening in the larynx.

laryngotracheal   associated with the larynx and trachea.

larynx   the organ of voice situated below and in front of the pharynx and at the upper end of the trachea.

laser (Light Amplification by Stimulated Emission of Radiation)   a tube in which stimulated emission takes place and the light produced oscillates in a regular pattern to produce a high-energy, coherent, parallel beam of light. Energy is transmitted as heat which can coagulate tissue. Used in the production of modern radiographic images by exposing a film to laser light. Has many therapeutic uses that include: endometrial ablation, detached retina, skin lesions and cancer. Precautions must be taken by those using lasers as eye damage can occur.

laser back pointer   mounted in the counterbalance of the gantry of radiotherapy equipment and projects a sheet of light in the direction of the axis of rotation of the gantry and the axis of rotation of the diaphragm system indicating the entry and exit point of the radiation beam.

laser printer   characters or images are built up by the image being scanned by a laser and then toner is fused onto the paper to produce the final print.

laser printing film   a single-sided emulsion used with imaging plates.

latent image   the image produced on a film after exposure but prior to development.

latent period   the time between the exposure to a carcinogenic agent and the clinical appearance of disease.

lateral   at or belonging to the side; away from the median line.

lateral decubitus radiograph   the patient lies on their side and the central ray passes from the anterior to the posterior aspect of the body. The projection is named after the side of the body that is uppermost.

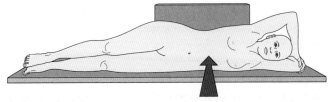

Lateral decubitus. From Pocketbook of radiographic positioning, 2nd edn, Ruth Sutherland, 2003, Churchill Livingstone, Edinburgh, with permission.

lateral radiograph   the patient is either erect or lying with the side of their body nearest the film. The projection is named after the side of the body nearest the film.

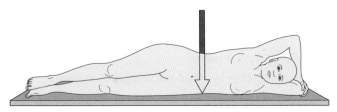

Lateral projection. From Pocketbook of radiographic positioning, 2nd edn, Ruth Sutherland, 2003, Churchill Livingstone, Edinburgh, with permission.

lateral resolution   in ultrasound, the ability to see small structures that lie along the beam, this is equal to the effective beam width and is best at the focus and reduces the further away from the focus the object is.

latex allergy   an allergic reaction to natural latex or one of the components used in production of latex equipment such as medical gloves and catheters. Latex allergy is becoming increasingly common in healthcare workers due to the increased use of gloves following the rise in the incidence of blood-borne viruses.

latissimus dorsi   muscle of the back.

latitude   the range of useful exposures a film will tolerate. *See also* **useful exposure range**.

latitude emulsions   a film with a reduced average gradient of 2.2 to enable a large range of densities to be recorded.

laughing gas   nitrous oxide (N_2O).

lavage   irrigation of or washing out a body cavity.

law of conservation of energy   energy can neither be created nor destroyed but can be changed from one form to another. The amount of energy in a system is therefore constant.

law of conservation of matter   matter is neither created nor destroyed, but it may change its chemical form as a result of chemical reaction.

law of conservation of momentum   the total linear or rotational momentum in a given system is constant.

laxatives (aperients)   drugs used to prevent or treat constipation. Administered orally, or rectally as suppositories or by enema. They may be: bulking agents that retain water and form a large, soft stool; faecal softeners that lubricate or soften the faeces; osmotic laxatives that increase fluid in the bowel lumen; stimulants that increase peristalsis, and combined softeners and stimulants.

lead equivalence a method of comparing protection barriers by calculating the thickness of lead required to have the same absorption to an exposure to radiation.

lead poisoning caused by excessive intake of lead, radiographically, dense transverse lines appear at the shafts of long bones.

lead shielding shielding blocks of lead placed on a tray below the radiotherapy tube to shape the radiation beam so that it accurately covers the treatment area and/or shields organs at risk. Alternative products may be used, usually alloys of bismuth or cadmium. *See also* **MCP block**.

lead strip a contouring device formed by placing a lead strip round the patient and the skin markings are transferred to the lead using marker pen, the markings are then copied onto papers giving the patient contour.

leakage radiation unwanted radiation that is emitted from an X-ray tube in directions other than the useful beam, it is reduced by the addition of lead round the X-ray tube.

lecithins a group of phospholipids found in animal tissues, mainly in cell membranes. They are present in surfactant. ***lecithin-sphingomyelin ratio*** a test which assesses fetal lung maturity. Below 2.0 is indicative of a higher risk of neonatal respiratory distress syndrome.

Leeds test objects a number of different test objects produced by the University of Leeds, used for quality control in radiology, to test, for example, film-screen combinations, television systems and CT scanners, etc.

left anterior oblique a radiographic projection with the patient either erect or semi prone at 45° to the film with the left side of the body closest to the film and the right side away from the film.

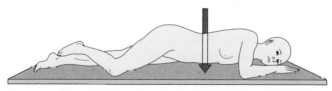

Left anterior oblique (LAO). From Pocketbook of radiographic positioning, 2nd edn, Ruth Sutherland, 2003, Churchill Livingstone, Edinburgh, with permission.

left colic (splenic) flexure is situated at the junction of the transverse and descending parts of the colon. It lies at a higher level than the right (hepatic) flexure.

left posterior oblique a radiographic projection with the patient either erect or semi supine at 45° to the film with the left side of the body closest to the film and the right side away from the film (see figure on p. 232).

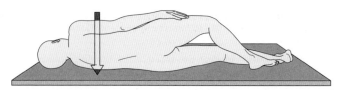

Left posterior oblique (LPO). From Pocketbook of radiographic positioning, 2nd edn, Ruth Sutherland, 2003, Churchill Livingstone, Edinburgh, with permission.

left ventricular assist device (LVAD)   mechanical pump used to increase the output of blood from the left ventricle of the heart. May be used in the short term to support critically ill patients, those waiting for a heart transplant, or to give the heart time to recover from disease.

leg   lower limb.

Legionella   a type of small Gram-negative bacillus associated with infected water supplies.

legionnaires' disease   a severe and often fatal pneumonia caused by *Legionella pneumophila*; there is pneumonia, dry cough, and often non-pulmonary involvement such as gastrointestinal symptoms, renal impairment and confusion. A cause of both community- and hospital-acquired pneumonia, it is associated with an infected water supply in public buildings such as hospitals and hotels. There is no person-to-person spread.

leg length discrepancy   a difference of up to 1 cm in true length is considered to be within a normal variation. The effects of discrepancy may either cause a compensatory pelvic tilt and secondary spinal scoliosis, or will force the person to walk on their toes in order to lengthen the leg. The latter will, in time, result in shortening of the Achilles tendon.

leimyoma   a benign tumour of smooth muscle.

leiomyosarcoma   a sarcoma which contains large spindle cells of unstriated muscle.

Leksell unit   a stereotactic radiotherapy unit containing a hemispherical array of 201 collimated, cobalt sources. It is usually used for the delivery of single fractions of radiation to intracranial targets.

lens   the small biconvex crystalline body which is supported by the suspensory ligament immediately behind the iris of the eye. On account of its elasticity, the lens can alter in shape, enabling light rays to focus exactly on the retina. A glass or plastic used to correct refractive errors (spectacles or contact lens) or in optical instruments.

Lenz's law   the direction of the induced current in a conductor caused by a changing magnetic flux is such that its own magnetic field opposes the changing magnetic flux. The law only applies in closed circuits.

leptomeningeal disease   a vascular abnormality of the skin described as resembling a port wine stain. Inflammation of the pia mater and arachnoid membranes of the brain and spinal cord.

lesion   pathological change in a bodily tissue.

lesser omentum   a smaller fold, passing between the transverse fissure of the liver and the lesser curvature of the stomach.

leucocytes   generic name for white blood cells. They are nucleated, mobile and are all involved with body defences, e.g. some are phagocytic and others produce antibodies. There are two main groups: (a) *polymorphonuclear cells* or *granulocytes* (neutrophils, basophils and eosinophils) – these have a many-lobed nucleus and granules in their cytoplasm; (b) *monocytes* and *lymphocytes* – these generally have no granules, but some lymphocytes are granular.

leucocytolysis   destruction and disintegration of white blood cells.

leucocytosis   increased number of leucocytes in the blood. Often a response to infection.

leucopenia   decreased number of white blood cells in the blood.

leucoplakia   *see* **leukoplakia**.

leucopoiesis   formation of white blood cells from stem cells.

leukaemia   a progressive, malignant disease of the blood-forming organs, with, most commonly, abnormal proliferation of white cells (leucocytes). Uncontrolled proliferation of the leukaemic cells causes secondary suppression of other blood components, and anaemia and a reduction in the number of platelets in the blood (thrombocytopenia) result. The lack of mature white cells increases the risk of infection, thrombocytopenia increases the risk of bleeding, and anaemia is also characteristic. Causes include ionizing radiation, previous chemotherapy, retroviruses, chemicals, genetic anomalies (e.g. Down's syndrome). The classification is according to cell type – lymphocytic or myelocytic, and the course acute or chronic. The chronic leukaemias may enter a 'blast crisis' or acute phase. Therapeutic options include chemotherapy, radiotherapy, interferon alpha, monoclonal antibodies and bone marrow transplantation, either using the patient's bone marrow (autologous) or that of a donor (allograft). *See also* **myeloproliferative disorders**.

leukoplakia   chronic inflammation characterized by white, thickened patches on the mucous membranes, particularly on the tongue, gums and inside the cheeks. Usually patchy and often premalignant. *See also* **kraurosis vulvae**.

leukotrienes   regulatory lipids derived from arachidonic acid (fatty acid). They function as signalling molecules in the inflammatory response and in some allergic responses.

levator   a muscle which acts by raising a part. An instrument for lifting a depressed part.

Lhermitte's sign   an electric shock-like symptom radiating down the spine and into the limbs.

Lhermitte's syndrome   flexion of the neck. A syndrome characterized by lymphoblastic infiltrations of the peripheral nervous system – associated with paresis.

lien   the spleen.

lienculus   a small accessory spleen.

lienorenal   associated with the spleen and kidney. *See also* **splenorenal**.

Li-Fraumeni syndrome   familial breast cancer affecting young women and associated with soft-tissue sarcomas and other cancers in close relatives.

ligament   a band of fibrous tissue binding joints together and connecting the articular surfaces to allow movement. A layer of serous membrane extending from one organ to another, for example, the peritoneum.

ligate   to tie off blood vessels, etc., at operation.

ligation   tying off; usually reserved for ligation of the uterine (fallopian) tubes, a method of sterilization.

ligature   the material used for tying vessels or stitching the tissues. *See also* **suture**.

light adaptation   adjustments made by the eye in bright light. The pupils constrict, rhodopsin breakdown reduces retinal sensitivity and cone activity increases. *See also* **dark adaptation**.

light beam diaphragm   a light source, incorporated in the tube housing to visually indicate the area covered by the radiation emitted from the X-ray tube.

light pen   a device, shaped like a pen, which interfaces with a computer screen and enables the computer to know which part of the screen is being pointed to.

Likert scale   a scale used in questionnaire surveys. Participants are asked to specify their degree of agreement with a particular statement, i.e. strongly agree, agree, unsure, disagree and strongly disagree.

liminal   of a stimulus, of the lowest intensity that can be perceived by human sense organs. *See also* **subliminal**.

line defects   edge dislocation when an extra plane of atoms extends into the crystal lattice.

linea   a line.

linea alba   the white line visible after removal of the skin in the centre of the abdomen, stretching from the ensiform cartilage to the pubis, its position on the surface being indicated by a slight depression.

lineae albicantes   white lines which appear on the abdomen after reduction of tension as after childbirth, tapping of the abdomen, etc. *See also* **striae**.

linea nigra   pigmented line from umbilicus to pubis which appears in pregnancy.

linear accelerator   radiotherapy equipment where electrons produced by an electron gun pass through a waveguide and are accelerated and fed into a treatment head to produce high-energy X-rays or an electron beam used in the treatment of various cancers.

linear array   in ultrasound, a set of elements mounted in line and pulsed electronically in sequence to produce a rectangular field of view.

linear attenuation coefficient (μ)   measures the probability of photon interaction along the path of an X-ray beam, that is the fraction of X-rays removed from a beam per unit thickness of the attenuating medium. Differences in the linear attenuation coefficient are responsible for radiographic image contrast and it is a series of these measurements which are used to produce the image in CT. It is dependent upon the beam energy, and the structure and density of the material traversed.

linear energy transfer   the energy that a particle dissipates, per unit length of its path, as it travels through absorbing medium.

linear expansivity   is a measure of thermal expansion and is defined as the change in unit length per unit change in temperature in degrees Kelvin.

linear measurement   the measurement of a straight line between two points.

linear scanner   in radionuclide imaging the crystal moves backwards and forwards across an organ, the images are then recorded as a photoscan or a dot diagram. The equipment has been superseded by gamma cameras.

linear sources   several collinear tubes mounted in an applicator and used in intercavitary therapy to treat line sources, for example the uterine canal.

lingua   the tongue.

lingual   next to the tongue.

linitis plastica   a form of gastric cancer which infiltrates throughout the gastric wall. This leads to diffuse thickening and failure to inflate at endoscopy and barium examinations.

lipase   any fat-splitting enzyme, such as pancreatic lipase. They convert fats into fatty acids and glycerol.

lipogenesis   a metabolic process where amino acids and glucose are converted to triglycerides (triacylglycerols) prior to storage in adipose tissue. It is stimulated by insulin.

lipoma   a benign tumour of fatty tissue, which develops in connective tissue.

lipoprotein   lipids combined with a protein that transport triglycerides (triacylglycerols) and cholesterol around the body in the blood. They are classified as: *high-density lipoproteins* (HDLs), *low-density lipoproteins* (LDLs) or *very-low-density lipoproteins* (VLDLs). A high level of LDL in the blood is associated with arterial disease whereas HDLs are considered to be protective. A high HDL:LDL is associated with a decreased risk of arterial disease.

liposarcoma   a malignant tumour of the fat cells.

liquid crystal display   a form of flat screen imaging monitor using liquid crystals and a back light to produce the image. In colour monitors each pixel is subdivided into three colours, red, blue and green by the use of filters, each of which can be activated independently to produce the colour image.

liquid scintillation process   a method of detecting radionuclides which decay solely by beta decay. The solution used contains a solvent, a scintillation solute and a secondary solute in which is dissolved a radionuclide.

liquor   a solution. *liquor amnii* fluid surrounding the fetus.

Lisfranc injury   dislocation of the third, fourth and fifth metatarsals with a fracture through the base of the second metatarsal.

LISP (LISt Processor language) a high-level computer language.

literature review   a methodical and wide-ranging examination of the papers relevant to a topic. Research methods and results are analysed and presented critically. The literature review includes how the search was carried out, e.g. bibliographical databases such as Medline.

lithiasis   any condition in which there are calculi.

litholapaxy (lithopaxy)   crushing a stone within the urinary bladder and removing the fragments by irrigation.

lithotripsy   destruction of calculi by crushing using high-powered ultrasound.

lithotriptor   a machine which sends shock waves through renal calculi, causing them to fragment and be passed naturally in the urine.

lithotrite   an instrument for crushing a stone in the urinary bladder.

litmus   a vegetable pigment used as an indicator of alkalinity (blue) or acidity (red). Often stored as paper strips: red litmus paper turns blue when exposed to an alkali; blue litmus paper turns red with an acid.

liver   the largest gland in the body, the weight in adults is within the range 1.2–1.5 kg. The liver is situated in the right upper part of the abdominal cavity. It is vital to homeostasis and its functions include: breakdown of red blood cells with the production of bile, detoxification of drugs and hormones, nutrient metabolism, protein synthesis and storage of glycogen, vitamins and minerals. The liver is the site of considerable heat generation.

liver function tests   blood tests used to assess liver function including: alanine aminotransferase, alkaline phosphatase, aspartate aminotransferase, coagulation tests, gamma-glutamyltransferase, serum bilirubin and serum proteins.

liver transplant   liver failure may be treated by surgical transplantation of a liver from a suitable donor.

lobe   a rounded section of an organ, separated from neighbouring sections by a fissure or septum, etc.

lobectomy removal of a lobe, for example lung or liver.

lobule a small lobe or a subdivision of a lobe.

local anaesthetic a drug used to render a specific area of the body insensitive to pain.

localization the method of delineating the exact clinical target volume in a patient prior to radiotherapy treatment.

localize to limit the spread. To determine the site of a lesion.

local rules rules outlining safe working practices of employees working with or coming into contact with radiation.

locomotor can be applied to any tissue or system used in movement. Most usually refers to nerves and muscles. Sometimes includes the skeletal system.

locomotor ataxia the disordered gait and loss of sense of position (proprioception) in the lower limbs, which occurs in tabes dorsalis.

locoregional referring to a specific part of the body.

loculated divided into numerous cavities.

loculation the presence of many small spaces or cavities.

logarithm the logarithm of a number to a given base, is the power by which the base must be raised to give the number. For example the logarithm of 100 to the base 10 is 2 as $10^2 = 100$.

log It curve *see* **characteristic curve**.

loin that part of the back between the lower ribs and the iliac crest; the area immediately above the buttocks.

long bones these have a shaft of compact bone with a central medullary cavity, the ends are expanded, for example, the femur, the radius.

longitudinal magnetization (M$_z$) part of the macroscopic magnetization vector, parallel to the main magnetic field (B$_o$). Following radio frequency excitation it returns to its equilibrium value (M$_o$) due to the characteristic time constant (T$_1$) of the tissues that have been excited.

longitudinal relaxation time (T$_1$, spin-lattice relaxation time, T$_1$ relaxation time) in magnetic resonance imaging, the time taken for the spins to give the energy obtained from the initial radio frequency impulse, back to the surrounding environment and return to equilibrium. It represents the time required for the longitudinal magnetization (M$_z$) to go from 0 to 63% of its final maximum value.

longitudinal study research study where data are collected on more than one occasion, such as the study of a group of people over time. *See also* **cohort study**.

loopography the radiographic investigation of an ileal conduit, a Foley catheter is inserted and dilated to block the conduit and contrast agent is injected under fluoroscopic control and plain films are taken.

Looser's zones   pseudo (or false) fractures.

LOP (left occipitoposterior)   used to describe the position of the fetus in the uterus.

lordoscoliosis   lordosis complicated by the presence of scoliosis.

lordosis   an exaggerated forward, convex curve of the lumbar spine.

lordotic radiograph   a chest projection where the patient is positioned for a routine PA chest and leans backwards, towards the X-ray tube by approximately 30–40°, taken to demonstrate a right middle lobe collapse or an interlobular pleural effusion.

low back pain   the commonest cause seems to be posteriolateral prolapse of the intervertebral disc, putting pressure on the dura and cauda equina and causing the localized pain of lumbago. It can progress to trap the spinal nerve root, causing the nerve distribution pain of sciatica.

low birthweight   term used to indicate a weight of 2.5 kg or less at birth, whether or not gestation was below 37 weeks. *See also* **small for gestational age**.

low-density lipoprotein (LDL)   *see* **lipoprotein**.

low energy X-ray beam   radiotherapy beam in the order of 50–160 kV, very low energy beam 8–50 kV.

lower motor neuron   a specialist nerve cell where the cell is in the anterior horn of the spinal cord and the axon passes to skeletal muscle.

lower respiratory tract infection (LRTI)   pneumonia.

low spatial frequency algorithm   in CT scanning an algorithm used to provide high contrast resolution. Frequently used in soft-tissue studies to demonstrate inherently low contrast tissues in close proximity.

low temperature chemistry   radiographic processing chemicals with a higher concentration of hydroquinone, a different restrainer and a higher concentration of preservative which have a working temperature range of 26–33°C and a pH of about 10.00.

LSI (Large Scale Integration)   a means of packing large numbers of electronic circuits into small chips.

LSP (Local Service Provider)   a company that supplies computer networking, for example, NHS PACS has five LSPs to deliver the system countrywide.

lubb-dupp   words descriptive of the heart sounds as heard on auscultation.

lubricants   faecal softeners that also lubricate and facilitate easy and painless defecation. *See also* **laxatives**.

lumbago   incapacitating pain low down in the back.

lumbar   associated with the loin for example lumbar nerve, lumbar vertebrae.

lumbar puncture (LP) the withdrawal of cerebrospinal fluid (CSF) through a hollow needle inserted into the subarachnoid space in the lumbar region of the spine. The CSF obtained is examined for its chemical (e.g. glucose) and cellular (e.g. white blood cells) constituents and for the presence of microorganisms; CSF pressure can be measured by the attachment of a manometer. Contrast agent can be introduced to demonstrate the subarachnoid space, spinal cord, nerve roots, ligaments, and associated structures.

lumbocostal associated with the loin and ribs.

lumbosacral associated with the loin or lumbar vertebrae and the sacrum.

lumen the space inside a tubular structure.

luminescence is caused when a material absorbs short wave length radiation and therefore lower energy photons are released, usually in the visible or near visible spectrum.

luminosity the measure of the amount of light emitted from an object.

lumpectomy the surgical excision of a tumour with removal of minimal surrounding tissue. Increasingly used, with radiotherapy and chemotherapy, for treatment of breast cancer.

lunate one of the eight carpal bones found in the wrist.

lungs the two main organs of respiration which occupy the greater part of the thoracic cavity; they are separated from each other by the heart and other contents of the mediastinum. They are concerned with gas exchange – the oxygenation of blood and excretion of carbon dioxide. *lung transplantation* may be single, double, *heart–lung transplants*, or sometimes in the case of child recipients, live-related *lobar transplants*.

lung ventilation the passage of air in the lungs studied by the inhalation of a radioactive gas.

lunula the semilunar pale area at the root of the nail.

luteinizing hormone (LH) a gonadotrophin secreted by the anterior pituitary gland. In females high levels in mid menstrual cycle stimulate ovulation and formation of the corpus luteum. The same hormone in males is called interstitial-cell stimulating hormone (ICSH); it stimulates the production of testosterone by the testes.

luxation partial dislocation.

lymph the fluid contained in the lymphatic vessels. It is formed from interstitial (tissue) fluid and is similar to plasma. Unlike blood, lymph contains only one type of cell, the lymphocyte. *lymph circulation* that of lymph collected from the tissue spaces; it then passes via capillaries, vessels, nodes and ducts to be returned to the blood. *lymph nodes* accumulations of lymphatic tissue at intervals along lymphatic vessels. They mainly act as filters. They provide a site for B and T lymphocyte/cell proliferation and the production of immunoglobulins.

lymphadenectomy   excision of one or more lymph nodes.

lymphadenitis   inflammation of a lymph node.

lymphadenopathy   any disease of the lymph nodes.

lymphangiectasis   dilation of the lymph vessels.

lymphangiography   lymphography.

lymphangioma   a simple tumour of lymph vessels frequently associated with similar formations of blood vessels.

lymphangioplasty   any plastic surgery on lymph vessels, such as those used to improve drainage. *See also* **lymphoedema**.

lymphangitis   inflammation of a lymph vessel.

lymphatic   associated with, conveying or containing lymph.

lymphoblast   an immature lymphocyte. Present in the blood and bone marrow in conditions such as acute lymphoblastic leukaemia (ALL).

lymphocyte   one variety of white blood cell. The lymphocytic stem cells undergo transformation to T lymphocytes/cells (in the thymus), which provide cellular immunity involved in destroying cancer cells, virus-infected cells and transplanted cells (graft), or B lymphocytes/cells, which form immunoglobulins (antibodies) and provide humoral immunity. The transformation is usually complete a few months after birth.

lymphocytosis   an increase in lymphocytes in the blood.

lymphoedema   excess fluid in the tissues from abnormality or obstruction of lymph vessels that blocks or interrupts lymph drainage. There is swelling of (usually) a limb and increased risk of cellulitis. It may occur, for example, after lymph node resection and/or radiotherapy; most common in breast cancer. Treated by compression bandaging.

lymphoepithelioma   rapidly growing malignant pharyngeal tumour. May involve the tonsil. Often has metastases in cervical lymph nodes.

lymphography   the radiographic investigation of the lymphatic system following the direct injection of contrast agent into a lymphatic vessel of the foot. Generally replaced by CT scanning.

lymphoid   associated with lymph. ***lymphoid tissue*** tissue similar to lymph nodes, situated in a variety of locations, bone marrow, gut, liver, spleen, thymus and tonsils.

lymphokines   a term applied to cytokines produced by stimulated T lymphocytes. They function during the immune response as intercellular chemical mediators.

lymphoma   a group of neoplastic diseases developing in lymphoid tissue. Lymphoma is characterized by lymph node enlargement, night sweats/ swinging pyrexia, pain from splenic enlargement/infarction, hepatomegaly, weight loss, malaise or recurrent infection. Causes include viral infections but most are idiopathic. Classified according to histological appearances to either ***Hodgkin's lymphoma*** or ***non-Hodgkin's*** lymphoma (NHL). Staging depends on sites involved – location and number, as well as associated 'secondary' symptoms. Therapy may be radiotherapy alone for the earliest stages, and/or chemotherapy. Bone marrow transplantation may also be necessary. *See also* **Burkitt's lymphoma**.

lymphosarcoma obsolete term for some types of lymphoma.

lysis the gradual decline of a disease, the destruction of cells.

lysozyme an antibacterial enzyme present in many body fluids such as tears and saliva.

lytic lesion disintegration or breakdown usually of bone cells.

. . . .

mA   the average electrical current passing through an X-ray tube during an exposure measured in milliamperes.

machine code   the language the computer can understand directly; all instructions are written in binary.

machine tank developer   the initial developer used in automatic processing machine and consists of developer replenisher and starter solution.

MacMillan nurses   nurses based both in hospitals and in the community who provide advice on symptom control and provide psychological support for cancer patients and their families.

macrocephaly   large head, not caused by hydrocephalus.

macrocyte   a large red blood cell. Occurs in megaloblastic anaemia (for example, pernicious anaemia) and in association with excess alcohol intake, liver disease and hypothyroidism.

macrocytosis   an increased number of macrocytes.

macrodactyly   excessive development, enlargement, of the fingers or toes.

macroglossia   an abnormally large tongue.

macrophages   mononuclear cells, which destroy foreign bodies and cell debris by phagocytosis. Part of the monocyte–macrophage (reticuloendothelial) system, they are derived from monocytes. *See also* **histiocytes**.

macroscopic   visible to the unaided eye; gross. *See also* **microscopic**.

macula   a spot.

macula densa   special cells of the nephron. Forms part of the juxtaglomerular apparatus.

macula lutea (yellow spot)   area of the retina responsible for clearest central vision.

magic angle artefact   in magnetic resonance imaging of a joint, if a tendon lies at an angle of 55° to the static magnetic field it appears brighter on T_1 and proton density weighted images but has a normal low signal on T_2 weighted images, and therefore can be potentially confused with pathology.

magnesium (Mg)   a metallic element needed in the body for many enzyme-catalysed reactions. Magnesium is an intracellular positively charged ion (cation) and is present in bone, and its metabolism is linked to that of calcium.

magnesium oxide   used at the back of the crystal in scintillation counters to direct light back towards the sodium iodide crystal.

magnet   a substance containing a north and a south pole.

magnetic disk   an 8-inch double-sided, double-density disk for storing images of up to 1.2 Mbytes.

magnetic domain   an area of a substance when all the atoms are pointing in the same direction.

magnetic field   exists when a point of force is experienced by a magnetic pole placed at the point.

magnetic flux   the lines of force through a magnetic field.

magnetic induction   if a substance contains magnetic atoms and is placed in a magnetic field and the poles of the atoms become aligned magnetizing the substance.

magnetic moment   a measure of the magnitude and direction of the magnetic properties of an object or particle that cause it to align with the static main field and form its own local magnetic field.

magnetic resonance   the absorption of the emission of the electromagnetic energy by nuclei in a static magnetic field following excitation by a radio frequency pulse. The resonant frequency of the pulse and the emitted signal are proportional to the strength of the magnetic field.

magnetic resonance imaging (MRI; nuclear magnetic resonance (NMR))   a non-invasive technique that does not use ionizing radiation. It uses radiofrequency radiation in the presence of a powerful magnetic field to produce high-quality images of the body in any plane.

magnetic resonance signal   the electromagnetic signal produced by the precession of the transverse magnetism of the spins which induce a voltage in the receiver coil which is then amplified by the receiver to form the signal.

magnetic susceptibility (χ)   the ability of a substance to become magnetized or to distort a magnetic field. *See also* **diamagnetic, paramagnetic, superparamagnetic, ferromagnetic**.

magnetic tape   tape that can store 180 Mbytes of information.

magnetization transfer contrast   in magnetic resonance imaging when the image contrast is manipulated by selectively saturating a pool of protein bound water. By applying an off-resonance pulse (1000–2000 Hz) these proteins are suppressed. As the protein bound water and the bulk water protons are in rapid exchange the saturation is transferred to the bulk phase of the water protons leading to a reduction in signal from the bulk water. Used to demonstrate small peripheral vessels and aneurysms in the brain and the detection of early demyelination or protein destruction.

magneto-optical disk   a disk used to store computer data by a combination of a magnetic field on the disk and the use of a laser to write or read the information thus enabling a large quantity of data to be stored on the disk.

magnetron   a piece of equipment that contains an anode and a cathode in a vacuum which are placed in a uniform magnetic field which causes the electrons to travel in a spiral, curved path from the cathode to the anode to produce radiowaves. A high-power radiofrequency oscillator used to power some linear accelerators.

magnitude   size.

magnum   large or great, as foramen magnum in occipital bone.

mainframe   a large computer, usually the centre of a system. Intelligent peripherals can then be attached.

major accident procedure   a detailed management plan allocating staffing, resources and areas of responsibility, used in incidents where more than 15 casualties are expected.

mal   disease.

mal de mer   seasickness.

malabsorption   defective absorption of nutrients from the digestive tract.

malabsorption syndrome   loss of weight and fat in the faeces (steatorrhoea), varying in severity. Caused by: (a) disease of the small intestine; (b) lack of digestive enzymes or bile salts; (c) surgical operations.

malalignment   faulty alignment, for example, bones after a fracture.

malar   relating to the cheek.

malformation   abnormal shape or structure; deformity.

malignant   virulent and dangerous.

malignant growth (tumour)   one that demonstrates the capacity to invade adjacent tissues/organs and spread (metastasis) to distant sites; often rapidly growing and with a fatal outcome. *See also* **cancer, sarcoma**.

malignant hyperpyrexia   a rare inherited condition which presents in response to certain anaesthetic drugs and neuroleptic (antipsychotic) drugs; there is progressive increase in body temperature and, if untreated, may be fatal.

malignant lymphoma   a malignant carcinoma of the thyroid gland which may spread to the lymph nodes or recur in the gastrointestinal tract.

malignant melanoma   malignant cutaneous mole or freckle (usually); it is the most dangerous of all skin cancers. Related to overexposure to ultraviolet radiation (sunburn); most common in fair-skinned, blond/red-haired people. It is characterized by change in colour, shape, size of mole or with bleeding or itching in a mole. The prognosis depends on Breslow thickness; staging involves lymph node status, with sentinel node biopsy (SNB) now becoming an integral part along with computed tomography (CT) scan. Surgery is the only curative treatment with chemotherapy and radiotherapy of limited effectiveness.

malignant pustule   virulent skin lesion. *See also* **anthrax**.

malignant tumour   a growth which is not encapsulated, infiltrates adjacent tissue, causes metastases which spread to other parts of the body and may ultimately result in the death of the patient. *See also* **cancer, sarcoma**.

malleolus   a part or process of a bone shaped like a hammer. ***external malleolus*** at the lower end of the fibula. ***internal malleolus*** situated at the lower end of the tibia.

mallet finger   a fracture where the dorsal base of a phalanx is torn away.

malleus   the hammer-shaped lateral bone of the middle ear. *See also* **incus, stapes**.

malocclusion   any deviation from the normal occlusion of the teeth, often associated with an abnormal jaw relationship. *See also* **orthodontics**.

malposition   any abnormal position of a part.

malpractice   improper or injurious medical or nursing treatment. Professional practice that falls below accepted standards and causes harm. It may be negligence, unethical behaviour, abuse or criminal activities.

malrotation   a congenital abnormality of the bowel when the distal limb of the mid gut fails to rotate on returning to the abdomen. Identified on ultrasound by looking at the placement of the blood vessels supplying the bowel.

maltase (α-glucosidase)   an enzyme found in intestinal juice. It converts maltose to glucose.

maltoma   low-grade β-cell lymphoma of the mucosa-associated lymphoid tissue. It may be related to *Helicobacter pylori* infection which, when eradicated, may lead to regression of disease.

malunion   the union of a fracture in a poor position.

mamma   the breast.

mammaplasty   any plastic operation on the breast. *See also* **augmentation, implant, reduction**.

mammilla   the nipple. A small papilla.

mammography   radiographic demonstration of the breast by use of specially low-penetration (long-wavelength) X-rays. Used in the diagnosis of or screening for breast conditions including cancer.

mandible   the bone forming the lower jaw.

manipulation   using the hands skilfully as in reducing a fracture or hernia, or changing an abnormal fetal position to facilitate a vaginal delivery.

Mann–Whitney test   a non-parametric statistical test comparing two sets of unmatched data using a table of values for U. If the results are less than the values in the table the results are significant. It is a substitute to Student's t test for independent groups.

manometer an instrument for measuring the pressure exerted by liquids or gases. Used for example for measuring the pressure exerted by the cerebrospinal fluid during lumbar puncture, or for measuring central venous pressure.

mantle technique so called because the treatment area represents a cloak, the field dimensions are larger than the patient and therefore shielding of the lungs is required, used to treat Hodgkin's disease. Consists of anterior and posterior parallel pair, shielding of the spinal cord may be required from the posterior field.

manual evacuation digital removal of faeces from the rectum.

manubrium a handle-shaped structure; the upper part of the sternum.

marble bones *see* **osteopetrosis**.

march fracture a type of stress fracture caused by an increase in physical activity which may so stress a metatarsal (usually the second) to produce an undisplaced self-healing hair-line crack. Management usually involves moderate rest with supportive padding and strapping for a few weeks but sometimes a walking plaster is required.

marginal cost the cost of providing the extra resources required to carry out activity above a baseline number.

marrow *see* **bone marrow**.

mAs the average electrical current passing through an X-ray tube during an exposure multiplied by the exposure time in seconds.

mass the amount of matter in a body.

mass attenuation coefficient is the linear attenuation coefficient divided by the density of the medium the beam passes through and is used to describe the probability of an interaction occurring between the X-ray beam and the tissue.

mass number the total mass of neutrons and protons within an atom.

mastalgia pain in the breast.

mast cells basophils (type of leucocyte) that have migrated to the tissues. They are located around small blood vessels and bind to IgE before producing chemicals such as histamine that are involved in inflammation and anaphylaxis.

mastectomy the surgical removal of one or both breasts due to malignant disease or the prevention of malignant disease. *simple* only breast tissue is removed. *radical* some of the muscles of the chest are removed along with the breast and axillary lymph nodes. *See also* **lumpectomy**.

mastication chewing.

mastitis inflammation of the breast. *chronic mastitis* the name formerly applied to the nodular changes in the breasts now usually called fibrocystic disease.

mastoid   nipple-shaped.

mastoid air cells   extend in a backward and downward direction from the antrum.

mastoid antrum   the air space within the mastoid process, lined by mucous membrane continuous with that of the tympanum and mastoid cells.

mastoid process   the prominence of the mastoid portion of the temporal bone just behind the ear.

mastoidectomy   drainage of the mastoid air-cells and excision of diseased tissue. *cortical mastoidectomy* all the mastoid cells are removed making one cavity which drains through an opening (aditus) into the middle ear. The external meatus and middle ear are untouched. *radical mastoidectomy* the mastoid antrum, and middle ear are made into one continuous cavity for drainage of infection. Loss of hearing is inevitable.

mastoiditis   inflammation of the mastoid air-cells.

matrix   the foundation substance in which the tissue cells are embedded. In digital imaging, the rows and columns of pixels on a display used to form a digital image.

maxilla   the upper jaw.

maxillary sinuses   two, pyramidal shaped cavities which lie on either side of the nasal cavity.

maxillofacial   associated with the maxilla and face.

maxillofacial surgery   branch of surgery concerned with the surgical management of developmental disorders and diseases of the facial structure.

maximum density (D Max)   the maximum density which can be reached on a film under set exposure and processing conditions, determined using a characteristic curve. *See also* **characteristic curve**.

maximum intensity projection   a volume rendering technique used to visualize high-intensity structures within a data acquisition. Achieved by a step by step process for producing projections from a two-dimensional or three-dimensional volume data set which is processed along selected angles. The highest data value for each pixel taken from a specific viewing angle is displayed. Used to demonstrate vascular structures in CT scanning and also in MR scanning.

McMurray's osteotomy   division of femur between lesser and greater trochanter. Shaft displaced inwards beneath the head and abducted. This position maintained by a nail plate. Restores painless weight bearing. In developmental dysplasia of the hip, deliberate pelvic osteotomy renders the outer part of the socket (acetabulum) more horizontal.

MCP block (LMPA, low melting-point alloy block)   an alloy of lead, bismuth, cadmium and zinc which can be formed into individually shaped shielding blocks. These can be mounted below the head of the radiotherapy machine providing customized shielding of normal tissue.

mean   the average. *arithmetic mean* a figure arrived at by dividing the sum of a set of values by the number of items in the set. *See also* **central tendency statistic, median, mode**.

mean dose point   in radiotherapy, the central dose point when all the doses are plotted by increasing or decreasing size.

mean window level   the average range of pixel values in an image.

meatus   an opening or channel.

mechanical ventilation   *see* **intermittent positive pressure ventilation**.

Meckel's diverticulum   a blind, pouch-like sac sometimes arising from the free border of the lower ileum. Occurs in 2% of the population: usually symptomless. May cause gastrointestinal bleeding or intussusception.

media   the middle coat of a vessel. Nutritive jellies used for culturing bacteria. *See also* **medium**.

medial   associated with or near the midline, or to the middle layer of a structure.

median   the middle. A central tendency statistic; the midway or middle value in a set of scores when placed in increasing order. *See also* **mean, mode**.

median line   an imaginary line passing through the centre of the body from a point between the eyes to between the closed feet.

median plane   a vertical plane that divides the body into right and left halves. Also called the *midsagittal plane, median sagittal plane*.

median sagittal plane   an imaginary plane passing vertically through the mid line of the body dividing it into right and left halves.

mediastinoscopy   a minor endoscopic surgical procedure for visual inspection of the mediastinum. May be combined with biopsy of the lymph nodes for histological examination, and diagnosis or staging in the case of cancer.

mediastinum   the space between the lungs. Contains the heart, great vessels and the oesophagus.

medical audit   systematic and critical review of medical care, including diagnosis and treatment, outcomes and quality of life.

medical ethics   a set of moral values and principles of conduct for professionals working with patients.

medical jurisprudence   *see* **forensic medicine**.

medical shock   shock caused by the loss of circulating blood volume as a result of dehydration, haemorrhage, vomiting, diarrhoea or severe burns. Now called *hypovolaemic shock*.

medication   a therapeutic substance or drug, administered orally or by injection intra-arterially, subcutaneously, intramuscularly, intravenously, or rectally, topically, transdermally or sublingually.

medicinal   associated with a medicine.

medicine   science or art of healing, especially as distinguished from surgery and obstetrics. A therapeutic substance. *See also* **drug**.

mediolateral   associated with the middle and one side.

medium   a substance used in bacteriology for the growth of microorganisms.

Medline   computerized database of medical science and associated literature.

medulla   the marrow in the centre of a long bone. The internal part of organs, for example, kidneys, adrenals and lymph nodes, etc. ***medulla oblongata*** the lowest part of the brainstem where it passes through the foramen magnum to become the spinal cord. It contains the nerve centres controlling various vital functions, for example, cardiac centres.

medullary   associated with the medulla.

medullary carcinoma   a malignant carcinoma of the thyroid gland which is slow growing and may have calcium present, it spreads to the lymph nodes and mediastinum.

medullary cavity   the hollow centre of a long bone, containing yellow bone marrow or medulla.

medullated   containing or surrounded by a medulla or marrow, particularly referring to myelinated nerve fibres.

medulloblastoma   malignant, rapidly growing tumour occurring in children; usually in the midline of the cerebellum.

megacephalic (macrocephalic, megalocephalic)   large headed.

megacolon   of the colon. ***acquired megacolon*** associated with chronic constipation of any cause, or may occur in acute severe colitis of any cause (***toxic megacolon***). ***congenital megacolon*** (***Hirschsprung's disease***) due to absence of ganglionic cells in a distal segment of the colon with loss of relaxation resulting in dilatation of the normal proximal colon.

megakaryocyte   large multinucleated cells of the marrow that produce platelets (thrombocytes).

megaloblastic anaemia   an anaemia caused by a deficiency of vitamin B_{12} or folate. It results in the formation of large red blood cells called megaloblasts.

megalocephalic   *see* **megacephalic**.

megavoltage radiotherapy units   radiotherapy units operating in the range of 4–25 megavolts, for example linear accelerators, used for external beam radiotherapy treatments.

meibomian glands   sebaceous glands lying in grooves on the inner surface of the eyelids, their ducts opening on the free margins of the lids.

Meigs syndrome   a benign, solid ovarian tumour associated with ascites and hydrothorax.

meiosis   a stage of reduction cell division when the chromosomes of a gamete are halved in number ready for union at fertilization.

melaena   black, tar-like stools. Evidence of gastrointestinal bleeding.

melanin   a brown/black pigment found in hair, skin and the choroid of the eye.

melanocytes   cells in the skin that produce melanin when stimulated by the pituitary hormone *melanocyte stimulating hormone* (MSH).

melanoma   a malignant tumour arising from the pigment-producing cells (melanocytes) of the skin, or of the eye. *See also* **malignant melanoma**.

melatonin   a hormone produced by the pineal body (gland) in response to the amount of light entering the eye. Influences sexual development and is involved in reproductive function. Also influences mood and various circadian rhythms, such as body temperature and sleep.

membrane   a thin lining or covering substance. *See also* **basement membrane, hyaloid membrane, mucous membrane, serous membrane, synovial membrane, tympanic membrane**.

menarche   when menstrual cycles commence.

meninges   the surrounding membranes of the brain and spinal cord. They are the *dura mater* (outer), *arachnoid membrane* (middle) and *pia mater* (inner). *See also* **meningitis**.

meningioma   a slowly growing fibrous tumour arising in the meninges.

meningism (meningismus)   a condition describing irritation and inflammation of the meninges due normally to infection or haemorrhage and consisting of neck stiffness and photophobia.

meningitis   inflammation of the meninges around the brain and spinal cord that can be due to an acute bacterial (for example, *meningococcal meningitis*) or viral infection, chronic infective and inflammatory conditions and occasionally malignancy.

meningocele   protrusion of the meninges through a bony defect. It forms a cyst filled with cerebrospinal fluid. *See also* **spina bifida**.

meningoencephalitis   inflammation of the brain and the meninges.

meningomyelocele (myelomeningocele)   protrusion of a portion of the spinal cord and its enclosing membranes through a bony defect in the spinal canal. It differs from a meningocele in being covered with a thin, transparent membrane which may be granular and moist.

meniscectomy   the removal of a semilunar cartilage of the knee joint, following injury and displacement. The medial cartilage is damaged most commonly.

meniscus   semilunar cartilage, particularly in the knee joint. The curved upper surface of a column of liquid.

menopause   the ending of menstruation. A period of time during which ovarian activity declines and eventually ceases (the climacteric). It normally occurs between the ages of 45 and 55 years. *artificial menopause* an earlier menopause caused by surgery or radiotherapy.

menorrhagia   an excessive regular menstrual flow.

menses   fluid discharged from the uterus during menstruation; menstrual flow.

menstrual   relating to the menses. *menstrual* or *uterine cycle* the cyclical changes that occur as the endometrium responds to ovarian hormones. There are three phases: proliferative, secretory, and menstrual in which bleeding occurs for about 5 days. The cycle is repeated approximately every 28 days (21–35 days), except during pregnancy, from the menarche to the menopause.

menstruation   the flow of blood and endometrial debris from the uterus once a month in the female. It usually starts at the age of 12–13 years in developed countries, and ceases around 50 years of age.

mentoanterior   forward position of the fetal chin in the maternal pelvis in a face presentation.

mentoposterior   backward position of the fetal chin in the maternal pelvis in a face presentation.

menu   a set of choices presented in a computer program.

mesencephalon   the midbrain.

mesenchymoma   a neoplasm composed of two or more cellular elements which are not usually associated with each other and fibrous tissue.

mesentery   a large sling-like fold of peritoneum passing between a portion of the intestine and the posterior abdominal wall. Contains nerves, lymphatics and blood vessels.

mesial   towards the front or the mid line.

mesoderm   middle layer of the three primary germ layers of the early embryo. It gives rise to the cardiovascular system, lymphatic system, bone, muscles, blood, the dermis, pericardium, pleura, peritoneum, urogenital tract, gonads and the adrenal cortex. *See also* **ectoderm, endoderm**.

mesothelioma   a rapidly growing tumour of the pleura (commonly), pericardium or peritoneum; usually associated with asbestos exposure at least 20 years previously. Industrially related, therefore compensation usually appropriate as few are operable and the median survival post-diagnosis is about 8 months. Therapy is almost universally palliative; generally chemo- and radioresistant.

mesovarium   a double fold of peritoneum that attaches the ovary to the broad ligament.

meta-analysis   a statistical summary of several research studies using complex quantitative analysis of the primary data.

metabolic   associated with metabolism. ***basal metabolic rate*** (BMR) the expression of basal metabolism in terms of kJ per m^2 of body surface per hour.

metabolic accumulation   the concentration of a substance in the body through the metabolic process, for example, iodine in the thyroid gland.

metabolism   the continuous series of chemical processes in the living body by which life is maintained. Nutrients and tissues are broken down (***catabolism***), new substances are created for growth and rebuilding (***anabolism***) and energy is released in catabolism and utilized in anabolism and heat production. *See also* **adenosine diphosphate, adenosine triphosphate, basal metabolism**.

metabolite   any product of or substance taking part in metabolism. An ***essential metabolite*** one that is necessary for normal metabolism, for example, vitamins.

metacarpophalangeal   associated with the metacarpal bones and the phalanges.

metacarpal bones   the five bones which form that part of the hand between the wrist and fingers.

metachronous   subsequent.

metal exchange   a method of silver recovery when the fixer solution passes through a base metal which is replaced by the silver and base metal ions are released into the solution which then goes to waste.

metaphysis   in a long bone, the side of the epiphyseal plate which is nearest the shaft and is the site of the production of bone during childhood. *See also* **epiphysis**.

metaplasia   a change from one type of tissue to another.

metastable state   when a nucleus is decaying and the length of time it takes can be measured.

metastasis   the secondary spread of malignant tumour cells from one part of the body to another. Either by the lymphatic route to the lymph nodes or to distant organs via the haematogenous (blood) route or can be transplanted during surgery. Most solid tumours are not curable if metastasis has occurred.

metatarsal bones   the five bones of the foot between the ankle and the toes.

metatarsophalangeal   associated with the metatarsus and the phalanges.

metatarsus adductus   a deformity where the forefoot is deviated towards the midline of the body in relation to the hindfoot.

methicillin-resistant *Staphylococcus aureus* (MRSA)   strains of *Staphylococcus aureus* that are resistant to methicillin (not used clinically) and flucloxacillin.

Causes serious and sometimes fatal infections in hospitals, and patients with MRSA are increasingly encountered outside hospital. Treatment involves vancomycin or teicoplanin, or various combinations of rifampicin, sodium fusidate and ciprofloxacin. Topical mupirocin is used to eliminate nasal or skin carriage. Infection control measures that include strict adherence to hand washing, proper environmental cleaning and isolation or patient cohorting are vital in controlling MRSA. Epidemic strains (**EMRSA**) have developed resistance to most antibiotics except glycopeptides, i.e. vancomycin and teicoplanin.

metritis inflammation of the uterus.

metrorrhagia uterine bleeding between the menstrual periods such as after intercourse or examination.

micelle tiny globules of fat and bile salts formed during fat digestion. Fatty acids and glycerol are transported into the intestinal cells (enterocytes) in this form, leaving the bile salts behind in the lumen of the bowel.

microcephaly an abnormally small head.

microcirculation blood flow through the arterioles, capillaries and venules. Damage to these vessels is a cause of pressure ulcers.

microcolon a small colon.

microglial cells a type of macrophage of the central nervous system.

micrognathia failure of the development of the lower jaw forming a receding chin.

microgram (μg) one millionth of a gram.

micrometre (μg) also still called a **micron**. One millionth of a metre.

micron *see* **micrometre**.

microorganism (microbe) a microscopic cell. Often synonymous with bacterium but includes virus, protozoon, rickettsia, chlamydia and fungus.

microprocessor an integrated circuit that can be pre-programmed to perform a variety of tasks.

microvilli microscopic projections from the free surface of cell membranes whose purpose is to increase the exposed surface of the cell for absorption, for example, intestinal epithelium.

micturating cystogram radiographic examination that can be used to investigate urinary incontinence. Following intravenous injection of a contrast agent or, more commonly, after contrast is introduced into the bladder via a urinary catheter until micturating begins. A series of radiographs are taken during the act of passing urine.

micturition (urination) passing urine.

midbrain that section of the brain that connects the cerebrum with the pons and cerebellum.

midriff the diaphragm.

midsagittal plane   *see* **median plane**.

milligram (mg)   one thousandth part of a gram.

millilitre (ml)   one thousandth part of a litre. Equal to a cubic centimetre.

millimetre (mm)   one thousandth part of a metre.

millimole (mmol)   one thousandth part of a mole.

Milwaukee brace   an orthotic device used in the corrective treatment of spinal curvature (scoliosis). It applies fixed traction between the occiput and the pelvis.

MIME (Multipurpose Internet Mail Extensions)   a method of sending binary objects by email.

mineralocorticoid   a group of corticosteroid hormones produced by the adrenal cortex. Involved in the regulation of electrolyte and water balance. *See also* **aldosterone**.

miscarriage   spontaneous loss of pregnancy before 24 completed weeks of gestation (previously referred to as abortion). *See also* **complete miscarriage, incomplete miscarriage, inevitable miscarriage, missed miscarriage, recurrent miscarriage, septic miscarriage, spontaneous miscarriage, threatened miscarriage, tubal miscarriage**.

missed abortion   a condition when a dead fetus or embryo remains in the uterus for 2 months or more before 24 weeks of age.

missed miscarriage   the early signs and symptoms of pregnancy disappear and the fetus dies but is not expelled for some time. *See also* **carneous mole**.

Mitchell theory   theory of latent image formation states that free silver ions come near to a shallow electron trap and deepens it, while this trap is deepened it attracts another electron and a free silver ion to form a silver atom called the pre-image centre. This then dissociates into a silver ion and an electron, the silver atom must attract a second silver ion to form a latent sub-image centre, this attracts further electrons causing a build up of silver atoms which eventually destroy the crystal lattice and allows development to take place. *See also* **Gurney Mott theory**.

mitosis   nuclear (and usually cell) division, in which somatic cells divide. It involves the exact replication of chromosomes, which results in two 'daughter' cells that are genetically identical to the cell of origin.

mitral   mitre-shaped, as the valve between the left atrium and ventricle of the heart (bicuspid valve).

mitral regurgitation (incompetence)   a defect in the closure of the mitral valve whereby blood tends to flow backwards into the left atrium from the left ventricle.

mitral stenosis   narrowing of the mitral orifice, usually due to rheumatic fever.

mitral valvulotomy (valvotomy)   an operation to correct a stenosed mitral valve.

mixing valve   a method of controlling the water and temperature of a unit by mixing the hot and cold water supplies together, found in automatic film processors.

M mode   motion modulation in ultrasound imaging when a linear scan is held while a time position graph of any motion builds up. Stationary parts are shown as straight lines and moving parts as oscillations, used in cardiac work to assess distances and the movement of objects.

modal dose   the most frequently occurring dose value in a chart.

mode   the most frequent (common) value in a series of scores. *See also* **central tendency statistic, mean, median**.

modem (MOdulator-DEModulator)   a device, also known as an acoustic coupler, which allows the computer to transmit data down a conventional telephone line.

modulation transfer function (MTF)   the assessment of an imaging system's performance at different object sizes.

Mohs' micrographic surgery   a surgical technique for microscopically controlled excision usually of a malignant skin tumour.

moist gangrene   death of part of the tissues of the body, occurs when venous drainage is inadequate so that the tissues are swollen with fluid.

molar tooth   multi-cusped posterior grinding tooth, placed fourth and fifth from the midline in the primary dentition, and sixth, seventh and eighth in the secondary dentition. The upper molars have three roots and the lower molars have two roots.

molar pregnancy   when a hydatidiform mole develops from the placental (trophoblastic) tissue of the early embryo, it is associated with raised human chorionic gonadotrophin (HCG) and may be benign or malignant.

mole   one of the seven base units of the International System of Units (SI), the measurement of amount of substance which contains as many elementary particles as there are atoms in 0.012 kilograms of carbon 12. A pigmented area on the skin, usually brown, they may be flat, some are raised and occasionally have hairs growing from them, alterations in shape, colour, size, or bleeding may be indicative of malignant changes.

molecular distortion   when the electron orbits are deformed relative to the atomic nucleus.

molecular weight   the sum of the atomic weights of atoms in a molecule.

molecule   combination of two or more atoms to form a specific chemical substance. The smallest part of a compound that can exist on its own and retain all the properties of the compound.

mollities   softness.

molluscum   a soft tumour.

molluscum contagiosum   an infectious condition common in infants caused by a virus. Tiny translucent papules with a central depression are formed.

molluscum fibrosum   the superficial tumours of von Recklinghausen's disease.

momentum   the product of the mass and the velocity of the body.

monarticular   relating to one joint.

monitor   a device similar to a television, but which receives video signals directly from the computer, rather than RE-modulated signals, giving much more accurate resolution. An anglicized version of the Rush Medicus quality assurance programme for use in hospitals.

monitor photography   the imaging of the video output from CT, MRI or ultrasound unit via a camera system.

monitoring   sequential recording. Term usually reserved for automatic visual display of measurements such as temperature, pulse, respiration and blood pressure. In management, looking at an activity in relation to a specification or target.

monoamine oxidase   an enzyme that breaks down monoamines, such as dopamine, 5-hydroxytryptamine (serotonin) and noradrenaline (norepinephrine) in the brain.

monoarthritis   arthritis affecting a single joint.

monochromatic emulsions   are film emulsions that are unable to detect any colours apart from the blue part of the visible spectrum, tend to be used with calcium tungstate screens.

monocyte   a phagocytic white blood cell. It migrates to the tissues to become a macrophage.

monocyte–macrophage system (reticuloendothelial system)   a widely disseminated system of specialized phagocytes in the bone marrow, liver, lymph nodes, spleen, and other tissues. Functions include blood cell and haemoglobin breakdown, formation of bile pigments, removal of cell breakdown products and as part of the defences against microorganisms.

monoenergetic   single energy.

mononuclear   describes a cell with a single nucleus such as a monocyte.

mononucleosis   an increase in the number of circulating monocytes (mononuclear cells) in the blood.

monoplegia   paralysis of only one limb.

mons veneris   the eminence formed by the pad of fat which lies over the pubic bone in the female.

Monteggia fracture-dislocation   fracture of the ulna associated with dislocation of the radial head.

morbidity   the state of being diseased. *standardized morbidity ratio* (SMBR) the degree of self-reported limiting long-term illness indirectly standardized for variations in age and gender.

moribund   in a dying state.

mortality number or frequency of deaths. ***mortality rate*** the death rate; the ratio of the total number of deaths to the total population. There are several specialized mortality rates and ratios including: ***childhood mortality*** (children aged 1–14 years), ***infant mortality*** (first year of life), ***maternal mortality*** (deaths associated with pregnancy and childbirth), ***neonatal mortality*** (first four weeks of life), ***perinatal mortality*** (stillbirths plus deaths in the first week of life), stillbirth rate. *See also* **standardized mortality rate, standardized mortality ratio**.

mortality rate the number of deaths per 1000 or other unit, of the population occurring annularly from a certain disease or condition.

Morton's neuroma a benign tumour of the nerve cells, which typically occurs between the third and fourth toes, characterized by a thickening of the tissue that surrounds the digital nerve.

mother board the main circuit board in a computer.

motile able to move spontaneously.

motor associated with action.

motor agraphia inability to express thoughts in writing, usually due to left precentral cerebral lesions.

motor neuron the nerve cell (or neuron) that supplies the electrical input to muscles. This can be either the ***lower motor neuron*** that directly innervates the muscles and originates in the brainstem and spinal cord or the ***upper motor neuron*** that originates from the motor cortex part of the brain and innervates the lower motor neuron.

motor neuron disease a group of neurodegenerative disorders affecting the nerves that supply the muscles leading to weakness and eventually death.

motor skill the ability to perform a particular task which involves significant movement of one or more joints of the body, for example, as part of a sports skill.

motor unit a lower motor neuron and all of the muscle fibres it innervates.

mottle the granular appearance in areas of even density on a radiographic image. *See also* **film grain, quantum mottle, structure mottle**.

mouse a device for making the computer more 'user friendly'. Instead of accessing the computer via a keypad, the mouse is used by rolling the device across a desktop, this moves a cursor to icon displays on the screen.

Mousseau-Barbin Tube a plastic intubation tube which is pulled through an oesophageal tumour by the use of a string or guidewire and is attached to the stomach with a suture. Used to maintain a free passage of food and fluid.

movement unsharpness blurring on an image due to movement of the equipment or the person which can be either voluntary or involuntary, for example heart beat.

mucin glycoprotein constituent of mucus.

mucinolysis breakdown of mucin.

mucocutaneous associated with mucous membrane and skin. ***mucocutaneous lymph node syndrome*** (MLNS) a disease affecting mainly babies and children. It is an inflammatory vasculitis characterized by fever, dry lips, red mouth and strawberry-like tongue. There is a rash on the trunk, and erythema with desquamation affecting the extremities. There is cervical lymphadenopathy, polymorphonuclear leucocytosis and a raised ESR. Also known as ***Kawasaki disease***.

mucosa a mucous membrane.

mucositis inflammation of the mucous membrane such as the lining of the mouth and throat.

mucous associated with or containing mucus, for example, mucous membrane.

mucous membrane contains glands which secrete mucus. It lines the cavities and passages that communicate with the exterior of the body.

mucous polyp a growth (adenoma) of mucous membrane which becomes pedunculated.

mucus viscid secretion of mucous glands.

multiaxial joints a joint which has movement round more than two axes, for example, the hip joint.

multicellular having many cells.

multi-leaf collimation (MLC) a method of customized beam shaping in radiotherapy without the use of lead blocks.

multilobular possessing many lobes.

multiplanar reconstruction in CT scanning, the formation of an image in any plane from the acquired axial data set.

multiple myeloma a form of bone marrow cancer resulting from the accumulation of malignant plasma cells.

multisection CT a CT scanner using multiple rows of detectors to enable several slices to be obtained at the same time thus increasing the speed of image acquisition.

multi-slice spiral CT scanner CT scanners that collect up to 64 slices (2006) of data during a spiral scan.

multivariate statistics analysis of three or more variables simultaneously. Used to clarify the association of two variables after allowing for other variables.

Munchausen syndrome a condition characterized by frequent requests for treatment or hospitalization for a symptomatic but imaginary illness. The patient may logically and convincingly present the symptoms and history of a real disease.

Munchausen syndrome by proxy (MSP) a condition when a parent or carer frequently fabricates or induces illness in a child with the intent of keeping them in hospital or in contact with doctors.

mural   associated with the wall of a structure.

murmur (bruit)   abnormal sound heard on auscultation of heart or great vessels, presystolic murmur characteristic of mitral stenosis.

muscle   one of the four basic tissues. Composed of specialized contractile tissue formed from excitable cells. There are three types. *cardiac muscle* makes up the middle wall of the heart; it is involuntary, striated and innervated by autonomic nerves. *skeletal muscle* is voluntary, striated and innervated by the peripheral nerves of the central nervous system. *red muscle, white muscle. smooth* or *involuntary muscle* is non-striated and involuntary and is innervated by the autonomic nerves.

muscle fibre   a muscle cell. Skeletal muscle fibres are classified according to type of action and metabolism: *muscle fibre type I* (*slow twitch*) fibres are characterized by relatively slow contraction time and high aerobic capacity. They are well suited to long duration activities. *muscle fibre type IIa* (*fast oxidative glycolytic*) fibres that are classed as fast-twitch but have some of the aerobic characteristics of slow-twitch fibres. *muscle fibre type IIb* (*fast twitch glycolytic*) fibres characterized by very fast contraction time and high anaerobic capacity. *muscle fibre type FT type C* fibres are thought to function at the extreme end of the anaerobic metabolic range.

musculature   the muscular system, or any part of it.

musculocutaneous   associated with muscle and skin.

musculoskeletal   associated with the muscular and skeletal systems.

mutation   a gene or chromosome alteration that results in genetic changes that alter the characteristics of the affected cell. The change is transmitted through succeeding generations. Mutations may be spontaneous, or induced by agents such as ionizing radiation that alter the chromosomal DNA.

mutual induction   when a changing current is passed through one conductor and produces a changing magnetic field, if another conductor is placed in the field an electromotive force will be formed in the second conductor.

myasthenia   muscle weakness.

mycosis fungoides   a malignant skin tumour from T-lymphocytes.

mycotoxins   poisons produced from fungi.

myelin   the white, fatty substance that covers and insulates some nerve fibres. *See also* **white matter**.

myelitis   inflammation of the spinal cord.

myeloablative   describes the therapy (for example, radiotherapy, chemotherapy) given intentionally to completely 'knock out' the bone marrow. Used in leukaemia and often precedes a bone marrow transplant.

myeloblasts   the early precursor cells of the polymorphonuclear granulocytic white blood cells.

myelocele   an accompaniment of spina bifida wherein development of the spinal cord itself has been arrested, and the central canal of the cord opens on the skin surface discharging cerebrospinal fluid.

myelocytes   precursor cells of polymorphonuclear granulocytic white blood cells.

myelography   radiographic examination of the spinal canal by injection of a contrast agent into the subarachnoid space. Superseded by CT and MRI.

myeloid   associated with the bone marrow. Associated with the granulocyte precursor cells in the bone marrow. *See also* **leukaemia**.

myelomatosis (multiple myeloma)   a tumour of the bone marrow.

myelopathy   disease of the spinal cord. Can be a serious complication of cervical spondylosis.

myeloproliferative disorders   condition where there is proliferation of one or more of the cellular components of the bone marrow such as myelofibrosis, primary proliferative polycythaemia and thrombocythaemia. *See also* **leukaemia**.

myelosclerosis   a generalized increase in bone density.

myocardial infarction   death of a part of the myocardium (heart muscle) from deprivation of blood following occlusion (blockage) of a coronary artery, for example from thrombosis. The patient experiences a 'heart attack' with sudden intense chest pain which may radiate to arms and lower jaw. Management includes: aspirin, thrombolytic therapy, pain relief, antiemetics, oxygen therapy, bed rest, observations including continuous ECG and later mobilization and cardiac rehabilitation. Patients should be cared for in a coronary care unit for 12–24 hours because of the risk of life-threatening arrhythmias such as ventricular fibrillation, and the need for skilled staff to monitor the effects of thrombolytic therapy. *See also* **angina pectoris, cardiac enzymes, coronary heart disease**.

myocardium   the middle layer of the heart wall. Formed from highly specialized cardiac muscle. *See also* **muscle**.

myofibri   bundle of fibres contained in a muscle fibre.

myogenic   originating in or starting from muscle.

myoglobin (myohaemoglobin)   a haem-protein molecule of skeletal muscle. It is involved with the oxygen released by the red blood cells, which it stores and transports to muscle cell mitochondria where it is used to produce energy. Myoglobin escapes from damaged muscle and appears in the urine in 'crush syndrome'.

myoma   a tumour of muscle tissue.

myometrium   the specialized muscular wall of the uterus.

myoneural   associated with muscle and nerve.

myosarcoma   a malignant tumour derived from muscle.

myositis   inflammation of muscle tissue.

myotome   the muscles supplied by a single spinal nerve.

myxoedema   a condition caused by hypothyroidism, characterized by the swelling of the hands, face, feet and periorbital tissue.

myxoma   a connective tissue tumour composed largely of mucoid material.

myxosarcoma   a malignant tumour of connective tissue with a soft, mucoid consistency.

naevus (mole) a circumscribed lesion of the skin arising from pigment-producing naevus cells or due to a developmental abnormality of blood vessels.

nanogram (ng) one thousandth part of a microgram. 10^{-9} of a gram.

nanometre (nm) one thousandth part of a micrometre. 10^{-9} of a metre.

nape (nucha) back of the neck.

narcotic a drug causing abnormally deep sleep.

nares (choanae) the nostrils. ***anterior nares*** the pair of openings from the exterior into the nasal cavities. ***posterior nares*** the pair of openings from the nasal cavities into the nasopharynx.

nasal associated with the nose.

nasal cavity that in the nose, separated into right and left halves by the nasal septum.

nasal conchae irregular bones which lie on the lateral walls of the nasal cavity.

nasal speculum used for examination of the nose and for treatments, such as nasal cautery and packing to stop bleeding.

nasal tube a catheter inserted into the nasal passages to permit the administration of oxygen therapy.

nasoduodenal associated with the nose and duodenum, as passing a naso-duodenal tube via this route, for feeding. *See also* **enteral**.

nasogastric (NG) associated with the nose and stomach, as passing a naso-gastric tube via this route, usually for aspiration, or feeding.

nasojejunal associated with the nose and jejunum, usually referring to a tube passed via the nose into the jejunum for feeding.

nasolacrimal associated with the nose and lacrimal apparatus.

naso-oesophageal associated with the nose and the oesophagus.

nasopharynx the portion of the pharynx above the soft palate.

National Framework for Assessing Performance a framework that includes six areas for the assessment of NHS performance: effective delivery of appropriate health care; efficiency; fair access; health improvement; health outcomes and the patient/carer experience. *See also* **Performance Indicators**.

National Institute for Clinical Excellence (NICE)   a Special Health Authority that generates and distributes clinical guidance based on evidence of clinical and cost effectiveness.

National Service Frameworks (NSFs)   evidence-based frameworks for major care areas and particular groups of disease, e.g. diabetes, older people, that state what patients/clients can presume to receive from the NHS.

nausea   a feeling of impending vomiting.

navel   *see* **umbilicus**.

navicular   boat-shaped, like a canoe, such as the bone in the foot.

nebulizer   an apparatus for converting a liquid into a fine spray. It is used to deliver medicaments for application to the respiratory tract or the skin. A very common method of drug delivery used in the management of asthma.

neck   a constricted section, the part of the body that connects the head with the trunk, the area below the head of a bone as in the neck of humerus, the neck of femur, the part of a tooth where the root merges with the crown. The constricted section of an organ as in the neck of uterus.

necrosis   localized death of tissue.

necrotizing fasciitis   rare infection caused by some strains of group A *Streptococcus pyogenes*. There is very severe inflammation of the muscle sheath and massive soft-tissue destruction. The mortality rate is high.

needle biopsy   the removal of tissue from a lesion, for analysis by using a needle; the needle is rotated and the tissue remains in the lumen.

needlestick injury   an injury caused when the skin is pierced by a hypodermic needle. Risk is greatest when the needle is contaminated with blood from a person infected with a blood-borne virus such as hepatitis B or C or HIV.

needs assessment   estimating the need (quantifying) for services in a population. ***normative***, or assessed, need is need defined by the expert or professional in any given situation; ***felt need***, or want, perceived by the individual; ***expressed need*** or operationalized felt need; ***comparative need*** using the characteristics of a population receiving a service to define those with similar characteristics as in need. ***needs assessment*** uses broad, non-specific indicators of need obtained through repeated health surveys of the general population (e.g. General Household Survey, Health Survey for England) and more specific indicators based on surveys of particular groups (e.g. survey of disabled people, urinary incontinence). The weighted capitation formula for resource allocation uses the characteristics of populations using hospital services as indicators of need.

negative correlation   in statistics, when information is linked and an increase in one item will result in a decrease in the other and an increase in one item will result in an decrease in the other.

negative number   a number with a value of less than zero.

negatron   a negative beta particle.

negligence   a form of professional malpractice which includes the omission of acts that a prudent health professional would have done or the commission of acts that a prudent health professional would not do. It is a professional duty to avoid patient/client injury or suffering caused in this way. It can become the basis of litigation for damages. *See also* **Bolam test, duty of care**.

Nelaton's line   an imaginary line joining the anterior superior iliac spine to the ischial tuberosity. The great trochanter of the femur normally lies on or below this line.

neoadjuvant therapy   preliminary cancer treatment such as chemotherapy or radiation that usually precedes another phase of treatment, for example, to reduce tumour size before surgery.

neonatal   relating to the first 28 days of life.

neonatal herpes   acquired during vaginal delivery from a mother actively shedding herpes simplex virus. It is a devastating illness with a 75% mortality rate and a high incidence of severe neurological pathology among survivors.

neonatal mortality   the death rate of babies in the first month of life.

neonatal unit (NNU/NICU/SCBU)   usually reserved for preterm and small-for-dates babies between 700 and 2000 g in weight, mostly requiring the use of high technology which is available in these units.

neonate   a newborn baby up to 4 weeks of age.

neoplasia   literally, the formation of new tissue. The new or abnormal development of cells that may be benign or malignant.

neoplasm   a new growth of cells forming a tumour that is either cancerous or non-cancerous.

nephrectomy   surgical removal of a kidney.

nephritis   non-specific term for inflammation within the kidney.

nephroblastoma   the most common solid tumour of the kidney arising from immature or undifferentiated embryonic cells, usually presents as an abdominal mass. Also known as **Wilms' tumour**.

nephrocalcinosis   calcification within the kidney.

nephrolithiasis   stone, disease affecting the kidney.

nephrolithotomy   removal of a stone from the kidney by an incision through the kidney substance. **percutaneous nephrolithotomy** a minimally invasive technique where the kidney pelvis is punctured using X-ray control. A guide wire is inserted through which the stone is removed using a nephroscope (endoscope).

nephrology   study of diseases of the kidney.

nephron   the functional unit of the kidney, comprising a glomerulus and renal tubule. The tubule has a Bowman's capsule, proximal and distal convoluted tubules, loop of Henle and a collecting tubule that drains urine from many nephrons to the renal pelvis.

nephronophthisis   rare disorder involving the growth of many small cysts in the medulla of the kidney; often leads to renal failure.

nephropathy   any disease of the kidney in which inflammation is not a major component.

nephroptosis   downward displacement of the kidney. The word is sometimes used for a *floating kidney*.

nephroscope   an endoscope for viewing kidney tissue. It can be designed to create a continuous flow of irrigating fluid and provide an exit for the fluid and accompanying debris.

nephrostomy   a surgically established fistula from the pelvis of the kidney to the body surface.

nephroureterectomy   removal of the kidney along with a part or the whole of the ureter.

nerve   an elongated bundle of fibres which serves for the transmission of impulses between the periphery and the nerve centres. *See also* **afferent nerve, efferent nerve, nerve growth factor**.

nerve growth factor (NGF)   protein required for nerve growth and maintenance.

nervous   relating to nerves or nerve tissue. Referring to a state of restlessness or timidity. *nervous system* the structures controlling the actions and functions of the body; it comprises the brain and spinal cord (central nervous system), and the peripheral nerve fibres and ganglia. *See also* **autonomic nervous system, peripheral nervous system, parasympathetic, sympathetic nervous system**.

network   a system, usually connected by telephone line, which interconnects a number of computers so that they can share information and hardware, for example, printers.

neural   associated with nerves.

neural canal   the cavity within the vertebral column that houses the spinal cord.

neural tube   formed from fusion of the neural folds from which the brain and spinal cord are formed.

neural tube defect   any of a group of congenital malformations involving the neural tube including anencephaly, hydrocephalus and spina bifida.

neuralgia   pain in the distribution of a nerve.

neurilemma   the thin membranous covering of a nerve fibre surrounding the myelin sheath.

neurinoma   a tumour arising from peripheral nerves. The most common is the *acoustic neuroma* arising from the 8th cranial nerve. The main symptom is deafness.

neuroblast   a primitive nerve cell.

neuroblastoma malignant tumour of immature nerve cells most often arising in the very young, and is most common in the adrenal medulla from tissue of sympathetic origin.

neurofibroma a tumour arising from the connective tissue of nerves resulting from the abnormal spread of Schwann cells.

neurogenic originating within or forming nervous tissue.

neurogenic incontinence overflow incontinence, dribbling of urine from an overfull bladder.

neurogenic shock shock caused by the loss of vascular tone and therefore dilatation of the blood vessels as a result of severe pain or fright. Now called *vasovagal shock*.

neuroglia (glia) the supporting tissue of the central nervous system (brain and cord). *See also* **astrocytes, ependymal cells, microglial cells, oligodendrocytes**.

neurologist a specialist in neurology or a medically qualified person who specializes in diagnosing and treating diseases of the nervous system.

neurology the science and study of nerves – their structure, function and pathology. The branch of medicine dealing with diseases of the nervous system.

neuromuscular associated with nerves and muscles.

neuron(e) a nerve cell. The basic unit of the nervous system comprising fibres (dendrites) which convey impulses to the nerve cell; the nerve cell itself, and the fibres (axons) which convey impulses from the cell. They are specialized excitable cells that are able to transmit an action potential. *See also* **motor neuron disease, lower motor neuron, upper motor neuron**.

neuropeptides neurotransmitters, including endorphins.

neuroplasticity the ability of nerve cells to regenerate.

neuroplasty surgical repair of nerves.

neurosis abnormal anxiety.

neurosurgery surgery of the nervous system.

neurothekeoma a soft-tissue tumour of the nerve sheath cells.

neutron a particle within the nucleus of an atom that has no electrical charge.

neutron number (N) the number of neutrons within the nucleus of an atom.

neutropenia reduction in the number of neutrophils in the blood.

neutrophil the most common form of white blood cell. It is a phagocytic polymorphonuclear cell with granules.

newton (N) a unit of force. Derived SI unit (International System of Units).

Newton's laws of motion   *Law 1*. A body will remain at rest or will travel with constant velocity unless acted upon by a net external force. *Law 2*. The rate of change of momentum of a body is proportional to the applied force. *Law 3*. The action of one body on a second body is always accompanied by an equal and opposite action of the second body on the first.

NEX   in magnetic resonance imaging the number of signal excitations repeated in a given acquisition. This is a way of increasing signal to noise ratio by increasing the time.

NHS Trusts   public accountable bodies that provide NHS health care to the population, either as a hospital or community trust.

night splinting   the passive night time use of external devices such as splints to maintain corrected deformities produced dynamically during walking. This may be an additional silicone digital device to maintain correction in bed, or a night splint to maintain ankle extension at 90° where there is tightening of the Achilles tendon. Night splints for the management of hallux valgus are often used as the only corrective measure.

night sweat   profuse sweating, usually during sleep; typical of tuberculosis or lymphoma.

nipple   the conical eminence in the centre of each breast, containing the outlets of the milk ducts.

nitric oxide (NO)   an internal substance that alters the transmission of nerve impulses. It is involved with processes that include memory, learning, gastric emptying, the response to painful stimuli and penile erection. May be used therapeutically for patients with acute respiratory distress syndrome.

nitrogen (N)   an almost inert gaseous element; the chief constituent of the atmosphere (78–79%), but it cannot be utilized directly by humans. However, certain organisms in the soil and roots of legumes are capable of nitrogen fixation. It is a vital constituent of many complements of living cells, e.g. proteins. The essential constituent of protein foods.

nitrogen balance   is when a person's daily intake of nitrogen from proteins equals the daily excretion of nitrogen: a negative balance occurs when excretion of nitrogen exceeds the daily intake. Nitrogen is excreted mainly as urea in the urine: ammonia, creatinine and uric acid account for a further small amount. Less than 10% total nitrogen is excreted in faeces.

nitrous oxide (N_2O)   an inhalation anaesthetic ensuring a brief spell of unconsciousness. Known colloquially as *laughing gas*.

nociceptors   receptors that respond to harmful stimuli that cause pain, such as trauma and inflammation.

nocturia   passing urine at night.

node   a protuberance or swelling. A constriction, for example, *node of Ranvier* the constriction in the neurilemma of a nerve fibre. Any computer equipment that communicates on a network.

nodule   a small node.

no fault liability   acknowledgement that compensation is payable without the requirement to prove a failure in fulfilling the duty of care.

noise   in imaging, the extraneous random visible grain on an image, although this detracts from the image quality, there is an acceptable amount of noise within a diagnostic image. Eliminating noise requires an increase in exposure which may be unnecessary to achieve the aims of the examination.

noise equivalent quanta (NEQ)   in a system is the square of the signal to noise ratio and indicates the flux density of X-ray quanta that forms the image.

nominal data   categorical data where the classes have no particular value or order, such as road names or colours. *See also* **ordinal data**.

nominal scale   a number given to objects that are similar to each other, a method of classification.

nominal standard dose   the tolerance of normal tissues (D) can be related to the overall treatment time (T) and the number of fractions (N) by the formula: $D_N = (NSD)T^{0.11} \times N^{0.24}$.

nomogram   graph with several variables used to determine another related variable, such as body surface area from weight and height.

non-accidental injury (NAI)   physical maltreatment, usually of children by their parents, carers, other adults, or even other children. The injuries cannot be attributed to natural disease processes or simple accident. The injuries are often multiple and typically include bruising, shaking injuries, fractures and burns, and involve the head, soft tissues, long bones and the thoracic cage. There may be evidence of neglect and usually there is associated psychological harm. *See also* **abuse**.

noncoplanar treatment   a treatment that is given in one or more planes. The rationale for this type of treatment is to avoid overlap of beam entrance and exit points.

non-Hodgkin's lymphoma (NHL)   tumour of lymphoid tissue. More common in older people. The cure rate is less good than that for Hodgkin's disease. *See also* **lymphoma**.

non-insulin dependent diabetes mellitus (NIDDM)   *see* **diabetes mellitus**.

non-invasive   describes any diagnostic or therapeutic technique that does not require penetration of the skin or of any cavity or organ.

non-invasive intermittent positive pressure ventilation (NIPPV)   a type of respiratory support that uses a nasal or full-face mask rather than an endotracheal or tracheostomy tube.

non-maleficence   ethical principle of doing no harm.

non-parametric tests   statistical test that makes no presupposition about the distribution of data. *See also* **parametric tests**.

non-small-cell lung carcinoma (NSCLC) commonest type of lung cancer accounting for approximately 80% of tumours. The histological subtypes include squamous, adenocarcinoma and large cell. The doubling time is approximately 130 days. Clinical presentation may be with cough, haemoptysis, recurrent pneumonia, increasing breathlessness, weight loss or may be an incidental finding on chest X-ray. Therapy may include surgery (in approximately 20%), chemotherapy and/or radiotherapy.

non-steroidal anti-inflammatory drugs (NSAIDs) a group of drugs that control pain, sickness and inflammation, examples include aspirin and ibuprofen.

noradrenaline (norepinephrine) a catecholamine neurotransmitter released from adrenergic nerve endings and in small amounts from the adrenal medulla. Its physiological effects include vasoconstriction and a rise in blood pressure. *See also* **adrenaline (epinephrine)**.

norm a measure of a phenomenon generally accepted as an ideal against which all other measures of the phenomenon can be measured, i.e. a standard against which values are measured.

normal distribution curve in statistics. When scores are plotted they form a symmetrical bell-shaped curve that has the mean, median and mode in the centre. *See also* **skewed distribution**.

normal population a normal distribution curve is produced when the data are plotted.

normal tissue tolerance the dose of radiation given to a specific organ or tissue, that gives a certain probability of a particular complication.

normoblast a normal-sized nucleated red blood cell, the precursor of the erythrocyte.

normotonic normal strength, tension, tone, by convention referring to muscle tissue. Antispasmodic drugs induce normotonicity in muscle, and can be used before radiography.

nostrils the anterior openings into the nose.

notch a large groove.

notifiable describes incidents or occurrences and diseases that must by law be made known to the appropriate agency. For example diseases such as tuberculosis, food poisoning and measles must be reported to the relevant department.

N-type semiconductor a device where the majority of carriers are the electrons in the conduction band and the minority carriers are the holes in the valence band. *See also* **P-type semiconductors**.

nuchal translucency scan an ultrasound scan done to measure from the cervical vertebrae to the posterior skin surface of the fetus. A measurement of greater than 3 mm at 11–14 weeks means that there could be an increased risk of aneuploidy (a variation in the number of chromosomes).

nucha the nape of the neck.

nuclear energy levels   the discrete energy levels occupied by nucleons in the nucleus of an atom.

nuclear force   the force present in the nucleus of an atom which contains the particles inside the nucleus. The nuclear binding energy is different in different elements but is about 8 MeV per nucleon.

nuclear magnetic resonance (NMR)   *see* **magnetic resonance imaging**.

nuclear medicine   the use of radionuclide techniques for the diagnosis, treatment and study of disease.

nuclear reactor   a method of producing electricity through controlled nuclear fusion which produces heat which turns water to steam which drives electric generators.

nuclear spin   a property of nuclei which have an odd number of neutrons and/or protons which gives them angular and magnetic momentum. The spins of the nuclei have characteristic fixed values. Nuclei of paired neutrons and protons align to cancel out their spins and therefore do not resonate.

nucleated   possessing one or more nuclei.

nucleon   the protons and neutrons within the nucleus of an atom.

nucleus   the central part of an atom that contains neutrons and protons. The membrane-bound cellular structure which contains the genetic material (chromosomes). A confined accumulation of nerve cells in the central nervous system associated with a particular function.

nucleus pulposus   the soft core of an intervertebral disc which can prolapse into the spinal cord and cause back pain or sciatica.

nuclide   an individual atom of given atomic number and mass number.

null hypothesis   a statement which asserts that there is no relationship between the dependent and independent variables.

numbers needed to treat   a method of stating the benefits of a therapeutic intervention. The number of subjects who need to receive treatment before one subject has a positive outcome.

nyastin suspension   antifungal antibiotic.

nymphae   the labia minora.

Nyquist frequency   the frequency equal to or greater than twice the highest frequency in an analogue signal.

Nyquist limit   the maximum frequency that can be handled to enable an accurate reconstruction to take place, for example, in pulsed wave Doppler imaging, above this level aliasing occurs. *See also* **aliasing**.

Nyquist theorem   states that an analogue signal waveform may be reconstructed without error from a sample which is equal to, or greater than, twice the highest frequency in the analogue signal, for example, to digitally convert a 2 MHz signal a sample must be taken at 4 MHz.

oat cell carcinoma   histological subtype of small cell carcinoma most commonly of bronchogenic epithelium. It accounts for approximately 20% of all lung cancers and is characterized by rapid growth (doubling time approximately 29 days). The highest incidence is in smokers. The lung primary may present with cough, haemoptysis, recurrent pneumonia, increasing breathlessness and weight loss or may be an incidental finding on chest X-ray. Therapy generally does not include surgery, but 90% are sensitive to chemotherapy, which is usually the treatment of choice.

obese   excessively overweight.

objective   associated with things external to oneself.

objective signs   those which the observer notes, as distinct from the symptoms of which the patient complains.

oblique   a slanting direction.

oblique fracture   a break in bone continuity that is at an angle to the main shaft of the bone.

oblique incidence   when a radiotherapy beam enters the patient at an angle other than 90° due to the curvature of the skin surface.

observational study   research in which the researcher observes, listens and records the events of concern. Where the researcher participates and has a role it is termed a participant observational study. May be used in qualitative social science research.

obstetrician   a qualified doctor who practices the science and art of obstetrics.

obstetrics   the science dealing with the care of the pregnant woman during the antenatal, parturient and puerperal stages; midwifery.

obturator   that which closes an aperture.

obturator foramen   the opening in the innominate bone which is closed by muscles and fascia.

occipital   associated with the back of the head.

occipital bone   the bone forming the back and part of the base of the skull, characterized by a large hole through which the spinal cord passes.

occipitoanterior   describes a presentation when the fetal occiput lies in the anterior half of the maternal pelvis.

occipitofrontal   associated with the occiput and forehead.

occipitoposterior   describes a presentation when the fetal occiput is in the posterior half of the maternal pelvis.

occiput   the posterior region of the skull.

occlusal   biting edge of the teeth.

occlusal film   a radiographic film in a waterproof envelope which the patient bites on, used to demonstrate either upper or lower 321123 on a single film.

occlusion   the closure of an opening, especially of ducts or blood vessels. In dentistry, the contact of the upper and lower teeth in any jaw position. *See also* **centric occlusion, traumatic occlusion**.

occult blood   blood that is not obvious on examination, detected by a chemical test, microscopic or spectroscopic examination.

occupational disease   *see* **industrial disease**.

occupational exposure   job-related risk of exposure to carcinogens.

occupational health   the active and proactive management of health in the workplace.

OCR (Optical Character Recognition)   a means of the computer directly reading printed or written characters.

ocular   associated with the eye.

oculomotor   the third pair of cranial nerves which innervate four of the extrinsic muscles and the upper eye lid. They also alter the shape of the lens and control pupil size.

odontalgia   toothache.

odontoid   resembling a tooth.

odontoid process   a peg-like projection of the axis (second cervical vertebra).

oedema   abnormal infiltration of tissues with fluid. There are many causes, including reduced blood albumin, disease of the cardiopulmonary system, the urinary system and the liver. *See also* **angio-oedema, ascites**.

oesophageal   associated with the oesophagus.

oesophageal atresia   a narrowing of the oesophagus which is often associated with a tracheo-oesophageal fistula.

oesophageal ulcer   ulceration of the oesophagus due to gastro-oesophageal reflux caused by hiatus hernia.

oesophageal varices   varicosity of the veins in the lower oesophagus due to portal hypertension. These varices can bleed and may cause a massive haematemesis.

oesophagostomy   a surgically established fistula between the oesophagus and the skin in the root of the neck. May be used temporarily for feeding after excision of the pharynx for malignant disease.

oesophagus   the musculomembranous canal, 23 cm in length, extending from the pharynx to the stomach.

oestradiol (estradiol)   an endogenous oestrogen secreted by the corpus luteum.

oestriol (estriol)   an endogenous oestrogen. Produced by the fetus and placenta. Oestriol levels in maternal blood or urine can be used to assess fetal well-being and placental function.

oestrogens (estrogens)   a generic term referring to a group of steroid hormones, oestradiol, oestriol and oestrone. Produced by the ovaries, placenta, testes and, in smaller amounts, the adrenal cortex in both sexes. Oestrogens influence normal skeletal growth especially in puberty and are responsible for female secondary sexual characteristics and the development and proper functioning of the female genital organs. Used in the combined oral contraceptive and as hormone replacement.

oestrone (estrone)   an endogenous oestrogen.

off-centre field of view   in magnetic resonance imaging a field of view that is not centred at the isocentre of the magnet.

ohm   the unit of electrical resistance equal to the resistance between two points on a conductor when a potential difference of one volt between the points, produces a current of one ampere.

Ohm's law   the current flowing through a conductor is proportional to the potential difference which exists across it providing other physical conditions remain constant.

olecranon process   the large process at the upper end of the ulna; it forms the point of the elbow when the arm is flexed.

olfactory   associated with the sense of smell.

olfaction   the sense of smell.

olfactory nerve   the first pair of cranial nerves. They carry sensory impulses from the olfactory epithelium of the nose to the brain.

olfactory organ   the nose.

oligodactyly   a developmental absence of one or more digits (fingers or toes). There is total absence of all parts of the digit, for example, metatarsals and all phalanges.

oligodendrocyte   a neuroglial cell of the central nervous system.

oligodendroglioma   a slow-growing tumour most commonly of the frontal lobe of the brain, may become more aggressive after many years.

oligospermia   a diminished output of spermatozoa.

omentum   a sling-like fold of peritoneum. The functions of the omentum are support and protection, limiting infection and fat storage. ***greater omentum*** the fold which hangs from the lower border of the stomach and covers the front of the intestines. ***lesser omentum*** a smaller fold, passing between the transverse fissure of the liver and the lesser curvature of the stomach.

omphalocele congenital herniation of the gut through the abdominal wall around the umbilicus which is associated with chromosomal abnormality.

oncogene an altered gene that contributes to cancer development.

oncogenic capable of tumour production.

oncology the scientific study and therapy of neoplastic growths.

one-tailed hypothesis a theory that predicts a particular outcome.

oocyte an immature ovum.

oogenesis the formation of oocytes in the ovary. *See also* **gametogenesis**.

oophorectomy the surgical removal of an ovary.

oophoron an ovary.

oophoropexy the surgical fixation of a displaced ovary to the abdominal wall or the inferior body of the uterus, can be done prior to radiotherapy treatment so that the ovary can be protected from receiving a large dose of radiation.

opacity the incident light over the transmitted light and is a measure of the effect the radiograph has on the original light shining on it.

open (compound) fracture there is a wound permitting communication of broken bone end with air.

open reduction the realigning of fractures using a surgical procedure.

operational management the management of the day-to-day activities (operations) of an organization such as a district general hospital. *See also* **strategic management**.

ophthalmic applicator equipment which is sutured to the eye to hold the radioactive, source iodine-125, when treating the eye. The applicator should be handled with rubber-tipped forceps to prevent damage to the thin, active window, other radiation sources can be used.

ophthalmology the science that deals with the structure, function, diseases and treatment of the eye.

ophthalmoscope instrument for examining the interior of the eye, consisting of a mirror with a hole in it through which the observer looks. The retina is illuminated by light reflected from the mirror.

opportunity cost when a resource is used in a particular way, the opportunity to use it for another purpose is lost. This includes money, time and the activities which cannot be undertaken. An example in health care would be the decision to use money for an expensive cancer drug leading to a lost opportunity to spend the money for another service such as cataract surgery.

opportunistic infection a serious infection with a microorganism which normally has little or no pathogenic activity but causes disease where patient resistance is reduced by a serious disease, invasive treatments or drugs.

opposition describes the position of the thumb and fingers when objects are picked up or grasped between thumb and fingers.

opsins   protein part of visual pigments found in cones and rods.

opsonin   complement protein or an antibody which coats an antigen.

optic   associated with sight.

optic atrophy   pathological whitening of the optic nerve head with loss of nerve axons.

optic chiasma   the meeting of the two optic nerves; where the fibres from the medial or nasal half of each retina (supplying half the visual field in either eye) cross the middle line to join the optic tract of the opposite side.

optic disc   the point where the optic nerve enters the eyeball.

optic nerves   second pair of cranial nerves. They convey impulses from the rods and cones in the retina to the brain.

optic neuritis   inflammation in the optic nerve that can be the first sign of multiple sclerosis.

optic neuropathy   disease of the optic nerve.

optical aberration   imperfect focus of light rays by a lens.

optical disk   a disk, usually a DVD or a CD that uses light in the form of a laser to burn data onto the disk and also to read information from the disk.

optical sensitizing   increasing the spectral sensitivity of the film by adding impurities to the film emulsion, because it is done by adding coloured dyes and therefore can be called *dye sensitizing, colour sensitizing* or *spectral sensitizing*.

oral   associated with the mouth.

oral cavity (buccal cavity)   the mouth.

oral cholecystography   the radiographic investigation of the biliary tract following the ingestion of a contrast agent, now superseded by ultrasound techniques.

oral medicine   branch of dentistry concerned with the management of diseases of the oral mucosa and related structures, including oral manifestations of systemic diseases.

oral rehydration solution (ORS)   a solution for the treatment of diarrhoeal dehydration. It contains glucose and electrolytes such as sodium chloride.

oral rehydration therapy (ORT)   administration of oral rehydration solution by mouth to correct dehydration.

oral surgery   branch of dentistry concerned with minor surgery to the teeth and jaws.

orbicular   resembling a globe; spherical or circular.

orbit   the bony socket containing the eyeball and its appendages.

orbitomeatal baseline   a line joining the outer canthus of the eye to the mid point of the external auditory meatus (see figure on p. 278).

orchidectomy the surgical removal of a testis.

orchis the testis.

ordinal data categorical data that can be ordered or ranked, for example, general condition – good, fair or bad, or size in general terms, as in 'smaller than'. *See also* **nominal data**.

ordinal scale the numbers allotted to the ranking or ordering data in a rough sequence.

organ an assembly of different tissues to form a distinct functional unit, for example, liver, uterus, able to perform specialized functions.

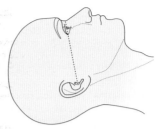

Orbitomeatal baseline. From Pocketbook of radiographic positioning, 2nd edn, Ruth Sutherland, 2003, Churchill Livingstone, Edinburgh, with permission.

organ of Corti sited in the cochlea of the internal ear it contains the auditory receptors of the cochlear branch of the vestibulocochlear nerve.

organism a living cell or group of cells differentiated into functionally distinct parts which are interdependent.

organs at risk the organs of the body that are more sensitive to radiation and therefore may influence treatment planning or prescribed dose, for example eyes, spinal cord and gonads.

orifice a mouth or opening.

origin the commencement or source of anything. ***origin of a muscle*** the end that remains relatively fixed during contraction of the muscle.

ornithine an amino acid, obtained from arginine during the urea cycle.

orogenital associated with the mouth and the external genital area.

oropharyngeal associated with the mouth and pharynx.

oropharyngeal airway a flexible oval tube, such as a Guedel airway, which can be placed along the upper surface of the tongue to prevent a flaccid tongue from resting against the posterior pharyngeal wall, thereby obstructing the airway, and is commonly used during general anaesthesia. Also used during cardiopulmonary resuscitation.

oropharynx that portion of the pharynx which is below the level of the soft palate and above the level of the hyoid bone.

orthochromatic emulsions film emulsions that have a spectral sensitivity up to and including the green part of the visible spectrum tend to be used with rare earth intensifying screens.

orthodontic device device used to move teeth by the controlled application of force. May be removable, myofunctional (functional) or fixed.

orthodontics a branch of dentistry concerned with the prevention and correction of irregularities and malocclusion of the teeth.

orthognathic surgery surgery aimed at correcting abnormalities in position of the jaw to improve function and appearance.

orthogonal radiographs radiographs taken at 90 degrees to one another to localize the treatment area or to verify the relative positions of radioactive sources with reference to the associated anatomy.

orthopaedics formerly a specialty devoted to the correction of deformities in children. It is now a branch of surgery dealing with all conditions affecting the locomotor system.

orthopantomograph specialist dental, tomographic equipment for imaging the upper and lower teeth on one projection.

orthosis external device utilized to correct, control or counteract the effect of an actual or developing deformity. They include braces, callipers and splints.

Ortolani's sign a test performed shortly after birth for the diagnosis of developmental dysplasia of the hip (congenital dislocation of the hip). It should always be undertaken by an experienced clinician. Often used in conjunction with Barlow's sign/test.

os a mouth. For example, external os, the opening of the cervix into the vagina, internal os, the opening of the cervix into the uterine cavity.

oscilloscope an instrument with a cathode ray tube, which displays a visual representation of electrical variations produced by a beam of electrons hitting the screen.

Osgood–Schlatter disease *see* **Schlatter's disease**.

osmosis the passage of pure solvent across a semipermeable membrane under the influence of osmotic pressure. It is the movement of a dilute solution into a more concentrated solution.

osseous relating to or resembling bone.

ossicles small bones, particularly those contained in the middle ear; the malleus, incus and stapes.

ossification the conversion of cartilage, etc. into bone. Also known as *osteogenesis*.

osteitis inflammation of bone.

osteitis deformans *see* **Paget's disease**.

osteitis fibrosa cavities form in the interior of bone. The cysts may be solitary or the disease may be generalized. This second condition may be the result of excessive parathyroid secretion and absorption of calcium from bone.

osteoarthritis sometimes termed degenerative arthritis, although the disease process is much more than simply 'wear and tear'; may be primary, or may follow injury or disease involving the articular surfaces of synovial joints. The articular cartilage becomes worn, osteophytes form at the periphery of the joint surface and loose bodies may result.

osteoarthropathy a condition where the bones of the forearms and shins become inflamed and painful, often associated with lung cancer.

osteoblast a bone-forming cell.

osteoblastoma a small, benign, tumour of poorly formed bone and fibrous tissue, seen in children and young adults.

osteochondritis originally an inflammation of bone cartilage. Usually applied to non-septic conditions, especially avascular necrosis involving joint surfaces, for example, osteochondritis dissecans in which a portion of joint surface may separate to form a loose body in the joint. *See also* **Scheuermann's disease, Köhler's disease**.

osteochondroma a benign bony and cartilaginous tumour.

osteochondrosis an idiopathic disease characterized by a disorder of the ossification of hyaline cartilage (endochondral). It encompasses a group of syndromes classified on the basis of their anatomical location. ***Primary articular epiphysis*** – Freiberg's disease and Köhler's disease. ***Secondary articular epiphysis*** – osteochondritis dissecans of the talus. ***Non-articular epiphysis*** (apophyseal injury) – Sever's disease. The osteochondroses occur during the years of rapid growth. Aetiology has been linked to hereditary factors, trauma, nutritional factors and ischaemia. The ***articular osteochondroses*** such as Freiberg's, Köhler's and osteochondritis dissecans are characterized by fragmentation with a centre of ossification.

osteoclasis the therapeutic fracture of a bone.

osteoclast cell that resorbs bone.

osteoclastoma a tumour of the osteoclasts. May be benign, locally recurrent, or malignant. The usual site is near the end of a long bone.

osteocyte a bone cell.

osteodystrophy faulty growth of bone.

osteogenesis bone formation. *See also* **ossification**.

osteogenesis imperfecta a hereditary disorder usually caused by an autosomal dominant gene. It may be present at birth or develop during childhood. The congenital form is much more severe and may lead to early death. The bones are extremely fragile and may fracture following minimal trauma.

osteogenic bone-producing. ***osteogenic sarcoma*** malignant tumour that originates from bone-producing cells.

osteolysis the degeneration and dissolution of bone caused by disease, infection and ischaemia.

osteolytic destructive of bone, for example, osteolytic malignant deposits in bone.

osteoma a benign tumour of bone which may arise in the compact tissue (ivory osteoma) or in the cancellous tissue. May be single or multiple.

osteomalacia   demineralization of the mature skeleton, with softening and bone pain. It is commonly caused by insufficient dietary intake of vitamin D or lack of sunshine, or both.

osteomyelitis   inflammation commencing in the marrow of bone.

osteonecrosis   the death of bone due to an impaired blood supply.

osteopathy   an established clinical discipline. It is concerned with the interrelationship between structure and function of the body. Osteopathy may be effective for the relief or improvement of a wide variety of conditions, for example, digestive disorders, as well as mechanical problems. Osteopathy is one of only a few complementary therapies to have achieved statutory self-regulation on a par with healthcare professions such as medicine.

osteopetrosis (Albers–Schönberg disease, marble bones)   a congenital abnormality giving rise to very dense bones which fracture easily.

osteophyte   a bony outgrowth or spur, usually at the margins of joint surfaces, for example, in osteoarthritis.

osteoplasty   reconstructive operation on bone.

osteoporosis   loss of bone density caused by excessive absorption of calcium and phosphorus from the bone, due to progressive loss of the protein matrix of bone which normally carries the calcium deposits. Associated with ageing in both men and women. Common cause of fractures, particularly fractures of the wrist, crush fractures of the spine and neck of femur fractures.

osteosarcoma   a malignant tumour growing from bone cells (osteoblasts).

osteosclerosis   increased density or hardness of bone.

osteotomy   division of bone followed by realignment of the ends to encourage union by healing. *See also* **McMurray's osteotomy**.

ostium   the opening or mouth of any tubular structure.

otitis   inflammation of the ear.

otitis externa   inflammation of the skin of the external auditory canal.

otitis media   inflammation of the middle ear cavity. The effusion can be serous, mucoid or purulent. Non-purulent effusions in children are often called *glue ear*. *See also* **grommet**.

otoliths   tiny calcareous deposits within the utricle and saccule of the internal ear.

otosclerosis   abnormal bone formation affecting primarily the footplate of the stapes. A common cause of progressive conductive deafness.

otoscope   an instrument for examining the ear, usually incorporating both magnification and illumination. Also called an *auriscope*.

outcome measures   scales developed to measure health outcome from clinical interventions: generic measures encompassing dimensions of physical, mental and social health; disease-specific scales detecting the effects of treatment of specific conditions. *See also* **quality adjusted life years**.

output   data and information leaving a computer, which can then be sent to a display screen, printer or another computer.

ova   the female gametes (reproductive cells). More correctly known as a secondary oocyte until penetration by a spermatozoon.

ovarian   relating to the ovaries.

ovarian cycle   the changes occurring in the ovary during the development of the follicle and oogenesis. It has two phases: *follicular* (days 1–14) when ovulation occurs, and *luteal* (days 15–28) when the corpus luteum develops. The cycle is controlled by follicle stimulating hormone and luteinizing hormone.

ovarian cyst   a tumour of the ovary, usually containing fluid – may be benign or malignant.

ovary   a female gonad. One of two small oval bodies situated on either side of the uterus on the posterior surface of the broad ligament. Controlled by pituitary hormones they produce oocytes and oestrogen and progesterones.

overheads   the cost of services that contribute to the general upkeep and running of the organization, for example, grounds maintenance, that cannot be linked directly to the core activity of a department.

oviduct   uterine or fallopian tubes.

ovulation   the maturation and rupture of a Graafian follicle with the discharge of an oocyte.

oxidation   the act of oxidizing or state of being oxidized. It involves the addition of oxygen, for example, formation of oxides, or the loss of electrons or the removal of hydrogen. A part of metabolism, whereby energy is released from fuel molecules.

oxidative phosphorylation   a mitochondrial energy-producing metabolic process, whereby adenosine diphosphate (ADP) is converted to adenosine triphosphate (ATP) by the addition of a phosphate group.

oxygen (O)   a colourless, odourless, gaseous element; necessary for life and combustion. Constitutes 20% of atmospheric air. Used therapeutically as an inhalation to increase blood oxygenation. Delivered as part of a general anaesthetic to maintain life. *See also* **hyperbaric**.

oxygen concentrator   a device for removing nitrogen from the air to provide a high concentration of oxygen for use by patients requiring many hours of oxygen therapy each day at home.

oxygen enhancement ratio   the ratio of radiation doses needed to produce a given biological effect in the presence or absence of oxygen.

oxygen mask   a facial mask which allows oxygen to be mixed with air before being administered to a patient.

oxygen tent a large plastic canopy that encloses the patient in a controlled environment used for oxygen therapy.

oxyhaemoglobin (oxygenated haemoglobin) an unstable compound formed from haemoglobin on contact with air in the alveoli.

oxyntic producing acid. *oxyntic cells* the cells in the gastric mucosa which produce hydrochloric acid.

oxytocin a hormone released from the posterior pituitary. It contracts the uterine muscle and milk ducts and is involved in reflex milk ejection.

P

pacemaker the region of the heart that initiates atrial contraction and thus controls heart rate. The ***natural pacemaker*** is the sinus node which is situated at the junction of the superior vena cava and the right atrium; the wave of contraction begins here, then spreads over the heart. *See also* **cardiac pacemaker**.

PACS (Picture Archiving and Communications Systems) a system which enables digital images to be stored electronically and then viewed on computer screens, and therefore allowing the transfer of images and data across the intranet.

PACS broker enables two computer systems to talk to each other by changing (translating) information into a common language.

paediatric advanced life support (PALS) the special techniques, drug doses and equipment appropriate to the body weight and surface area of the child being resuscitated.

paediatric dentistry the diagnosis, prevention and treatment of dental and related diseases in children.

Paget's disease (osteitis deformans) a chronic disease of bone where overactivity of the osteoblasts and osteoclasts leads to dense bone formation and areas or rarefaction. Sufferers are particularly susceptible to sarcoma of bone, if the vestibulocochlear (auditory) nerve is involved, there is impairment of hearing. Erosion of the nipple caused by invasion of the dermis by intraduct carcinoma of the breast.

pain unpleasant sensation experienced when specialist nerve endings (nociceptors) are stimulated. It is individual and subjective with a physiological and emotional component. Pain ranges from mild to agonizing, but individual responses are influenced by factors which include: information about cause, age, whether acute or chronic and pain tolerance.

pain management involves a holistic multidisciplinary approach, and in some healthcare settings there is a designated pain team or nurse specialist.

pain threshold the lowest intensity at which a stimulus is felt as pain. There is very little difference between people.

pain tolerance the greatest intensity of pain that the individual is prepared to put up with. There is substantial variation between people.

pair production when a photon with energy greater than 1.02 MeV collides with the nucleus of an atom sometimes giving up all its energy in the production of an electron and a positron.

palatal   next to the tongue.

palate   the roof of the mouth. *See also* **hard palate, soft palate**.

palatine   associated with the palate.

palatine arches   the bilateral double pillars or arch-like folds formed by the descent of the soft palate as it meets the pharynx.

palatine bones   irregular bones that lie on the posterior aspect of the nasal and orbital cavities.

palliate   relieve symptoms. Often refers to option where a patient is not curable and is fit only for treatment to prevent distress from symptoms. It may involve surgery, chemotherapy, radiotherapy, nerve block, and/or drugs (typically opioids).

palliative   (describes) anything that serves to alleviate but cannot cure a disease.

palliative care   the specialty of symptom relief.

palliative treatment   aims to relieve the symptoms of cancer or restrain the temporary growth of a tumour.

palm   the anterior or flexor surface of the hand.

palmar   associated with the palm of the hand.

palmar arches   superficial and deep, are formed by the anastomosis of the radial and ulnar arteries.

palpebra   an eyelid.

panarthritis   inflammation of all the structures of a joint.

panchromatic emulsions   are film emulsions that are sensitive to all wavelengths of the visible spectrum.

pancreas   a tongue-shaped glandular organ lying below and behind the stomach. Its head is encircled by the duodenum and its tail touches the spleen. It is about 18 cm long and weighs about 100 g. It secretes the hormones insulin and glucagon, and also alkaline pancreatic juice which contains digestive enzymes involved in the digestion of fats, carbohydrates and proteins in the small intestine.

pancreatitis   inflammation of the pancreas which may be acute or chronic. Most commonly caused by gallstones or alcohol.

pancreozymin   intestinal hormone identical to *cholecystokinin* (CCK). Previously both names were used.

panosteitis   inflammation of all constituents of a bone, the medulla, bony tissue and periosteum.

Papanicolaou test (Pap)   a smear of epithelial cells taken from the cervix is stained and examined under the microscope for detection of the early stages of cancer.

papilla   a minute nipple-shaped eminence.

papillary carcinoma a malignant tumour of the thyroid caused by irradiating the neck in childhood, it is characterized microscopically by having delicate finger-like cores of stroma lined by tumour cells.

papilloedema swelling of the optic disc, the white patch on the retina where the optic nerve emerges.

papilloma a benign tumour of epithelial cells characterized by being branching or lobular, generally viral warts.

papillomatosis the growth of benign papillomata on the skin or a mucous membrane. Removal by laser means fewer recurrences.

para-aortic near the aorta.

paracentesis usually applied to the surgical puncture of the abdominal cavity for the aspiration of fluid.

paradigm an example, model, or set of ideas or assumptions.

paradigm shift the changes that occur as the build-up of evidence causes a paradigm to be questioned and eventually replaced by a new set of ideas.

paradoxical respiration associated with injuries that result in the ribs on one side being fractured in two places, such as in flail chest. The injured side of the chest moves in (deflates) on inspiration and vice versa.

paraesthesia any abnormality of sensation such as tingling.

parallel-hole collimator gamma camera collimator made of a thick lead plate with several thousand parallel sided holes perpendicular to the plane of the plate, gives a 1:1 relationship between the object being recorded and the image produced.

parallel pair used in radiotherapy to describe two directly opposing treatment fields.

paralysis complete or incomplete loss of nervous function to a part of the body. This may be sensory or motor or both.

paralytic associated with paralysis.

paralytic ileus paralysis of the intestinal muscle so that the bowel content cannot pass onwards even though there is no mechanical obstruction. *See also* **aperistalsis**.

paramagnetic a substance that increases the strength of a magnetic field in which it is placed by aligning with the static magnetic field and therefore affecting the relaxation times of the tissues containing them. *See also* **diamagnetic, superparamagnetic, ferromagnetic**.

paramagnetism the influence of an applied magnetic field on the electrons orbiting the nuclei within the substance which results in the formation of an elementary bar magnet.

paramedian near the middle.

parametric tests statistical tests that presuppose the data are from a sample from a population that has a normal distribution curve, the data are interval and therefore the test is powerful. *See also* **non-parametric tests**.

parametrium   the connective tissues immediately surrounding the uterus.

paranasal   near the nasal cavities, as the various sinuses.

paraneoplastic   describes symptoms or signs associated with the presence of a malignant neoplasm but not directly from the situation of the primary or the metastases.

paraoesophageal   near the oesophagus.

paraparesis   loss of power in the legs.

paraplegia   paralysis of the lower limbs, usually including the bladder and rectum below the level of the spinal cord abnormality. *See also* **hemiplegia, monoplegia, tetraplegia**.

paraplegic   a person with paralysis of the lower limbs.

pararectal   near the rectum.

parasympathetic   describes the part of the autonomic nervous system having craniosacral outflow. It is concerned with the normal at rest body processes and opposes the action of the sympathetic nervous system.

parathormone   parathyroid hormone. *See also* **parathyroid glands**.

parathyroid glands   four small endocrine glands lying close to or embedded in the posterior surface of the thyroid gland. They secrete parathyroid hormone (PTH) a protein hormone that regulates calcium and phosphate homeostasis. It is released when serum calcium level is decreased.

paraurethral   near the urethra.

paravaginal   near the vagina.

paravertebral   near the spinal column.

paravertebral block   anaesthesia (more correctly, analgesia) is induced by infiltration of local anaesthetic around the spinal nerve roots as they emerge from the intervertebral foramina.

paravertebral injection   introduction of a local anaesthetic into sympathetic chain can be used as a test in ischaemic limbs to see if sympathectomy is indicated.

parenchyma   the essential, active cells of an organ as distinguished from its vascular and connective tissue.

pareneoplastic syndrome   a collection of general effects associated with cancer, for example, infection, fever, cachexia, anaemia.

parent radionuclide   a nucleus before it has decayed. *See also* **radioactive decay**.

parenteral   not via the alimentary tract. Therapy such as fluid, drugs, or nutrition administered by a route other than the alimentary tract.

paresis   partial or slight paralysis; weakness of a limb.

parietal   associated with a wall.

parietal bones   the two bones which form the sides and vault of the skull.

Parinaud's syndrome   conjunctivitis that is usually unilateral, follicular and followed by enlargement of the preauricular lymph nodes and tenderness.

Paris system   a method of introducing radioactive sources during brachytherapy using Iridium:-192

Parkinson's disease   an incurable neurodegenerative condition in which there is a relatively selective loss of dopamine nerve cells in the brain caus-ing a resting tremor, bradykinesia (slowness of movement) and rigidity in the limbs. Some people differentiate between Parkinson's disease and parkinsonism, the causes of which are multiple and include repeated brain trauma (as in boxing), stroke, atherosclerosis, various toxic agents, viral encephalitis and neuroleptic drugs (typical).

parotid gland   the salivary gland situated in front of and below the ear on either side.

parous   having borne a child or children.

Parrot's nodes   bossing of frontal bones in congenital syphilis.

pars interarticularis   the area between the superior and inferior articular processes in the spinal column, deficient in spondylolisthesis.

particle range   the distance from its point of origin that a charged particle no longer reacts with the material it is travelling through.

particle theory   the basic concept of quantum physics and considers that electromagnetic radiation of short wavelength and high velocity con-sists of particles or quanta or photons each having a discrete amount of energy.

PASCAL   a high-level language for computers.

passwords   entry is forbidden into many computer-controlled systems unless a particular password has been entered. Passwords are frequently graded, so that limited access to the system is allowed by some passwords but unlim-ited access is provided by other passwords.

patella   a triangular, sesamoid bone; the **kneecap**.

patent   open; not closed or occluded.

patent ductus arteriosus   failure of ductus arteriosus to close soon after birth, so that an abnormal shunt between the pulmonary artery and the aorta is preserved. **patent interventricular septum** a congenital defect in the divid-ing wall between the right and left ventricle of the heart.

Paterson-Parker system   a method of introducing radioactive sources during brachytherapy for gynaecological applications using ^{137}caesium needles and tubes.

pathogen   an agent capable of producing disease.

pathological fracture   a fracture caused by underlying disease.

patient advice and liaison service (PALS)   an advice service to patients in NHS and Primary Care Trusts, representing their concerns and complaints to the relevant department within the trust.

patient contour   the shape of a cross-section of a patient when they are initially positioned prior to radiotherapy treatment. *See also* **contouring device**.

patient dosimetry   the measure of dose delivered to the clinical target volume.

patient immobilization   equipment to enable a patient to remain still during treatment or examination including, patient shells, effervescent materials, vacuum bags, bite blocks, breast boards, foam pads, sandbags.

patients' forum   a statutory and independent body comprising patients who will represent the views of patients about how their local NHS services are run.

patient shell   a clear plastic structure which is worn by the patient to enable accurate localization, patient position, patient contour, beam exit and entry points and a base for additional build-up material and shielding.

pattern of distribution   in statistics looks at the frequency that a qualitative result occurs.

peak bone density (PBD) or mass (PBM)   the greatest bone density achieved by an individual, usually achieved in the 30s.

peak sensitivity   the range of wavelengths that a film emulsion is the most sensitive to.

peak value   the maximum value of either positive or negative current or voltage that occurs on an alternating current waveform.

peau d'orange   appearance of (usually) the breast when a cancer results in lymphatic obstruction and dimpling at the hair follicles causing the breast to look (literally) like orange skin; usually a sign of locally advanced disease.

pectoral   associated with the breast.

pectus   the chest.

pectus carinatum   *see* **pigeon chest**.

pectus excavatum   *see* **funnel chest**.

pedal   associated with the foot.

pedal pulse   the dorsalis pedis artery palpated on the dorsum of the foot.

pedicle   a stalk, for example, the narrow part by which a tumour is attached to the surrounding structures.

peduncle   a stalk-like structure.

peer support support from other members of a group to which one belongs. For example, new patients perceive established patients as providing support. Likewise, health professionals use their peer groups to gain and provide support, particularly in stressful circumstances.

Pel–Ebstein fever a recurrent high temperature having a cycle of 15–21 days, which occurs in cases of lymphadenoma.

pellagra a syndrome caused by a diet deficient in niacin and in patients suffering from alcoholism and drug addiction.

pelvic relating to the pelvis.

pelvic cavity that formed by the pelvic bones, more particularly the part below the iliopectineal line.

pelvic floor a mainly muscular partition with the pelvic cavity above and the perineum below. In the female, weakening of these muscles can contribute to urinary incontinence and uterine prolapse.

pelvic girdle the bony pelvis comprising two innominate bones, the sacrum and coccyx.

pelvimetry the measurement of the dimensions of the pelvis.

pelvis a basin-shaped cavity, for example, pelvis of the kidney. The large bony basin-shaped cavity formed by the innominate bones and sacrum, containing and protecting the bladder, rectum and, in the female, the organs of generation. ***contracted pelvis*** one in which one or more diameters are smaller than normal; this may result in difficulties in childbirth. ***false pelvis*** the wide expanded part of the pelvis above the brim. ***true pelvis*** that part of the pelvis below the brim.

penis the male organ of copulation.

penumbra the area at the edge of a beam of radiation that receives some but not all of the main beam because it is not practically possible to produce an X-ray beam from a point source. *See also* **geometric unsharpness**.

pepsin a proteolytic enzyme secreted by the stomach, as the precursor pepsinogen, which hydrolyses proteins to polypeptides. It has an optimum pH of 1.5–2.0.

pepsinogen a proenzyme secreted mainly by the chief cells in the gastric mucosa and converted to pepsin by hydrochloric acid or existing pepsin.

peptic associated with pepsin or to digestion generally. ***peptic ulcer*** a non-malignant ulcer in those parts of the digestive tract that are exposed to the gastric secretions; hence usually in the stomach or duodenum but sometimes in the lower oesophagus or with a Meckel's diverticulum.

peptidase an enzyme that breaks down proteins into amino acids. *See also* **aminopeptidases, dipeptidases**.

peptides organic compounds that yield two or more amino acids on hydrolysis; for example, dipeptides and polypeptides. ***peptide bond*** a chemical bond formed during a dehydration reaction when two amino acids form peptides.

percentage depth dose   in radiotherapy, the ratio of the absorbed dose at any given point to the absorbed dose on the beam axis at the depth of maximum dose expressed as a percentage.

perceptibility   the point at which an image can be clearly seen, when contrast is equal to, or greater than the contrast threshold.

perceptibility curve   a curve produced from measurable data after a phantom has been radiographed and a number of people have recorded the contrast observed at various exposure levels.

percutaneous   through the skin.

percutaneous endoscopic gastrostomy (PEG)   gastrostomy tube inserted endoscopically through the abdominal wall to allow feeding and the passage of drugs.

percutaneous myocardial revascularization   a treatment for angina. A catheter with laser energy source is introduced into the heart via the femoral artery. The laser is used to produce channels through to the myocardium, thus allowing more oxygenated blood to reach the myocardium.

percutaneous nephrolithotomy   *see* **nephrolithotomy**.

percutaneous transhepatic cholangiography (PTC)   *see* **cholangiography**.

percutaneous transluminal angioplasty   a balloon is passed into a stenosed artery (for example, coronary artery) and inflated with contrast agent; it presses the atheroma against the vessel wall, thereby increasing the diameter of the lumen.

percutaneous transluminal coronary angioplasty (PTCA)   a procedure used in the treatment of angina. A balloon-tipped catheter is used to dilate a stenosed coronary artery.

perforation   a hole in a previously intact sheet of tissue. Used in reference to perforation of the tympanic membrane, or the wall of the stomach or gut, constituting a surgical emergency.

performance indicators (PIs)   quantitative measures of the activities and resources used in healthcare delivery. High-level performance indicators, for example, deaths from all causes (people aged 15–64), early detection of cancer, day case rate, cancelled operations, and clinical indicators, for example, deaths in hospital after surgery, a heart attack or hip fracture, are used to assess the six areas of the National Framework for Assessing Performance.

perfusion   the passage of fluid through tissue, a specific organ or body part.

perianal   surrounding the anus.

periapical film   a small radiographic film in a waterproof envelope that is placed inside the mouth to radiograph individual teeth.

periarterial   surrounding an artery.

periarthritis   inflammation of the structures surrounding a joint. Sometimes applied to frozen shoulder.

periarticular   surrounding a joint.

peribulbar   around the eyeball inside the orbit.

pericardial effusion   a collection of pericardial fluid in the heart restricting cardiac movement, producing signs and symptoms of heart failure.

pericarditis   inflammation of the pericardium of the heart.

pericardium   the double serous membranous sac which envelops the heart. The layer in contact with the heart is called visceral (or epicardium); that reflected to form the sac is called parietal. Between the two is the pericardial cavity, which normally contains a small amount of serous fluid.

perichondrium   the membranous covering of cartilage.

pericolic   around the colon.

pericranium   the periosteal covering of the cranium.

perifollicular   around a follicle.

perilymph   the fluid contained in the internal ear, between the membranous and bony labyrinth.

perimetrium   the peritoneal covering of the uterus.

perinephric   surrounding the kidney.

perineum   the wedge-shaped structure situated between the rectum and the external genitalia.

perineurium   connective tissue enclosing a bundle of nerve fibres.

period   the number of seconds taken to complete one cycle of alternating current. In ultrasound the length of time required for one oscillation to occur.

periodic table   a list of the 103 elements with the number of electron shells shown horizontally and the chemical properties, that is the number of electrons in the outer shell grouped vertically.

periodontal disease   gum disease. In the early stages it presents as gingivitis and later causes loosening of the teeth.

periodontal membrane   a membrane that attaches a tooth to the socket in the maxilla or mandible.

periodontics   branch of dentistry concerned with prevention and treatment of diseases of the supporting tissues of the teeth.

periodontitis   inflammatory disease of the periodontium, resulting in destruction of the periodontal ligament.

periodontium   collective name given to the tissues supporting a tooth and comprising the gingiva, periodontal ligament, cementum and surrounding alveolar bone.

perioral   around the mouth.

periosteum   the membrane which covers a bone. In long bones only the shaft as far as the epiphysis is covered. It protects and allows regeneration.

periostitis inflammation of the periosteum. *See also* **diffuse periostitis, haemorrhagic periostitis**.

peripheral relating to the outer parts of any structure. Any device attached to a computer, e.g. a printer or modem.

peripheral nervous system (PNS) describes that part of the nervous system outside the brain or spinal cord. Usually applied to those nerves which supply the musculoskeletal system and surrounding tissues to differentiate from the autonomic nervous system.

peripheral resistance (PR) the force exerted by the arteriolar walls which is an important factor in the control of normal blood pressure.

peripheral vascular disease (PVD) any abnormal condition arising in the blood vessels outside the heart, the main one being athcrosclerosis, which can lead to thrombosis and occlusion of the vessel, resulting in gangrene.

peripheral venography the radiographic investigation of the venous system of a limb following the direct injection of contrast agent into a vein.

peripheral vision that surrounding the central field of vision.

periportal surrounding the hepatic portal vein.

peristalsis a rhythmic wave-like contraction and dilatation occurring in a hollow structure, for example, ureter, gastrointestinal tract. In the intestine it is the movement by which the contents (food and waste) are propelled along the lumen. It consists of a wave of contraction preceded by a wave of relaxation.

peritoneal cavity a potential space between the parietal and visceral layers of the peritoneum.

peritoneal effusion a collection of serous fluid in the peritoneal cavity.

peritoneum the delicate serous membrane which lines the abdominal and pelvic cavities (parietal layer) and also covers some of the organs (visceral layer) contained in them.

peritonitis inflammation of the peritoneum, usually secondary to disease of one of the abdominal organs.

periumbilical surrounding the umbilicus.

perivascular around a blood vessel.

permanent teeth adult teeth, 32 in number, which are numbered 12345678 in each quadrant of the mouth.

permeability the measure of the response of a material to a magnetic field. It is the ratio of the magnetic flux induced in the material to the strength of the applied magnetic field. In physiology, the extent to which substances dissolved in the body fluids are able to move through cell membranes or layers of cells (for example, the walls of capillaries or absorptive tissues).

permittivity   absolute permittivity is the ratio of the electrical displacement to the electrical field at the same point. *relative permittivity* (or *dielectric constant*) of a capacitor is the ratio of its capacitance with the specific dielectric between the plates to its capacitance with air between the plates.

pernicious anaemia   results from the inability of the bone marrow to produce normal red cells because of the lack of a protein, released by gastric parietal cells, called the intrinsic factor, which is necessary for the absorption of vitamin B_{12} from food. An autoimmune mechanism may be responsible.

peromelia   a teratogenic malformation of a limb.

persistent (patent) ductus arteriosus   a congenital heart defect.

perspiration   the excretion from the sweat glands through the skin pores. *See also* **insensible perspiration, sensible perspiration**.

Perthes' disease (pseudocoxalgia)   avascular degeneration of the upper femoral epiphysis occurs in children; revascularization occurs, but residual deformity of the femoral head may subsequently lead to arthritic changes.

pes   a foot or foot-like structure.

pes cavus (high-arched foot, claw-foot)   a pathological elevation of the longitudinal arch caused by plantar flexion of the forefoot relative to the rearfoot. The medial longitudinal arch is most affected but the lateral longitudinal arch can also be elevated. There is dorsal humping of the midfoot and associated forefoot and rearfoot deformities. These may include clawing or retraction of the lesser toes, a trigger first toe, and a depressed first metatarsal with either heel varus or equinus. It may be acquired or congenital.

pes planus (flat-foot)   a generic term for a foot with an abnormally low arch. The medial longitudinal arch is depressed or absent, and the foot has an increased contact area with the ground. During weightbearing the foot appears to have no longitudinal arch. It may be congenital or acquired. When young children first stand the feet appear to be flat, as adipose tissue under the medial longitudinal arch is pressed close to the ground. Older children very frequently have flattening of the medial longitudinal arch on standing but the arch reappears on standing on tiptoe (a mobile flat foot). *flexible pes planus* is generally asymptomatic in children but may become a semi-rigid condition in adulthood. It has been linked with excess laxity of the joint capsule and the ligaments supporting the arch, which allows it to collapse when weight is applied. *rigid pes planus* in adults may be a progression from flexible to semi-rigid to rigid as part of the ageing process. Structural changes due to the existing abnormal position become fixed, as soft and osseous tissues adapt. Rigidity is increased where there are significant osteoarthritic changes or inflammatory arthritic destruction.

petit mal   a form of epilepsy where there is a brief alteration in consciousness.

petrous   resembling stone.

Peyer's patches aggregates of lymphatic tissue situated in the ileum. Function to prevent microorganisms entering the blood. Site of infection in typhoid fever.

pH hydrogen ion concentration, expressed as a negative logarithm and a quantitative method of measuring the acidity or alkalinity of a solution, on a log scale of 0 to 14, where pure water is 7. Below 7 is acid, and higher than 7 is alkaline. Developer has a pH of 9.6–10.6, and fixer a pH of 4.2–4.9.

pH meter a calibrated, electric meter used to take accurate pH readings of processor chemicals.

phaeochromocytoma (paraganglioma) a condition in which there is a tumour of the adrenal medulla, or of the structurally similar tissues associated with the sympathetic chain. It secretes adrenaline (epinephrine) and allied hormones and the symptoms are due to the excess of these substances. Results in hypertensive crises, with associated headache, flushing and tachycardia.

phagocyte a cell capable of engulfing bacteria and other particulate material.

phagocytosis the process by which phagocytes engulf particles such as bacteria.

phalanges the small bones of the fingers and toes.

phallus the penis.

phantom limb the sensation that a limb is still attached to the body after it has been amputated. Pain may seem to come from the amputated limb.

pharmacy medicines drugs which can only be sold if a pharmacist is present.

pharyngeal pouch pathological dilatation of the lower part of the pharynx.

pharyngolaryngeal associated with the pharynx and larynx.

pharyngotympanic tube (eustachian tube) a canal, partly bony, partly cartilaginous, connecting the pharynx with the tympanic cavity. It allows air to pass into the middle ear, so that the air pressure is kept even on both sides of the eardrum.

pharynx the cavity at the back of the mouth. It is cone-shaped and is lined with mucous membrane; at the lower end it opens into the oesophagus. The pharyngotympanic (eustachian) tubes pierce its lateral walls and the posterior nares pierce its anterior wall. The larynx lies immediately below it and in front of the oesophagus.

phase contrast angiography a two-dimensional or three-dimensional magnetic resonance imaging technique to distinguish flowing blood from static tissue. The magnitude image shows the blood vessels and the phase image shows the direction of flow.

phase encoding a technique used to locate a magnetic resonance signal by applying a series of varying phase-encoded, gradient pulses so that the phase of spin is altered prior to the signal readout. The spins retain the memory of the separate phase-encoded pulses.

phased array in ultrasound a sector field of view with multiple transducer elements, formed in precise sequence and under electronic control. This gives a wide field of view using a small transducer, for example, cardiac or paediatric head scans.

phenidone a developer agent.

phenotypic characteristic.

pheromones chemicals with a specific odour. They are present in the sweat produced by the apocrine sweat glands. They may influence sexual behaviour.

Philadelphia chromosome (Ph) an anomaly of chromosome number 22. It is found in the blood cells of most people with chronic myeloid leukaemia.

phimosis constriction of the prepuce so that it cannot be drawn back over the glans penis.

phlebography (venography) radiological examination of the venous system involving injection of an opaque medium. Mostly replaced by ultrasound.

phlegm (sputum) mucus expectorated (coughed up) from the bronchi.

phocomelia teratogenic malformation. Arms and feet attached directly to trunk giving a seal-like appearance. Many cases in the 1960s were associated with the use of thalidomide during pregnancy.

phonation the production of speech sounds.

phosphates salts of phosphoric acid.

phosphor a substance that has a characteristic light emission when stimulated by an electron beam.

phosphorescence is when a medium is irradiated and light is emitted, when the irradiation stops light continues to be emitted.

phosphor layer the suspension of phosphor crystals in a binder to form the layer of an intensifying screen that converts radiation to light.

phosphor storage plate *see* **imaging plate**.

phosphor type the higher the total efficiency of a phosphor the more light is produced and therefore the thinner the phosphor, rare earth phosphors are more efficient than calcium tungstate phosphors.

phosphorus (P) a poisonous element. Forms an important constituent (as phosphates) of nucleic acids, bone and all cells. *radioactive phosphorus* (^{32}P) is used in the treatment of thrombocythaemia.

phosphorylation   the process of attaching a phosphate group to a protein, sugar or other compound.

photocathode   a structure made of zinc cadmium which produces electrons in proportion to the amount of light falling on it. *See also* **image intensifier**.

photodynamic therapy   the administration of a tumour-localizing, photosensitizing drug which is activated by a laser light of a specific wavelength to damage tumour cells.

photoelectric absorption   when a photon collides with an orbiting electron and gives all its energy to the electron which is then ejected from the atom.

photofluorography   the recording of the image on the output phosphor of an image intensifier.

photographic dosimeter   a device containing a photographic film and several different filters that is worn over a period of time. The film is processed and the density on the film is measured. The density is proportional to the amount of radiation received by the wearer.

photographic unsharpness   blurring of a radiographic image due to the recording medium. *See also* **unsharpness**.

photomultiplier tube   equipment that produces an amplified current when exposed to electromagnetic radiation, photons hitting the cathode produce electrons which in turn hit other surfaces thus producing more electrons. Used in earlier CT scanner units.

photons   a quantum of electromagnetic radiation having an energy of hf, h equals Planck's constant and f is the frequency of the radiation.

photoscan   the image from a linear scanner recorded on radiographic film.

photo-thermographic printing   uses a film containing chemicals which are activated when an image is scanned by a laser onto the film, the film is then heated to produce the image, the chemicals remain in the film. *See also* **thermographic printing**.

phren   the diaphragm.

physical abuse   *see* **abuse, non-accidental injury**.

physical half-life   is the time required for the activity of a radioactive sample to decay to half its original value.

physiological   often used to describe a normal process or structure, to distinguish it from an abnormal or pathological feature (for example, the physiological level of glucose in the blood).

physiological advantage   a muscle's ability to shorten. Its greatest physiological advantage is when a muscle is at rest.

physiological saline   *see* **isotonic**.

physiological solution   a fluid isotonic with the body fluids and containing similar salts.

physiology   the science dealing with normal functioning of the body.

pia mater   the innermost of the meninges; the vascular membrane which lies in close contact with the brain and spinal cord.

picture archiving communications system (PACS)   in radiography, a networked system of viewing monitors connected to a central image database that allows integration of image and demographic information.

pie chart   in statistics, a circle divided into segments, each segment represents a number of results as a proportion of the whole.

pie lines   marks on a processed film which have been caused by chemicals drying on the surface of the automatic processor rollers.

piezoelectric crystal   a crystal which converts electrical impulses into sound waves and vice versa by deforming when a voltage is applied across it, for example, ceramic or quartz crystals.

piezoelectric effect   when an electric current is produced by certain materials when pressure is applied to their surface. *See also* **inverse piezoelectric effect**.

pigeon chest (pectus carinatum)   a narrow chest, bulging anteriorly in the breast bone region.

pilomotor nerves   tiny nerves that innervate the hair follicle, causing the hair to become erect and give the appearance of 'goose flesh'.

pilosebaceous   associated with the hair follicle and the sebaceous gland opening into it.

pilot study   an early smaller-scale study carried out before the main research project to evaluate viability and to identify problems with the research methodology.

pineal body (pineal gland)   a small reddish-grey conical structure on the dorsal surface of the midbrain. It secretes various substances which include 5-hydroxytryptamine and melatonin. The release of melatonin is connected to the amount of light entering the eye. Melatonin levels fluctuate during the 24 hours and appear to influence gonadotrophin secretion, diurnal rhythms such as sleep, and mood. *See also* **depression**.

pin-hole collimator   gamma camera collimator with a small hole, a few millimetres in diameter at the end of a lead cone which, due to the divergence of the gamma rays, give an enlarged image of a small object.

pinna   the auricle. That part of the ear which is external to the head.

pisiform   one of the eight bones of the wrist.

pitch   in CT scanning, is the ratio of table movement, during one 360° rotation.

pituitary fossa   a depression in the spenoid bone for the pituitary gland; if the gland becomes enlarged, the fossa becomes enlarged.

pituitary gland (hypophysis cerebri)   a small oval endocrine gland lying in the pituitary fossa of the sphenoid bone. The anterior lobe (adenohypophysis) produces and secretes several hormones; growth hormone, adrenocorticotrophic hormone, thyroid-stimulating hormone, luteinizing hormone, follicle stimulating hormone, prolactin and melanocyte stimulating hormone. The posterior lobe (neurohypophysis) stores and secretes oxytocin and vasopressin (antidiuretic hormone). These hormones are made by nerve fibres in the hypothalamus.

pivot joint   a synovial joint which allows rotation only, for example, the superior radio-ulnar joint.

pixel   picture cell, the dots which can be used by a character on a digital image display screen, the smaller the pixel the greater the image quality.

placebo   a harmless substance given as medicine. In a randomized placebo-controlled trial, an inert substance, identical in appearance with the material being tested. When neither the researcher nor the subject knows which is which, the trial is said to be double blind.

placebo effect   a therapeutic effect is observed after the administration of a placebo.

placenta   the afterbirth, a hormone-secreting vascular structure developed and functioning about the third month of pregnancy and attached to the inner wall of the uterus. Through it the fetus is supplied with nourishment and oxygen and through it the fetus gets rid of its waste products. In normal labour it is expelled, with the fetal membranes, during the third stage of labour. When this does not occur it is termed a ***retained placenta*** and may be an ***adherent placenta***. The placenta is usually attached to the upper segment of the uterus; where it lies in the lower uterine segment it is called a ***placenta praevia*** and usually causes placental abruption with painless antepartum bleeding.

placenta accreta   when the placenta invades the uterine muscles which makes separation from the placenta difficult and can result in bleeding during birth.

placenta praevia   when the placenta is attached to the lower part of the uterine wall and may cause antepartum haemorrhage.

placentography   radiographic examination of the placenta, now superseded by ultrasound.

planar implants   an interstitial implant to treat a volume of tissue of the same area to a thickness of 5 mm on either side.

Planck's constant   a constant that relates the quantum of energy (E) of a photon to the frequency (f) of the corresponding electromagnetic radiation. $E = hf$ where h is Planck's constant.

plane joint   a synovial joint that allows a gliding movement only, for example, the sacro-iliac joints.

planning target volume (PTV)   a tissue volume used to aid the selection of the appropriate beam sizes and arrangements to ensure that the prescribed dose of radiation is delivered to the clinical target volume during radiotherapy treatment.

plantar   associated with the sole of the foot.

plantar arch   the union of the plantar and dorsalis pedis arteries in the sole of the foot.

plantar flexion   downward movement of the big toe.

plaque   an elevated area of skin. In dentistry a soft deposit of bacteria and cellular debris formed when oral hygiene is poor. *See also* **dental plaque**.

plasma   the fluid part of blood.

plasma cell   an immune cell that produces antibodies. It is derived from B lymphocytes/cells.

plasmacytoma   a rare condition where a myeloma is confined to one or two bones only.

plasmin   proteolytic enzyme produced when plasminogen is activated. It breaks down fibrin clots when healing is complete. Also called *fibrinolysin*.

plasminogen   precursor of plasmin. Release of activators, for example, tissue plasminogen activator (t-PA), from damaged tissue promotes the conversion of plasminogen into plasmin.

plasticizer   an addition to the radiographic film emulsion to prevent it from becoming too brittle.

platelets (thrombocytes)   cellular fragments concerned with blood coagulation.

platelet plug   one of the four overlapping stages of haemostasis. Platelets aggregate and adhere to form a temporary plug at the site of blood vessel damage.

pleomorphism   differences between individual daughter cells or subclones.

pleura   the serous membrane covering the surface of the lung (*visceral pleura*), the diaphragm, the mediastinum and the chest wall (*parietal pleura*).

pleural cavity   is the potential space between the visceral and parietal pleurae which in health are in contact in all phases of respiration.

pleural effusion   inflammation of the pleura of the lungs with secretion of serous fluid into the pleural cavity.

pleurisy, pleuritis   inflammation of the pleura. May be fibrinous (dry), be associated with an effusion (wet), or be complicated by empyema.

pleuropulmonary   relating to the pleura and lung.

plexopathy   decreased movement or sensation in a joint caused by impaired function of the nerves that cause sensation and movement.

plexus   a network of vessels or nerves.

Plummer–Vinson syndrome   a rare disorder caused by oesophageal webs at the level of the cricoid cartilage.

PN junction   is formed by fusing together a P-type semiconductor and an N-type semiconductor.

pneumoconiosis (dust disease)   fibrosis of the lung caused by long-continued inhalation of dust in industrial occupations. The most important complication is the occasional superinfection with tuberculosis. *See also* **anthracosis, asbestosis, byssinosis, rheumatoid pneumoconiosis, siderosis, silicosis**.

pneumocytes   cells lining the alveolar walls in the lungs. Type I are flat. Type II are cuboidal and secrete surfactant.

pneumoencephalography   radiographic examination of cerebral ventricles after injection of air by means of a lumbar or cisternal puncture.

pneumonia   acute infection of the lung by an invading organism associated with new pulmonary shadowing on a radiograph. Can be subdivided into community-acquired, hospital-acquired, and pneumonia associated with profound immunosuppression.

pneumonitis   inflammation of lung tissue.

pneumoperitoneum   air or gas in the peritoneal cavity. Can be introduced for diagnostic or therapeutic purposes.

pneumothorax   air or gas in the pleural cavity separating the visceral from the parietal pleura so that lung tissue is compressed. Occurs spontaneously when an over-dilated pulmonary air sac ruptures, permitting communication of respiratory passages with the pleural cavity. Associated with many lung diseases, including asthma, bronchial cancer, COPD, congenital cysts, tuberculosis, trauma, and positive pressure ventilation. ***tension pneumothorax*** a valve-like wound or tear in the lung allows air to enter the pleural cavity with each inspiration, but not to escape on expiration, thus progressively increasing intrathoracic pressure and constituting an acute medical emergency. Signs are of hyperinflation, midline shift and increasing respiratory distress.

point defects   the loss of an atom from a structure. ***Frenkel defect*** forming an interstitial ion or atom. ***Schottky defect*** removing the atom completely.

polar graph paper   paper with a series of circular lines around a central point, intersected with radial lines from the same point forming 15° divisions, used in treatment planning.

polarized   describes the resting state of the plasma membrane of an excitable cell where there is no impulse transmission. The inside of the membrane is electrically negative relative to the outside. *See also* **depolarization**.

polar molecules   when an atom contains molecules that are not coincident to the nucleus resulting in a positive and a negative end to the atom.

polyarthralgia   pain in several joints.

polyarthritis   inflammation of several joints.

polycystic   composed of many cysts.

polycystic kidney diseases a number of conditions which have variable effects on kidney function. Many lead to end-stage renal failure and the need for dialysis. Often associated with cystic disease of other organs, especially the liver and meninges.

polycythaemia (rubra vera) an uncommon disease of the bone marrow, characterized by increased production of red blood cells, leucocytes and platelets.

polydactyly (polydactylism) having more than the normal number of fingers or toes. On the foot the extra digits may develop from one metatarsal or there may be duplication of metatarsal segments. Sometimes selective amputation at an early age is indicated. This ensures optimum foot function, thus facilitating shoe fitting in childhood and adult life.

polymorphonuclear having a many-shaped or lobulated nucleus, usually applied to the phagocytic leucocytes (granulocytes), neutrophils, basophils and eosinophils.

polyp (polypus) a pedunculated tumour arising from any epithelial surface, for example, cervical, uterine, nasal, intestinal. Usually benign but may be malignant. ***adenomatous polyps*** are premalignant. Tissue overgrowth underlying the epithelium may also be the cause of polyp formation.

polyposis a condition in which there are numerous intestinal polyps.

polyuria excess urine production, the urine contains sugar and is a sign of diabetes mellitus.

pons a bridge; a process of tissue joining two sections of an organ.

pons varolii part of the brainstem which serves to connect the various lobes of the brain.

POP (Post Office Protocol) an email system.

popliteal associated with the area behind the knee.

popliteal space the diamond-shaped depression behind the knee, bounded by muscles and containing the popliteal nerve and vessels (artery and vein).

popliteus a muscle in the popliteal space which flexes the leg and aids rotation.

population the pool of information from which statistics are drawn.

population inversion when half the atoms in a structure are in an excited state.

pore a minute surface opening. One of the mouths of the ducts (leading from the sweat glands) on the skin surface; they are controlled by fine papillary muscles, closing in the cold and opening in the presence of heat.

porphyrins group of organic compounds that form the basis of respiratory pigments, including haemoglobin. Naturally occurring porphyrins are uroporphyrin and coproporphyrin.

port   a connection point on a computer for input or output hardware.

porta   the depression (hilum) of an organ at which the vessels enter and leave.

porta hepatis   the transverse fissure through which the hepatic portal vein, hepatic artery and bile ducts pass on the under surface of the liver.

portacaval, portocaval   relating to the hepatic portal vein and inferior vena cava.

portacaval anastomosis   the hepatic portal vein is joined to the inferior vena cava with the object of reducing the pressure within the hepatic portal vein in cases of hepatic portal hypertension.

portal circulation   *see* **hepatic portal circulation**.

portal hypertension   more properly called *hepatic portal hypertension*. Increased pressure in the hepatic portal vein. Usually caused by cirrhosis of the liver; results in splenomegaly, with hypersplenism and alimentary bleeding. *See also* **oesophageal varices**.

portal imaging   methods of verifying the radiotherapy treatment area, using either radiographic film or digital imaging methods. The portal image of the treatment area is compared to the image taken at simulation. *See also* **therapy verification film, electronic portal imaging**.

portal vein   more properly called *hepatic portal vein*. That conveying blood into the liver; it is about 75 mm long and is formed by the union of the superior mesenteric and splenic veins.

portal venography   the radiographic investigation of the portal system following a direct injection of contrast agent into the spleen.

positive correlation   in statistics, when information is linked and an increase in one item will result in an increase in the other and a decrease in one item will result in a decrease in the other.

positron emission tomography (PET)   uses cyclotron-produced isotopes of extremely short half-life that emit positrons which are introduced into the patient. A specialist gamma camera is used that has multiple detectors lying in a circular gantry that surrounds the patient. The detectors detect the isotopes that decay through positron emission as this produces two photons of 511 keV which are emitted at 180° to each other. Only if two detectors are opposite each other, each registering a photon within nanoseconds of each other, are the photons recorded. PET scanning is used to evaluate physiological function of organs, for example, the brain.

positrons   positively charged particles that combine with electrons (negative charge), causing gamma rays to be emitted.

post anaesthesia   after anaesthetic and before full recovery.

postanal   behind the anus.

posterior   situated at the back. *See also* **anterior**.

posterior chamber   of the eye situated between the anterior surface of the lens and the posterior surface of the iris. *See also* **aqueous**.

posteroanterior radiograph   from the back to the front of the body.

postganglionic   situated distal to a collection of nerve cells (ganglion), as a postganglionic nerve fibre.

posthepatic   behind the liver.

postmortem   after death.

postnasal   behind the nose and in the nasopharynx.

postnatal   after childbirth.

postpartum   occurring after labour.

potassium bromide   a developer restrainer.

potassium hydroxide   a developer accelerator.

potassium metabisulphite   a developer preservative.

potassium sulphite   a fixing solution preservative.

Posteroanterior radiograph (PA). From Pocketbook of radiographic positioning, 2nd edn, Ruth Sutherland, 2003, Churchill Livingstone, Edinburgh, with permission.

potential difference   a measure of electrical work on a unit positive charge in moving it from one point to another in volts.

potential energy   represents the work done in raising a body to a height h. Work which can be performed due to the position or state of a system; unit: joule.

Pott's disease   spondylitis; spinal caries; spinal tuberculosis. The resultant necrosis of the vertebrae causes kyphosis.

Pott's fracture   a fracture-dislocation of the ankle joint. A fracture of the lower end of the tibia and fibula, 75 mm above the ankle joint, and a fracture of the medial malleolus of the tibia.

pouch   a pocket or recess. ***pouch of Douglas*** the rectouterine pouch.

power   is the rate at which work is done in joules per second. SI unit watt. In ultrasound the power of the ultrasound beam is the energy flow rate of the whole beam which must be kept to a minimum value due to the harmful effects of ultrasound.

power calculation   a measure of statistical power. The likelihood of the research study to generate statistically significant results.

Power Doppler   a measure of the amplitude of the Doppler signal when scanning very slow moving structures, for example, small blood vessels in the body, it will not show the velocity or direction of flow.

PR (per rectum)   describes the route used for examination of the rectum, or introduction of drugs or fluids into the body.

precancerous   pertaining to a stage of abnormal tissue growth that is likely to develop into a malignant tumour. *See also* **carcinoma in situ**.

precordial (praecordial)   relating to the area of the chest immediately over the heart.

precursor   forerunner.

pre-exposed step wedges   produced by film manufacturers that when processed, have a series of increased density steps which can be used to determine the consistency of the film processor.

prefrontal   situated in the anterior portion of the frontal lobe of the cerebrum.

preganglionic   proximal to a collection of nerve cells (ganglion), as a preganglionic nerve fibre.

preload   the degree of stretch present in the myocardial muscle fibres at the end of diastole. *See also* **afterload, stroke volume**.

premature   occurring before the proper time.

premature beat   *see* **extrasystole**.

premature birth   in English law, the birth of a baby after 24 weeks but before 37 weeks' gestation.

premedication   drugs given before the administration of another drug, for example, those given before a general anaesthesia to reduce anxiety.

premenstrual   preceding menstruation. ***premenstrual (cyclical) syndrome*** (PMS) a group of physical and mental changes occurring any time between 2 and 14 days before menstruation. They are relieved almost immediately when menstruation starts.

premolar tooth   permanent tooth with two cusps (bicuspid), placed fourth and fifth from the midline. They succeed the primary molars. They have either a single grooved root or two roots.

prenatal   associated with the period between the last menstrual period and birth of the child, normally 40 weeks or 280 days.

prepatellar   in front of the patella, as applied to a large bursa. *See also* **bursitis**.

prepubertal   before puberty.

prepuce   the foreskin of the penis.

prescription only medicines   drugs which must have a written prescription signed by a doctor, dentist or specialist nurse prescriber.

presenile dementia   occurring in people between 50 and 60 years of age. *See also* **Alzheimer's disease**.

preservative   in developer, a chemical, potassium metabisulphite that discourages oxidation and slows down the formation of discolouration products, in fixing solutions, for example, sodium sulphite or potassium sulphite is to prevent the breakdown of the fixing agent into sulphur particles.

pressure   force applied per unit area; unit pascal.

pressure areas   any body area subjected to pressure sufficient to compress the capillaries and disrupt the microcirculation. Usually occurs where tissues are compressed between a bone and a hard surface, for example, theatre table, trolley, bed, chair, splint, or where two skin surfaces are in contact such as under the breasts. Pressure areas include: head, spine, sacrum, shoulders, elbows, hips, buttocks, heels, ankles. *See also* **pressure ulcer**.

pressure point   a place at which an artery passes over a bone, against which it can be compressed, to stop bleeding.

pressure ulcer (decubitus ulcer, pressure sore)   previously called a ***bedsore***. Defined as an area of localized damage to the skin and underlying tissue caused by pressure, shear, friction, or a combination of these factors. Pressure ulcers develop when any area of the body is subjected to unrelieved pressure that leads to local hypoxia, ischaemia and necrosis with inflammation and ulcer formation. Shearing forces also disrupt the microcirculation when they cause the skin layers to move against one another. Shearing damages the deeper tissues and can lead to an extensive pressure ulcer. Friction from continual rubbing leads to blisters, abrasions and superficial pressure ulcers, and is made worse by moisture such as urine or sweat. Factors that increase the risk of pressure ulcer formation include: poor oxygenation, incontinence, age over 65–70, immobility, altered consciousness, dehydration and malnutrition.

presystole   the period preceding the systole or contraction of the heart muscle.

prevalence   total number of cases of a disease existing in a population at a single point in time.

prevalence rate   the number of cases of a particular disease which exist at a given point in time.

prevalence ratio   the prevalence of a disease, expressed as a ratio of population size.

preventive dentistry   the prevention of, and preventive treatment for, dental disease and the promotion of good oral health.

prima facie   'at first sight', or sufficient evidence brought by one party to require the other party to provide a defence.

primary   first in order.

Primary Care Trust (PCT)   in England a body that works with Social Services and other local government departments and other relevant bodies, for example, voluntary sector, to assess local health needs, plan, develop and provide community and primary healthcare services, and commission secondary services for the local population, in order to improve health, and reduce inequalities in health and improve access. They employ staff, run community hospitals, own property, and are responsible for public health. *See also* **Strategic Health Authority**.

primary collimation   indicates the maximum field size of an X-ray beam at a specific distance.

primary haemorrhage   bleeding that occurs at the time of the injury.

primary radiation   the main beam of radiation from a source which has not interacted with an object.

primary radiation barrier   the floor, walls and ceiling of a room which may be exposed directly to the primary beam of radiation from X-ray equipment.

primary site   the initial position of tumour growth.

primary solute   the main solute used in liquid scintillation counting as it fluoresces when electrons drop to their original low-energy state. *See also* **fluorescence**.

primary tumour   the neoplasm at the site of origin.

primigravida   a woman who is pregnant for the first time.

primipara   a woman who has given birth to a child for the first time.

Private Finance Initiative (PFI)   a joint venture between private and public sector to build a facility, for example, a hospital, using private finance. The NHS then leases the building. Some non-clinical services may also be provided under the lease agreement.

probability   the likelihood that something is going to occur.

probe (transducer)   a hand-held instrument composed of multiple elements of piezo-electric material each with its own electrodes, used in ultrasound imaging.

process   a prominence or outgrowth of any part.

proctitis   inflammation of the anus or rectum.

proctocolitis   inflammation of the anus, rectum and colon.

proctoscope   an endoscope with a light source used to visually inspect the rectum.

professional self-regulation   the professional quality and continuing professional development standards set by various professional regulatory bodies for health professionals, for example, General Medical Council (GMC), for professional practice, discipline and conduct.

profile   the image captured by the detector in CT scanning.

progesterone   a steroid hormone secreted by the corpus luteum, placenta and, in limited amounts, by the adrenal glands. Progesterone acts on the endometrium, myometrium, cervical mucus and breasts. It is important in the preparation for and maintenance of pregnancy.

progestogen   any natural or synthetic progestational hormone including progesterone.

progestogen-only pill   an oral contraceptive that is taken continuously and at regular time intervals to provide effective contraception.

prognosis   a forecast of the probable course and termination of a disease.

program   a set of written instructions for the computer.

prolactin (PRL)   a hormone secreted by the anterior pituitary, concerned with lactation and reproduction.

prolactinoma   prolactin-secreting pituitary adenoma of the pituitary gland. *See also* **hyperprolactinaemia**.

prolapse   descent; the falling of a structure.

prolapse of an intervertebral disc (PID)   protrusion of the disc nucleus into the spinal canal. Most common in the lumbar region where it causes low back pain and/or sciatica. ***prolapse of the iris*** iridocele. ***prolapse of the rectum*** the lower portion of the intestinal tract descends outside the external anal sphincter. ***prolapse of the uterus*** the uterus descends into the vagina and may be visible at the vaginal orifice.

proliferate   increase by cell division.

PROM (Programmable Read Only Memory)   a specially prepared computer chip which can be programmed.

promontory   a projection; a prominent part.

pronate   to place ventral surface downward, for example, on the face; to turn (the palm of the hand) downwards. *See also* **supinate**.

pronator   that which pronates, usually applied to a muscle. *See also* **supinator**.

prone   lying on the anterior surface of the body with the face turned to the side. Of the hand, with the palm downwards. *See also* **supine**.

Pronosco X-posure System™   specialist equipment for assessing bone mineral density.

propagate   in ultrasound to move forward through a medium, at an initial velocity and direction.

propagation speed   the speed at which a wave moves through a medium in metres per second.

prophylactic   an agent which prevents the development of a disease.

proprioception   appreciation of balance and the position of the body and individual body parts in relation to each other, especially as they change during movement.

proprioceptor   a sensory receptor located in a muscle, tendon, ligament or vestibular apparatus of the ears whose reflex function is locomotor or postural.

proptosis   protrusion or bulging of an organ – commonly describes forward displacement of the eyeball.

prospective study   research that deals with future data, moving forward in time. *See also* **retrospective study**.

prostacyclin   a substance formed by endothelial cells lining blood vessels. It inhibits platelet aggregation and is concerned with preventing intravascular clotting.

prostaglandins   a large group of regulatory lipids. Found in most body tissues where they regulate physiological functions including: smooth muscle contraction, inflammation, gastric secretion and blood clotting. Used pharmaceutically to terminate pregnancy, induce labour and for asthma and gastric hyperacidity.

prostate   a small conical gland at the base of the male bladder and surrounding the first part of the urethra. Adds alkaline fluid containing enzymes into the semen.

prostate specific antigen (PSA)   protein secreted by prostatic tissue. Acts as a tumour marker for prostate cancer, and its detection in the blood forms the basis for a screening test. Conditions other than prostate cancer can cause an increase in PSA level.

prostatic   relating to the prostate. ***benign prostatic hyperplasia*** (BPH) benign enlargement of the prostate gland occurring mainly in older men. Leads to urinary problems such as poor stream and retention. ***prostatic acid phosphatase***. *See also* **acid phosphatase**.

prostatitis   inflammation of the prostate gland.

prosthesis   an artificial substitute for a missing part, a device designed to improve function such as a pacemaker.

prosthetic dentistry   the restoration of the function and aesthetics of missing teeth using artificial dentures.

prosthetic services   provide prostheses, for example replacement breast, eye, nose, or wigs.

protease   an enzyme which digests protein (proteolytic).

protective barriers   methods of protecting the patients, staff and general public from unnecessary exposure to radiation using lead panelling and/or concrete.

protective isolation (reverse barrier nursing)   involves separating patients who are immunocompromised and susceptible to infection, either by disease or treatment. The type of patients needing protection from infection include those with leukaemia, those having immunosuppressant treatment for organ transplantation, chemotherapy or radiation or neutropenic patients. *See also* **containment isolation, source isolation**.

proteins   highly complex nitrogenous compounds found in all animal and vegetable tissues. They are built up of amino acids and are essential for growth and repair of the body. Those from animal sources are of high biological value because they contain the essential amino acids. Those from vegetable sources contain not all, but some of the essential amino acids. Proteins are hydrolysed in the body to produce amino acids, which are then used to build up new body proteins.

proteolysis the hydrolysis of the peptide bonds of proteins with the formation of smaller polypeptides.

proteolytic enzymes enzymes that promote proteolysis; they are used in the management of leg ulcers to remove slough.

prothrombin inactive precursor of the enzyme thrombin produced in the liver. Factor II in blood coagulation.

prothrombin time assesses the activity of the extrinsic coagulation pathway. It is the time taken for plasma to clot in vitro following the introduction of thromboplastin in the presence of calcium. It is inversely proportional to the amount of prothrombin present, a normal person's plasma being used as a standard of comparison. The prothrombin time is extended in people taking anticoagulant drugs and in some haemorrhagic conditions.

protocol written standards for a way of working or the transfer of information, for example, between different computers.

proton a positively charged particle found in the nucleus of an atom.

proton density weighted image a magnetic resonance image showing contrast related to the number of mobile protons in the structure and requires scanning parameters that minimize the effects of relaxation time (T_1 and T_2) to obtain the appropriate weighting.

proto-oncogene a gene with the potential to become a cancer-causing oncogene if stimulated by mutagenic carcinogens. *See also* **oncogene**.

protopathic the term applied to the somatic sensations of fast localized pain; slow, poorly localized pain; and temperature. *See also* **epicritic**.

protraction a forward movement such as thrusting out the jaw. *See also* **retraction**.

proximal nearest to the head or source. *See also* **distal**.

prune belly syndrome a condition when the muscles of the lower abdomen are defective and the recti muscles are absent. It is associated with undescended testes and dilated ureters and bladder, the skin on the abdominal wall appears wrinkled.

pseudoarthrosis a false joint, for example, due to ununited fracture; also congenital, for example, in tibia.

pseudocoxalgia *see* **Perthes' disease**.

pseudocyesis *see* **phantom pregnancy**.

pseudofractures (Looser's zones) narrow bands of decalcification indicating osteomalacia.

pseudogout an arthritis (usually monoarthritis) caused by crystals of calcium pyrophosphate dihydrate within the joint.

pseudohermaphrodite a person in whom the gonads of one sex are present, while the external genitalia comprise those of the opposite sex.

Pseudomonas a Gram-negative motile bacillus commonly found in decaying organic matter.

pseudopolyposis widely scattered polypi, usually the result of previous inflammation – sometimes ulcerative colitis.

pseudotumour a false tumour.

psoas muscles of the loin.

psoas abscess a cold abscess in the psoas muscle, resulting from tuberculosis of the vertebrae. The abscess appears as a firm smooth swelling which does not show signs of inflammation – hence the adjective 'cold'.

psoriasis inflammation of the skin, redden areas with white scales.

psoriatic arthritis arthritis occurring in association with psoriasis.

psychoactive substances and drugs that may alter mental processes.

psychometry the science involved with mental testing.

pterygium a triangular patch of fibrous tissue on the cornea that extends medially from the nasal border of the cornea to the outer canthus of the eye.

ptosis prolapse of an organ. Drooping of the upper eyelid due to paralysis of the third cranial nerve.

ptyalin *see* **amylase**.

P-type semiconductor a device where the majority carriers of electrons are the positive holes in the valence band and the minority carriers are the electrons which have sufficient energy to rise to the conduction band. *See also* **N-type semiconductors**.

puberty the period during which the reproductive organs become functionally active and the secondary sexual characteristics develop.

pubes the hair-covered area over the pubic bone.

pubis the pubic bone or os pubis. The two bones that meet at the symphysis pubis.

pudendum the external reproductive organs, especially of the female.

pulley a hand hold placed over a bed to enable patient's on traction to lift themselves up to give themselves exercise and make bedmaking easier.

pulmonary associated with the lungs.

pulmonary artery flotation catheter (PAFC) specialized balloon-tipped catheter which is 'floated' from the central veins, through the heart and into the pulmonary artery. Allows measurement of pulmonary artery pressure, pulmonary artery occlusion pressure and cardiac output.

pulmonary artery occlusion pressure (PAOP) pressure in the left atrium measured by inflating a balloon on the tip of a pulmonary artery catheter thereby temporarily occluding the pulmonary artery; also known as **wedge pressure**.

pulmonary artery pressure   blood pressure in the pulmonary artery usually measured using a pulmonary artery catheter.

pulmonary circulation   deoxygenated blood leaves the right ventricle to the pulmonary artery, flows through the lungs where it loses carbon dioxide, becomes oxygenated and returns to the left atrium of the heart.

pulmonary embolus (PE)   a blockage which occurs in the pulmonary arterial system in the lungs; most commonly as a result of deep vein thrombosis in the leg or pelvic veins. Prophylaxis includes deep breathing and foot exercises, early mobilization, antithromboembolic stockings with the administration of heparin in at-risk groups.

pulmonary emphysema   overdistension and subsequent destruction of alveoli and reduced gas exchange in the lungs. Associated with tobacco smoking, it is a form of chronic obstructive pulmonary disease (COPD). See also **bronchitis**.

pulmonary hypertension   raised blood pressure within the pulmonary circulation, due to increased resistance to blood flow within the pulmonary vessels. It may be primary (genetic), or secondary due to chronic lung disease or chronic pulmonary embolism.

pulmonary infarction   obstruction of a branch of the pulmonary artery resulting in death of lung tissue.

pulmonary oedema   fluid within the alveoli. The lungs are 'waterlogged' and gas exchange is reduced, such as in left ventricular failure, mitral stenosis, or fluid excess in renal failure.

pulmonary stenosis   narrowing of the pulmonary valve.

pulmonary tuberculosis   see **tuberculosis**.

pulmonary valve   semilunar valve situated between the pulmonary artery and right cardiac ventricle.

pulmonary ventilation (minute volume)   the amount of air moved in and out of the lungs in one minute.

pulp   the soft, interior part of some organs and structures. **digital pulp** the tissue pad of the finger tip.

pulp cavity   the central canal(s) of the tooth. See also **dental pulp**.

pulsation   beating or throbbing, as of the arteries or heart.

pulsativity index   a method of numerically determining the low diastolic blood flow (impedance) through a vessel using the equation systolic − diastolic/mean.

pulse height analyser   a device which can be adjusted to record input pulses within a specific range and then produce an electrical output, therefore can be used to detect different radionuclides.

pulse modulator   supplies high-voltage negative pulses to the magnetron or klystron in a linear accelerator.

pulse rate   the number of cardiac contractions per minute.

pulse repetition frequency   in ultrasound the number of pulses occurring in one second expressed in kilohertz (kHz).

pulsed dose-rate technique   the radiotherapy method of using high-dose-rate equipment to deliver a low-dose-rate treatment by repeating a programmed cycle at predetermined intervals such as 1 hour.

pulsed-wave Doppler   an ultrasound system which transmits bursts of ultrasound and then, after a preselected time, receives for a very short period of time, enabling a specific point within the beam to be examined.

pulser   the part of an ultrasound machine that generates electrical pulses which stimulate the transducer to produce ultrasound.

punctum   entrance to lacrimal drainage system on eyelid margin.

pupil   the opening in the iris of the eye, which allows the passage of light.

pupillary   relating to the pupil.

pupillary reflex   the reflex dilatation and constriction of the pupil in response to the amount of light entering the eye. Controlled by the oculomotor nerves (third cranial).

purgative   a strong drug to encourage complete bowel evacuation.

purines   nitrogenous bases needed as constituents of nucleoproteins. Uric acid is produced when purines are broken down. Increased uric acid in the blood is associated with disorders of metabolism and excretion of uric acid, and leads to the development of gout.

PV (per vaginam)   describes the route used for examination of the vagina, or the administration of drugs.

P **value**   in research, the symbol used to denote the probability of the results of a test occurring by chance. A *P* value is given in all inferential statistics. This is the probability that the results found have occurred by chance alone. The *P* value is measured on a scale of 0–1, so, for example, a *P* value of *P* =0.05 means 5%, or a 1 in 20 chance. A lower-case p is used for proportions.

pyarthrosis   pus in a joint cavity.

pyelography   *see* **urography**.

pyelonephritis   infection within the substance of the kidney, often derived either from the urine or from the blood.

pyloric stenosis   narrowing of the pylorus due to scar tissue formed during the healing of a peptic ulcer. Congenital hypertrophic pyloric stenosis due to a thickened pyloric sphincter muscle. *See also* **pyloromyotomy**.

pyloroduodenal   associated with the pylorus and the duodenum.

pylorus   region containing the opening of the stomach into the duodenum, controlled by a sphincter muscle.

pyopneumothorax   pus and gas or air within the pleural sac.

pyothorax   pus in the pleural cavity.

pyramidal   applied to some conical eminences in the body.

pyramidal cells (Betz cells)   nerve cells in the precentral motor area of the cerebral cortex, from which originate impulses to voluntary muscles.

pyramidal tracts   main motor tracts in the brain and spinal cord, which transmit impulses arising from the pyramidal cells. Most decussate (cross over) in the medulla.

pyrexia   body temperature above normal, usually between 37°C and 40/41°C. *pyrexia of unknown origin* where the reason for the raised body temperature is not known. *See also* **fever, hyperpyrexia**.

pyrimidines   nitrogenous bases needed as constituents of nucleic acids.

pyrogens   foreign proteins arising from previous bacteriological activity producing fever.

pyruvic acid   an important metabolic molecule. Converted to acetyl CoA which is used in the Krebs cycle, or forms lactic acid during anaerobic glucose metabolism.

quadriceps large four-part extensor muscle of the thigh, comprises the rectus femoris, vastus medialis, vastus lateralis and vastus intermedius.

quadriparesis weakness of all four limbs.

quadriplegia (tetraplegia) paralysis when all four limbs are affected.

qualitative relating to quality.

qualitative research research study based on observation and/or interviews to ascertain people's opinions, feelings or beliefs. Non-statistical methods often used in analysis. *See also* **quantitative research**.

qualitative tests tests which measure 'soft data' – feelings, opinions etc.

quality adjusted life years (QALYs) measure of years of life gained through a health intervention adjusted for the quality of life. For example, if an intervention prolongs life by 5 years, but at only half the quality of normal life, this produces 2.5 QALYs.

quality assurance systematic monitoring and evaluation of agreed levels of service provision which are followed by modifications in the light of the evaluation and/or audit. A process to evaluate whether system or service is being provided to a consistent standard. *See also* **benchmarking, clinical audit, performance indicators**.

quality audit the review of a quality system by recording and documenting the results.

quality circles an initiative to improve the quality of care in a specific area. The health professionals in a clinical area investigate a healthcare intervention systematically and relate it to good standards of practice.

quality control the checking of performance on a regular basis to ensure consistency of results.

quality correction cycle the identification of a problem and the steps taken to rectify the fault and prevent it happening again.

quality index an index used for comparison purposes in radiotherapy which is defined as: in a $10 \times 10\,\mathrm{cm}^2$ field at a 100-cm source-chamber distance where the ionization measured at a depth of 20 cm is divided by the ionization measured at a depth of 10 cm at the same source-chamber distance.

quality management the steps taken to ensure constant performance; they will include protocols for safe working, monitoring and checking.

quality of life (QoL)   is a patient-centred subjective outcome measure to complement clinical outcomes. Usually measures the presence or absence of symptoms (e.g. pain), side-effects of treatment (e.g. tiredness, loss of hair), feelings of well-being, impact on income, family, work and social life.

quality of radiation   is dependent of the kV used, the higher the kV the more penetrating the beam, but when the kV is sufficient to penetrate the body part any further increase decreases the difference in intensity of the emerging beam and therefore decreases the subject contrast.

quality policy   a set of written principles stating how people should act to provide consistent performance.

quality standard   a statement or target indicating the level of performance required by teams and individuals.

quality system   the management and organizational structures which underpin a high standard of working practice.

quantitative   relating to quantity.

quantitative research   research study based on the measurement and analysis of observations using statistical methods. *See also* **qualitative research**.

quantitative tests   measure actual, numerical results.

quantum conversion efficiency   the percentage of X-rays (quanta) falling on a phosphor which are changed to light photons.

quantum detection efficiency   the percentage of X-rays (quanta) falling on a phosphor which are stopped by the phosphor.

quantum mottle   uneven density on a film due to the random distribution of image-forming X-ray quanta producing a non-uniform light emission from intensifying screens.

racemose   resembling a bunch of grapes.

radial   associated with the radius. Applied to the nerve, artery and vein.

radiation   the process of heat loss from a body in the form of electromagnetic radiation; this is the only heat transfer process that can take place in a vacuum. Emanation of radiant energy in the form of electromagnetic waves, including gamma rays, infrared, ultraviolet rays, X-rays and visible light rays. Subatomic particles, such as neutrons or electrons, may also be radiated. Radiation may be non-ionizing or ionizing and has many diagnostic and therapeutic uses. *See also* **ionizing radiation**.

radiation dosimetry   the method of measuring the amount of radiation received by an individual. Also called *radiation monitoring*.

radiation nephritis   inflammation of the renal nephrons; *acute* associated with hypertension and proteinuria occurring 6–13 months after radiotherapy. *chronic* associated with urinary protein and casts, nocturia and loss of the ability to concentrate and occurs 1.5–4 years after radiotherapy.

radiation oncologist   medical specialist in the treatment of disease by X-rays and other forms of radiation.

radiation pneumonitis   inflammation of the lungs caused by the radiation dosage received by the patient.

radiation protection   equipment and rules to ensure that staff and patient's experience safe working practices. *See also* **local rules, dosimetry**.

radiation protection advisor   a suitably qualified and experienced person whose role is to advise staff on the safe use of ionizing radiation.

radiation protection supervisor   a person directly involved with ionization who is responsible for ensuring safe working practices in a specific department and is appointed by the radiation protection advisor.

radiation safety committee   a local group of radiation users, advisors and management who discuss matters related to radiation safety.

radiation sickness   tissue damage from exposure to ionizing radiation leads to diarrhoea, vomiting, anorexia and bone marrow failure.

radiation treatment planning   the method required to graphically display the isodose distribution that results when one or more radiation beams converge on the target volume in external beam therapy.

radical   associated with the root of a thing.

radical mastectomy   rarely performed operation that involves removal of the breast, pectoralis major muscle and clearance of the axillary lymph nodes.

radical surgery   usually extensive surgery which aims to be curative, not palliative.

radical treatment   aimed at attempting to kill or remove all malignant cells present.

radiculography   radiography of the spinal nerve roots after the introduction of a positive contrast agent via a lumbar puncture to locate the site and size of a prolapsed intervertebral disc. Superseded by CT and MRI.

radioactive   exhibiting   radioactivity.   Describes   an   unstable atomic nucleus which emits charged particles as it disintegrates. *See also* **radioisotope**.

radioactive decay   the process by which a nucleus of a radioactive atom spontaneously transforms by one or more discrete energy steps until a stable state is reached. *See also* **half-life**.

radioactive disintegration   when a stable nuclide, the parent, changes to another nuclide, the daughter, which may be either stable or unstable and therefore radioactive.

radioactive equilibrium   equilibrium reached, after radioactive disintegration, when the weight of each nuclide in the atom is inversely proportional to the half-life of the nuclide.

radioactive fallout   release of radioactive particles into the atmosphere. Results from industrial processes or accidents, and the testing or use of nuclear weapons.

radioactive source   a radioactive substance sealed, in a capsule, which, when inserted   into   the   body,   delivers   a   predetermined   dose   of radiation.

radiobiology   the study of the effects of radiation on living organisms. The use of radioactive tracers to study biological processes.

radiocarbon   a   radioactive   form   of   the   element   carbon,   such   as carbon-14 (^{14}C), used for investigations, for example, absorption tests and research.

radiodermatitis   skin inflammation caused by exposure to ionizing radiation.

radiograph   a photographic image formed by exposure to X-rays; the correct term for an 'X-ray'.

radiographer   there are two distinct professional disciplines within radiography, diagnostic and therapeutic; they are health professionals qualified in the use of ionizing radiation and other techniques, either in diagnostic imaging or radiotherapy.

radiographic contrast the photographic differences between two adjacent areas on a film.

radiography the use of X-radiation (a) to create images of the body from which medical diagnosis can be made (diagnostic radiography); or (b) to treat a person suffering from a (malignant) disease, according to a medically prescribed regimen (therapeutic radiography). *See also* **radiotherapy**.

radioimmunoassay the use of radioactive substances to measure the amount of concentration of an antigen, antibody or protein or substances such as hormones and drugs in the blood.

radioiodinated human serum albumin (RIHSA) used for detection and localization of brain lesions, determination of blood and plasma volumes, circulation time and cardiac output.

radioisotope (radionuclide) any isotope that is radioactive. Forms of an element which have the same atomic number but different mass numbers, exhibiting the property of spontaneous nuclear disintegration. When taken orally or by injection, can be traced by a Geiger counter.

radioisotope scan pictorial representation of the amount and distribution of radioactive isotope present in a particular organ.

radiolabel the modification of a substance to make it radioactive so that it can be used to target a particular organ or body part so that it can be detected in radionuclide imaging.

radiologist a medical specialist in diagnosis by using X-rays and other allied imaging techniques.

radiology the study of the diagnosis of disease by using X-rays and other allied imaging techniques.

radiolucent a substance that has minimal effect on an X-ray beam and therefore the beam does not change as it passes through the substance.

radiomimetic exerting effects similar to those of ionizing radiation, for example, nitrogen mustards.

radionecrosis tissue death caused by radiation.

radionuclide (radioisotope) any nuclide that is radioactive. Forms of an element which have the same atomic number but different mass numbers, exhibiting the property of spontaneous nuclear disintegration. When taken orally or by injection, can be traced by a Geiger counter.

radionuclide generator a system containing a long-lived parent radionuclide which decays to a short-lived daughter radionuclide.

radionuclide therapy the introduction of a radionuclide either orally or by injection; this is then taken up by a targeted organ which receives a calculated radiation dose to maximize the dose of radiation to the treatment area in a patient and minimize the dose to normal tissue.

radiopaque having the property of significantly absorbing X-rays, thus becoming visible on a radiograph. Barium and iodine compounds are used, as contrast agents, to produce artificial radiopacity.

radiosensitivity   the relative susceptibility of cells, tissues, organs, organisms, or any other substances to the effects of ionizing radiation.

radiosurgery (stereotactic radiotherapy)   a radiotherapy treatment based on a 3D coordinate system designed to achieve a high concentration of absorbed dose to an intracranial target.

radiotherapist (oncologist)   medical specialist in the treatment of disease by X-rays and other forms of radiation.

radiotherapy   a method of treating disease and eradicating tumour cells by aiming to deliver a therapeutic dose of radiation while preserving normal tissue function and structure.

radiotracer   the modification of a substance to make it radioactive so that it can be used to target a particular organ or body part so that it can be detected in radionuclide imaging.

radium (Ra)   a radioactive element occurring in nature.

radius   the lateral bone of the forearm.

radon seeds   capsules containing radon – a radioactive gas produced by the disintegration of radium atoms.

raised intracranial pressure (RIP)   an elevation in intracranial pressure is a serious situation. Causes include: tumours, intracranial haemorrhage, trauma causing oedema or haematoma and obstruction to the flow of cerebrospinal fluid. The features depend on the cause, but there may be headache, vomiting, papilloedema, fits, bradycardia, arterial hypertension and changes in the level of consciousness. *See also* **benign intracranial hypertension**.

RAM (Random Access Memory)   the part of the memory of a computer which can be accessed by the user; the amount of RAM available determines how much data can be stored by the user.

randomized controlled trial (RCT)   research study using two or more randomly selected groups: experimental and control. It produces high-level evidence for practice.

random sampling   in research. The selection process whereby every person in the population has an equal chance of being selected.

random variable   background factors such as environmental conditions that may affect any conditions of the independent variables equally. *See also* **independent variable**.

range   describes the span of values (lowest – highest) observed in a sample.

range of motion (ROM)   the movements possible at a joint.

rank   in statistics, the method of organizing data.

raphe   a seam, suture, ridge or crease.

rare earths   metals having two electrons in the outer shell and either 8 or 9 electrons in the penultimate shell; they are used for the phosphors in television monitors, lasers and modern intensifying screens. Examples include lanthanum, europium, gadolinium, terbium, yttrium.

rarefaction   less dense, as applied to diseased bone. In ultrasound the opposite of compression.

raster lines   the lines formed when a beam of electrons scans a phosphor to form an image. *See also* **phosphor**.

rating   the rating of an X-ray unit is the combination of exposure settings which can occur without unacceptably damaging the unit.

ratio data   measurement data with a numerical score, for example, height, that has a true zero of 0. It is interval data with an absolute zero. *See also* **interval data**.

raw data   original received information.

raw data matrix   in magnetic resonance imaging it is the initial image before analysis. The points at the centre of the matrix represent areas of low spatial frequencies and the frequencies become higher the further away from the centre.

Rayleigh scattering   *see* **coherent scattering**.

reactance   the opposition to current flow and is produced by capacitors and inductors but not by resistors.

reactionary haemorrhage   bleeding that occurs a few hours after an injury but within 24 hours; shock and/or drugs can inhibit the blood flow.

reactive arthritis (Reiter's syndrome)   arthritis that develops in response to infection, usually urogenital, gastrointestinal or throat infection. *See also* **sexually acquired reactive arthritis**.

real time   a computer controlling, or recording, events as they are actually happening.

real time scanning   a method of producing a moving image on a screen.

real-time ultrasonography   an ultrasound imaging technique involving rapid pulsing to enable continuous viewing of movement to be obtained, rather than stationary images.

reasonable doubt   to secure a conviction in criminal proceedings, the prosecution must establish beyond reasonable doubt the guilt of the accused.

receiver   the part of the ultrasonic transducer that detects returning sound waves and converts them to electrical signals.

receiver bandwidth   the measure of a range of frequencies within which a magnetic resonance system is tuned to receive the signal. Alteration affects the signal-to-noise ratio, by narrowing the bandwidth the ratio is increased and by broadening it the ratio is decreased.

receiver operating characteristics   a method of measuring the ability of an observer to make a diagnosis.

receptaculum   receptacle, often forms a reservoir.

receptor   sensory afferent nerve ending capable of receiving and transmitting stimuli. A protein situated on or inside a cell membrane which reacts with various molecules, drugs, hormones or cell mediators.

recipient   the individual who receives something from a donor such as blood, an organ such as a kidney or bone marrow.

reciprocity   the ability to produce an accurate range of densities over a film which reflect the structure being imaged.

reciprocity failure   seen with either very short exposures at high intensity or very long exposures at low intensity which do not produce the expected density on the film.

reciprocity law   the amount of density produced on a film is dependent only on the total amount of light energy available.

recognition acuity   the ability of an individual to recognize standard shapes.

reconstruction technique   a method of forming an image from a set of measurements; in CT imaging this includes automatic corrections. *See also* **iterative reconstruction algorithm**.

recovery position   a first aid measure in which a patient with an altered level of consciousness is positioned so that their airway is maintained and to prevent the inhalation of secretions or vomit.

rectified   made unidirectional, when alternating current is modified so that current only flows in a positive direction. ***half-wave rectification*** the negative half of the cycle is suppressed. ***full-wave rectification*** the negative half of the cycle is made positive by the use of rectifiers.

rectifier   a piece of equipment that allows current to flow in only one direction.

rectosigmoid   associated with the rectum and sigmoid colon.

rectouterine   associated with the rectum and uterus, as the rectouterine pouch.

rectovaginal   associated with the rectum and vagina.

rectovesical   associated with the rectum and bladder.

rectum   the lower part of the large intestine between the sigmoid flexure and anal canal.

rectus abdominis   abdominal muscle.

recumbent   lying or reclining.

recumbent position   lying on the back with the head supported on a pillow: the knees can be flexed and parted to facilitate inspection of the perineum.

recurrent (habitual) miscarriage   when miscarriage occurs in three successive pregnancies.

recurring costs regular and ongoing costs, such as planned maintenance and staff salaries.

red muscle describes muscle consisting mainly of slow-twitch fibres. The red colour is derived from the plentiful blood supply and myoglobin.

redistribution during fractionated radiotherapy those cells that are not killed become more resistant to radiation, they try to change to the mitotic stage of the cell cycle so that they can repopulate.

reductase an enzyme that starts the reduction of an organic compound.

Reed–Sternberg cell a large, abnormal multinucleated cell found in the lymphatic system in Hodgkin's disease.

referred pain pain occurring at a distance from its source, for example, pain felt in the upper limbs from angina pectoris; that from the gallbladder felt in the scapular region.

reflection to throw back light or radiation, X and γ radiation cannot be reflected.

reflective layer the layer between the base and the phosphor layer in an intensifying screen whose function is to reflect light towards the film.

reflex literally, reflected or thrown back; involuntary, not controlled by will.

reflex action an involuntary motor or secretory response by tissue to a sensory stimulus, for example, tendon stretch, sneezing, blinking, coughing. Reflexes may be postural or protective. Testing reflexes provides valuable information in the localization and diagnosis of neurological diseases. *See also* **accommodation reflex, conditioned reflex, corneal reflex**.

reflux backward flow. *See also* **vesicoureteric reflux**.

refraction the bending of light rays as they pass through media of different densities. In normal vision, this occurs so that the image is focused on the retina.

refresh rate the rate at which an electron beam scans the whole of a computer screen.

regional ileitis *see* **Crohn's disease**.

regression techniques various analytical methods used in multivariate statistics. Used to predict dependent variable(s) from independent variable(s).

regulation in a transformer is caused by resistance in the windings, if the electric load from the secondary winding is increased a higher current flows in the secondary winding but the potential difference across the secondary winding is decreased. ***percentage regulation*** a calculation to determine the efficiency of a transformer, the lower the percentage the more efficient is the transformer.

regurgitation   backward flow, for example, of stomach contents into, or through, the mouth, or blood through an incompetent (regurgitant) heart valve.

rehabilitation   to restore normal function.

Reiter's syndrome   sexually acquired reactive arthritis.

reject analysis   the examining of images that have been judged to be unacceptable to try to find out why the films have been rejected and whether it is due to equipment or operator problems.

related   in statistics the data are matched – each sample has a matched sample with one or more than one variable in common.

relaxant   a drug or technique that reduces tension. *See also* **muscle relaxant**.

relaxin   polypeptide hormone secreted by the placenta and ovaries to soften the cervix and loosen the ligaments in preparation for birth.

relay   an electrical switch in which one circuit is controlled by another ciruit.

reliability   in research, a term meaning consistency of results. The likelihood of achieving the same findings using the same research conditions over a period of time or with different researchers.

remark   instruction ignored by the computer, but enables the user to add comments in plain English.

remission   the period of abatement of a fever or other disease.

renal   relating to the kidney.

renal arteriography   the demonstration of the renal arteries following the injection of a contrast agent into the femoral artery.

renal calculus   stone in the kidney.

renal colic   *see* **colic**.

renal erythropoietic factor (REF)   a substance released by the kidneys in response to renal (and therefore systemic) hypoxia. Once secreted into the blood, it reacts with a plasma protein to produce erythropoietin.

renal failure   can be described as acute or chronic. ***acute renal failure*** (ARF) occurs when previously healthy kidneys suddenly fail because of a variety of problems affecting the kidney and its perfusion with blood. This condition is potentially reversible. ARF is treated by haemofiltration or haemodiafiltration until kidney function improves. ***chronic renal failure*** (CRF) occurs when irreversible and progressive pathological destruction of the kidney leads to end-stage renal disease (ESRD). This process usually takes several years but once ESRD is reached, death will follow unless the patient is treated with some type of renal replacement therapy such as dialysis, or renal transplant. *See also* **acute tubular necrosis, uraemia**.

renal function tests   kidney function tests.

renal glycosuria   occurs in patients with a normal blood sugar and a lowered renal threshold for glucose.

renal transplant   kidney transplant.

renal tubule   part of a nephron.

renin   an enzyme released by the kidney (juxtaglomerular apparatus) in response to low serum sodium or low blood pressure. Renin starts the angiotensin-aldosterone response. A plasma protein (angiotensinogen) is activated to produce angiotensin I, which in turn is converted into angiotensin II.

rennin   milk curdling enzyme found in the gastric juice of human infants and ruminants. It converts caseinogen into casein.

renogram   radioisotope study of the kidney.

renography   a method of assessing the output and function of the kidneys in radionuclide imaging by producing time–activity curves.

reoxygenation   the process when tumour cells gain access to oxygen which is released when cells are killed with low-energy transfer radiations – for example, between radiotherapy fractions. If the cells receive oxygen they are more likely to be killed during the next dose of treatment.

repair   cells injured during radiotherapy attempt to repair themselves; healthy tissue is quicker than tumour cells in achieving the repair.

repetition time   in magnetic resonance imaging, the time between the beginning of one radio frequency pulse sequence to the start of the next.

repetitive strain injury (RSI)   a misleading term used to describe diffuse pain and inflammation randomly occurring in the hand and forearm arising from repetitive activities in the workplace, aggravated by static posture.

replenishment   the addition of an amount of developer and fixer to the processing tank every time a film is processed to maintain the activity of the solutions.

repolarization   the process whereby the membrane potential returns from the depolarized state to its polarized resting (negative) state.

repopulation   the re-growth of tissue cells, during fractionated radiotherapy normal tissue cells can regenerate at a faster rate than the tumour cells therefore reducing the side effects of the treatment.

reproductive system   the structures necessary for reproduction. In the male it includes the testes, deferent ducts (vas deferens), prostate gland, seminal vesicles, urethra and penis. In the female it includes the ovaries, uterine tubes, uterus, vagina and vulva.

research   systematic investigation of data, reports and observations to establish facts or principles, in order to produce organized scientific knowledge.

research design   how a research study is to be undertaken such as data collection method, statistical analysis, etc.

residual   remaining.

residual air   the air remaining in the lung after forced expiration.

residual thiosulphate test   a method of assessing the archival permanence of a film by dropping a drop of solution on the film and comparing it with a colour chart.

residual urine   the volume of urine remaining in the bladder after micturition.

resistance   the impedance to the flow of electrons; it is measured in ohms.

resistivity index   the ultrasonic method of numerically determining the resistance of blood flowing through a vessel by using the equation systolic − diastolic/mean.

resistor   an object which opposes the flow of electrons; resistors in series are placed end to end, resistors in parallel are connected parallel to each other.

resolution   indicates the size of the smallest object that a system will record and the smallest distance that must exist between two objects before they are seen as two separate objects. It is expressed as line pair per millimetre. In ultrasound the ability to distinguish between two adjacent structures, the higher the frequency of the probe the better the resolution.

resonate   mechanically deform, vibrate.

resorption   the act of absorbing again, for example, absorption of (a) callus following bone fracture, (b) roots of the deciduous teeth, (c) blood from a haematoma.

respiration   the gaseous exchange between a cell and its environment. *See also* **abdominal breathing, Cheyne–Stokes respiration, paradoxical respiration**.

respirator   equipment to qualify the air breathed through it. A device for giving artificial respiration or to assist pulmonary ventilation.

respiratory failure   failure of the lungs to oxygenate the blood adequately.

respiratory quotient   the ratio between inspired oxygen and expired carbon dioxide during a specified time.

respiratory rate   number of breaths per minute, normally 20 in an adult.

respiratory system   deals with gaseous exchange. Comprises the nose, nasopharynx, larynx, trachea, bronchi and lungs.

restrainer   a chemical to improve the selectivity of a solution; in the developer solution either benzotriazole or potassium bromide is used to ensure low fog and high image contrast.

resuscitation   restoration to life of one who is collapsed or apparently dead. *See also* **cardiopulmonary resuscitation**.

retching   straining at vomiting.

retention of urine   inability to pass urine.

reticular resembling a net.

reticule a thin plastic tray holding lead markers which are positioned to delineate the geometry of the radiotherapy treatment field and a set treatment distance.

reticulocyte an immature circulating red blood cell which still contains traces of the nucleus. Accounts for up to 2% of circulating red cells.

reticulocytosis an increase in the number of reticulocytes in the blood indicating active red blood cell formation in the marrow. *See also* **reticulocyte**.

reticuloendothelial system (RES) *see* **monocyte–macrophage system**.

retina layer of tissue in the eye that converts light into electrical signals. Consists of a multiple-layer complex of neurosensory retina containing nerve cells including photoreceptors (rods and cones), and a layer of pigmented cells beyond the neurosensory retina.

retinoblastoma a rapidly growing, congenital, hereditary, malignant tumour arising from the retinal germ cells in the eye, occurs exclusively in children.

retinol also known as retinene. A light-absorbing molecule formed from vitamin A. It combines with a protein (opsin) to form rhodopsin (visual pigment).

retractile capable of being drawn back, i.e. retracted.

retraction a backward movement. *See also* **protraction**.

retrocaecal behind the caecum.

retroflexion the state of being bent backwards. *See also* **anteflexion**.

retrograde going backward. retrograde urography/pyelography. *See also* **urography**.

retrograde ejaculation a situation where semen is discharged backwards into the bladder. It may follow prostate surgery or be associated with diabetic neuropathy.

retrograde pyelograph the radiographic investigation of the renal tract when excretion urography has failed. A catheter is introduced into the renal pelvis via the urethra to enable the introduction of a contrast agent.

retroperitoneal behind the peritoneum.

retropharyngeal behind the pharynx.

retropubic behind the pubis.

retrospective study research that deals with past data, moving backwards in time. *See also* **prospective study**.

retrosternal behind the sternum.

retrotracheal behind the trachea.

retroversion turning backward. *See also* **anteversion**.

retroversion of the uterus tilting of the whole of the uterus backward with the cervix pointing forward.

revenue budget the budget allocation for day to day running costs, for example, salaries, telephone, electricity and drugs, etc. *See also* **capital budget**.

reverberation in ultrasound when multiple repeat echoes which are produced when two strong reflectors lie parallel to each other.

reverse barrier nursing (protective isolation) involves separating patients who are immunocompromised and susceptible to infection, either by disease or treatment. The type of patients needing protection from infection include those with leukaemia, those having immunosuppressant treatment for organ transplantation, chemotherapy or radiation or neutropenic patients. *See also* **containment isolation, source isolation**.

reverse bias is when a battery is connected across a PN junction, the potential barrier is raised as current flow is stopped until the barrier breaks down. Opposite forward bias.

RGB (Red, Green and Blue) input to a computer colour monitor.

rhabdomyosarcoma a highly malignant tumour derived from striated muscle cells.

rheumatic associated with rheumatism, a non-specific term.

rheumatic diseases a diverse group of diseases affecting connective tissue, joints and bones. They include: ***inflammatory joint disease***, for example, rheumatoid arthritis, septic arthritis and gout; ***connective tissue disease***, for example, systemic lupus erythematosus; ***non-articular/soft tissue rheumatism***, for example, fibromyalgia. rheumatic heart disease (RHD) chronic cardiac disease with valve damage resulting from rheumatic fever.

rheumatic fever an inflammatory disease which may be due to an inadequately treated infection, can affect the joints and can lead to long-term heart problems.

rheumatism a non-specific term embracing a diverse group of diseases and syndromes which have in common disorder or diseases of connective tissue and hence usually present with pain, or stiffness, or swelling of muscles and joints. Used colloquially to describe ill-defined aches and pains. *See also* **rheumatic diseases**.

rheumatoid arthritis a disease of unknown aetiology, characterized by polyarthritis usually affecting firstly the smaller peripheral joints, before extending to involve larger joints accompanied by general ill health and resulting eventually in varying degrees of joint destruction and deformity with associated muscle wasting. It is not just a disease of joints; and most body systems can be affected, for example, lung, peripheral nerves. Many rheumatologists therefore prefer the term 'rheumatoid disease'. There is some question of it being an autoimmune process.

rheumatoid factors autoantibodies found in most people with rheumatoid arthritis. It is not yet known whether they are the cause of, or the result of, arthritis.

rheumatoid pneumoconiosis fibrosing alveolitis occurring in patients suffering from rheumatoid arthritis. *See also* **anthracosis, asbestosis, byssinosis, siderosis silicosis**.

rheumatology the science or the study of the rheumatic diseases.

rhinosinusitis inflammation of the nose and paranasal sinuses.

rhodopsin the visual purple (pigment) found in the rods. Required for vision in low-intensity light. Its colour is maintained in darkness; bleached by daylight. Vitamin A is needed for its formation.

rhomboid diamond-shaped.

ribonuclease an enzyme that breaks down ribonucleic acid.

ribs the twelve pairs of bones which articulate with the twelve dorsal vertebrae posteriorly and form the walls of the thorax. The upper seven pairs are *true ribs* and are attached to the sternum anteriorly by costal cartilage. The remaining five pairs are the *false ribs*; the first three pairs of these do not have an attachment to the sternum but are bound to each other by costal cartilage. The lower two pairs are the *floating ribs* which have no anterior articulation. *cervical ribs* are an extension of the transverse process of the seventh cervical vertebra in the form of bone or fibrous tissue; this causes an upward displacement of the subclavian artery.

rickets bone disease caused by vitamin D deficiency during infancy and childhood (prior to ossification of the epiphyses) which results from poor dietary intake or insufficient exposure to sunlight. There is abnormal metabolism of calcium and phosphate with poor ossification and bone growth. There is muscle weakness, anaemia, respiratory infections, bone tenderness and pain and hypocalcaemia. Delays occur in motor development such as walking, eruption of teeth and closure of the fontanelles. Later there may be bony deformities, for example, bow legs. Rickets may be secondary to vitamin D malabsorption, or impaired metabolism, such as with chronic renal failure. The same condition in adults is known as osteomalacia.

rickety rosary a series of protuberances (bossing) at junction of ribs and costal cartilages in children suffering from rickets.

rider's bone a bony mass in the origin of the adductor muscles of the thigh, from repeated minor trauma in horse riding.

right anterior oblique a radiographic projection with the patient either erect or semi prone at 45° to the film with the right side of the body closest to the film and the left side away from the film (see figure on p. 332).

right colic (hepatic) flexure the bend between the ascending and transverse colon, beneath the liver.

right posterior oblique a radiographic projection with the patient either erect or semi supine at 45° to the film with the right side of the body closest to the film and the left side away from the film (see figure on p. 332).

rights the recognition in law that certain inalienable rights, such as the right to life, should be respected, for example, Human Rights Act 1998.

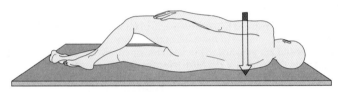

Right anterior oblique (RAO). From Pocketbook of radiographic positioning, 2nd edn, Ruth Sutherland, 2003, Churchill Livingstone, Edinburgh, with permission.

Right posterior oblique (RPO). From Pocketbook of radiographic positioning, 2nd edn, Ruth Sutherland, 2003, Churchill Livingstone, Edinburgh, with permission.

rigid pes planus in adults, abnormality of the foot may be a progression from flexible to semi-rigid to rigid as part of the ageing process. Structural changes due to the existing abnormal position become fixed, as soft and osseous tissues adapt. Rigidity is increased where there are significant osteoarthritic changes or inflammatory arthritic destruction.

ripple bed a mattress where alternate sections fill and then empty automatically to prevent decubitus ulcers.

RIS (Radiology Information System) a computer system specifically for imaging departments which enables the booking and planning of work for inpatients and outpatients, the identification of suitable tests, the management and reporting of images and the transmission of information back to the ward or individual requesting the services.

risk assessment a structured and methodical assessment of risk carried out for a particular area or activity. For example moving and handling patients in the operating theatre.

risk factors factors associated with an increase in the likelihood of ill health, disease, handicap or disability. Demonstration of the association has to fulfil Sir Austin Bradford Hill's eight criteria (for example, smoking and lung cancer): (a) biological plausibility—tobacco tar contains known carcinogens, the stages of tumour development following exposure are clearly demonstrated, (b) reversibility—smoking cessation reduces subsequent increase in risk of lung cancer by half in the first year, to nil after 10 years, (c) animal demonstration—model of beagles in laboratory experiments, (d) dose response—risk of lung cancer in smokers shown to increase progressively with the number of cigarettes smoked per day, (e) follows exposure—temporal relationship demonstrated, lung cancer always follows exposure to cigarettes with a time lag of 20 to 30 years, (f) over time and overseas—relationship consistent between different case series and different places (in the world), (g) experimental design—must be reliable. Randomized controlled trials most convincing, but may be unethical. Observational studies (case control, cohort) useful if correctly carried out. (h) strength of the effect—the larger increase in risk, the more likely the causal relationship.

risk management managing risk in healthcare settings involves: identification of the risk, analysis of the risk and controlling the risk.

ROA (right occipitoanterior) used to describe the position of the fetus in the uterus.

rodent ulcer a basal cell carcinoma often seen on the face which, although locally invasive, does not give rise to metastases.

rods photoreceptors in the retina for appreciation of coarse detail vision in low light conditions. They contain the visual pigment rhodopsin.

Rolando's fracture a fracture of the base of the first metacarpal.

ROM (Read Only Memory) the pre-programmed part of the computer which enables it to run programs.

root the part of a tooth that lies below the gum.

root filling the removal of the root of a tooth which is then filled and forms the base for an artificial crown.

rooting reflex a primitive reflex present in newborns. The infant will turn his or her head to that side when the cheek is touched.

ROP (right occipitoposterior) used to describe the position of the fetus in the uterus.

rotating anode part of an X-ray tube that is made of a molybdenum disc with a tungsten/rhenium focal tract embedded in it; the positive anode rotates during exposure to enable higher intensities of X-rays than a stationary anode tube due to the larger surface allowing more heat to be deposited and then dissipated.

rotating jig in radiotherapy, a method of determining the contour of a shell. The shell is supported on 4 pins and the 5th pin rotates around an axis at right angles to the plane and scaled in degrees of rotation and centimetres. The contour can then be plotted on polar graph paper.

rotation a limb movement around the axis down the centre of a long bone.

rotation therapy a technique when the source of the radiation is moved through an angle of 360° during treatment.

rotator a muscle that acts to turn a part.

rotator cuff four muscles; subscapularis, supraspinatus, infraspinatus and teres minor. Their tendons converge to form a cuff over the shoulder joint. Controls and produces rotation of the shoulder.

round ligaments uterine supports that run from the uterus, through the inguinal canal, to the labia majora.

router computer equipment that connects computer networks together; it is more powerful than a hub, for example, used to allow access to a single internet connection (phoneline).

RS 232 a type of standard interface between computer and peripheral, defining the plug and socket sizes and how the data are transmitted between the computer and peripheral.

rubor redness: one of the five classic local signs and symptoms of inflammation, the others being dolor, loss of function, calor and tumor.

ruthenium-90 an isotope contained in a silver applicator with a window thickness of 0.1 mm, attached to the sclera for 7–10 days and used to treat the eye.

S

saccular aneurysm a dilation of only a part of the circumference of an artery.

sacculation appearance of several saccules.

saccule a minute sac. A small fluid-filled sac in the membranous labyrinth of the inner ear. *See also* **utricle**.

sacral associated with the sacrum.

sacroanterior describes the position of the breech in the pelvis when the fetal sacrum is in the anterior part of the maternal pelvis.

sacrococcygeal associated with the sacrum and the coccyx.

sacroiliac associated with the sacrum and the ilium.

sacroiliitis inflammation of a sacroiliac joint. Involvement of both joints characterizes conditions such as ankylosing spondylitis, Reiter's syndrome and psoriatic arthritis.

sacrolumbar associated with the sacrum and the loins.

sacroposterior describes the position of the breech in the pelvis when the fetal sacrum is in the posterior part of the maternal pelvis.

sacrum the triangular bone lying between the fifth lumbar vertebra and the coccyx. It consists of five vertebrae fused together, and it articulates on each side with the innominate bones of the pelvis, forming the sacroiliac joints.

saddle joints synovial joints that allow flexion, extension, abduction, adduction and some axial rotation, for example, the first carpometacarpal joint.

safelights lights covered with optical filters to enable staff to work in a darkened room without the film emulsion being affected by the light.

sagittal resembling an arrow.

sagittal plane the anteroposterior plane of the body.

sagittal sinuses venous channels (sinuses) that drain blood from the brain.

sagittal suture the immovable joint between the two parietal bones.

saliva fluid secreted by the salivary glands. It contains water, mucus and salivary amylase.

salivary associated with saliva.

salivary calculus a stone formed in the salivary ducts.

salivary glands the glands which secrete saliva, i.e. the parotid, submandibular (submaxillary) and sublingual glands.

salpingitis acute or chronic inflammation of the uterine (fallopian) tubes. *See also* **hydrosalpinx**.

salpingogram radiological examination of tubal patency by retrograde introduction of contrast agent into the uterus and along the uterine tubes. Being superseded by ultrasound examination.

salpinx a tube, especially the uterine (fallopian) tube or the eustachian tube.

salvage therapy treatment given to a site where previous treatments have failed and the disease has recurred.

sample the particular subset chosen from a population.

saphenous apparent; manifest. The name given to two superficial veins in the leg, the great (long) and the small (short), and to the nerves accompanying them.

sarcoidosis a granulomatous disease of unknown aetiology in which histological appearances resemble tuberculosis. May affect any organ of the body, but most commonly presents as a condition of the skin, lymph nodes or the bones of the hand.

sarcoma malignant tumour of connective tissue, muscle, nerve, bone (osteosarcoma), usually first seen as a painless swelling. Treatment options include surgery, radiotherapy and chemotherapy usually in combination. *See also* **Ewing's tumour**.

sarcomatosis a condition in which sarcomata are widely spread throughout the body.

sartorius the 'tailor's muscle' of the thigh, since it flexes one leg over the other.

saturated fatty acids those fatty acids having no double bonds in their structure. Most originate from animal sources. High dietary intake is associated with arterial disease.

saturation in magnetic resonance imaging, a non-equilibrium state where equal numbers of spins are aligned with and against the magnetic field. This occurs immediately following a 90° radio frequency pulse with the longitudinal magnetization aligned in the transverse plane.

saturation analysis a technique to determine the concentration of a hormone or chemical in a small sample of blood or urine.

scald a burn caused by hot liquid or vapour.

scale a sequence of numbers.

scalp the hair-bearing skin which covers the cranium.

scalp cooling technique used to minimize or prevent alopecia associated with the administration of cytotoxic drugs such as doxorubicin.

scalpel a surgical knife.

scan an image built up by movement along or across the object scanned, either of the detector or of the imaging agent, to achieve complete coverage, for example, ultrasound scan.

scan delay the time between the start of the contrast agent injection and the onset of CT scanning.

scan limits start and end points of data acquisition.

scanners a device which enables documents, pictures, etc. to be held as a digital image.

scan time the time taken for data acquisition.

scaphoid boat-shaped, as a bone of the tarsus and carpus.

scaphoid fracture commonly occurs as a result of compression of the scaphoid, when there is a fall onto the outstretched hand in hyperextension. Commonly, if the fracture involves the proximal third of the scaphoid, there is a high risk of non-union and threat of avascular necrosis, due to the poor blood supply.

scapula the shoulder blade – a large, flat triangular bone.

scattered when photons hit an object and are deflected from their original path, they may or may not loose energy as a result.

scattergram in statistics, where two variables are represented by a single plot against an x and y axis.

scattering cross section the area of the patient, measured in cm^2 or barns, that lies in the X-ray field, the larger the area the higher the probability that the radiation will interact with the tissue.

Scheuermann's disease osteochondritis of the spine affecting the ring epiphyses of the vertebral bodies. Occurs in adolescents.

Schilling test estimation of absorption of radioactive vitamin B_{12} for investigation of the cause of vitamin B_{12} deficiency.

Schlatter's disease (Osgood–Schlatter disease) osteochondritis of the tibial tubercle.

Schlemm's canal a channel in the inner part of the sclera, close to its junction with the cornea. It drains excess aqueous humour and maintains normal intraocular pressure.

Schmorl's nodes erosion of the bodies of the vertebrae, due to pressure from the nucleus pulposus. Narrowing of the disc space may occur.

Schottky defect the result of removing an atom completely from a structure.

Schwann cells neuroglial cells of the peripheral nervous system. They are concerned with the production of the myelin sheath that surrounds some nerve fibres.

schwannoma a benign, encapsulated tumour arising from the neurilemma of the peripheral, cranial or autonomic nerves.

sciatica entrapment of the sciatic nerve during its course from the lower back to the leg causing pain which runs down the back of the leg to the heel and which can lead on to weakness such as foot drop and sensory loss in the lower leg.

scintillation counters   a device used to detect small quantities of X or γ radiation from a patient using either a detector in crystalline form or as a liquid scintillation material. Gamma rays from the patient strike the detector and are converted to photons, which pass through a photomultiplier producing a pulsed voltage corresponding to the original radioactivity.

scintillation detector   a device for measuring radiation emitted from a patient using a sodium iodide crystal and a photomultiplier tube.

scintillation efficiency   the percentage of quantal energy stopped by a phosphor which is changed to useful light photons.

scintillography (scintiscanning)   visual recording of radioactivity over selected areas after administration of suitable radioisotope.

sclera   the 'white' of the eye, the opaque bluish-white fibrous outer coat of the eyeball covering the posterior five-sixths; it merges into the cornea at the front.

sclerocorneal   associated with the sclera and the cornea, as the circular junction of these two structures.

sclerodactyly   deformity affecting the fingers. There is fixed, partial flexion of the fingers with subcutaneous calcification. Ulceration of the finger tips may occur. Associated with scleroderma.

scoliosis   lateral curvature of the spine, which can be congenital or acquired and is due to abnormality of the vertebrae, muscles and nerves.

score   in statistics, the total number of responses.

scotopic vision   dark-adapted vision.

screen asymmetry   the production of a pair of intensifying screens when the back screen is slightly faster than the front to compensate for any absorption that may have taken place which reduces the amount of energy reaching the screen.

screen contact test   a perforated metal sheet is placed on a radiographic cassette and an exposure of 55 kV at a 2-metre focus-film distance, the film is processed and when viewed at 4 metres any dark areas indicate loss of screen film contact.

screen unsharpness   blurring of an image due to the phosphor size and thickness, the presence of an absorption/reflective layer or if a dye is used in the intensifying screen construction. It can also be influenced by poor screen/film contact.

screening   a preventive measure to identify potential or incipient disease at an early stage when it may be more easily treated. It is carried out in a variety of settings, including primary care, hospitals, and clinics for antenatal care, and well babies, well men and well women clinics. Screening checks include: mammography, cervical cytology, blood pressure checks, checks for diabetes mellitus, faecal occult blood, prostatic specific antigen test for prostate cancer, ultrasound and triple blood test during pregnancy. The screening process may cause anxiety even when no abnormality is found (negative result).

scrolling   the movement of text or data on the display screen of a computer.

scrotum   the pouch of pigmented skin in the male which contains the testes.

scurvy   a lack of vitamin C, radiographically the periosteum is raised and osteoporosis is present.

search engine   a database of key words that internet users can access to find information on the web.

sebum   the secretion of the sebaceous glands; it contains fatty acids, cholesterol and dead cells.

secondary   second in order.

secondary care   health care indirectly accessed via primary care. Usually refers to specialist medical and surgical services provided in hospitals.

secondary collimation   a method of varying the radiation field size to suit individual treatment areas or diagnostic examinations. *See also* **applicators**.

secondary haemorrhage   occurs about 10 days after an injury and is always due to sepsis.

secondary radiation   the ejection of electrons from a substance after it has been bombarded with charged particles of sufficient energy.

secondary radiation barrier   a barrier that protects from the effects of scattered radiation or leakage from the X-ray tube or housing. *See also* **primary radiation barrier**.

secondary solute   used in liquid scintillation counting to absorb photons emitted by the primary solute and re-emit them as photons of a longer wavelength therefore increasing the efficiency of the detection by photomultiplier tubes.

secondary tumour   refers to a primary cancer that has spread to other distant sites in the body, such as colorectal cancer spreading to the liver. *See also* **metastasis**.

secretin   a hormone produced in the duodenal mucosa, which causes secretion of pancreatic juice, and with other regulatory peptides inhibits gastric secretion and motility.

secretion   a fluid or substance, formed or concentrated in a gland and passed into the gastrointestinal tract, the blood or to the exterior.

secretory   involved in the process of secretion: describes a gland which secretes.

sector probe   an ultrasound probe with a small footprint used for intercostal and cardiac imaging.

sedation   the production of a state of lessened functional activity.

sedative   an agent which reduces functional activity by its action on the nervous system. *See also* **anxiolytic**.

Seldinger catheter   a special catheter and guide wire for insertion into an artery, along which it is passed to, for example, the heart.

selection unit   remote-controlled unit for placing, for example, radioactive caesium-137 into body cavities.

selectivity   the ability of a developing agent to differentiate between exposed silver halide and unexposed silver halide and therefore only converting the exposed crystals to metallic silver. An agent which has no effect on either the metallic silver in the developed image or the gelatine in which it is suspended.

Selectron   a proprietary device which stores sealed radioactive sources of caesium, iridium or cobalt in a shielded container in readiness for intracavitary treatment in the uterus, cervix or vagina. In recent years extended to other body sites such as bronchus and oesophagus.

self induction   occurs when a current-carrying conductor induces a magnetic field in itself and the current changes.

sella turcica   pituitary fossa located on sphenoid bone.

semen   seminal fluid. Fluid ejaculated during coitus. It comprises spermatozoa from the testes and the secretions from the prostate gland, seminal vesicles and bulbourethral glands.

semicircular canals   three fluid-filled canals contained within the bony labyrinth of the internal ear. Orientated in the three planes of space they are part of the vestibular apparatus concerned with dynamic equilibrium and balance.

semiconductor   a solid device that contains a conduction band and valence band and allows current to flow in one direction only. ***Intrinsic semiconductors*** are chemically pure and have a perfect regulation of atoms in the crystal lattice, ***extrinsic semiconductors*** have impurities added to improve electrical conductivity. *See also* **diodes and triodes**.

semilunar   shaped like a crescent or half moon.

semilunar cartilages   the crescentic interarticular cartilages of the knee joint (menisci).

seminal   associated with semen.

seminal vesicle   two tubular accessory glands behind the male bladder. They produce a thick alkaline fluid, which forms some 60% of semen volume.

seminiferous   carrying or producing semen such as the seminiferous tubules, the site of spermatogenesis.

seminiferous tubule   coiled tube in the testis for carrying semen.

seminoma   a neoplasm of the testis that is highly radiosensitive; subtype of germ cell tumour.

semipermeable   describes a membrane which is permeable to some substances in solutions, but not to others.

senescence   normal physical and mental changes in increasing age.

sensible perspiration   the term used when there are visible drops of sweat on the skin.

sensitivity   the ability of a detector, for example a film or intensifying screen, to register very small quantities of radiation, the more sensitive the detector the wider the range of intensities can be detected. The counting efficiency of a gamma camera in counts per second per megabecqueral. The ability of a test to accurately identify a condition or disease in affected individuals, such as mammography screening for breast cancer.

sensitometer   an exposure device for printing a pre-determined image onto a film.

sensitometry   a method of measuring blackening on a film, plotting a characteristic curve, producing measurements from the curve and therefore comparing different films or film screen combinations. *See also* **characteristic curve**.

sensory   associated with sensation. *sensory nerves* those which transmit impulses from peripheral receptors to the brain and spinal cord.

sensory agraphia   inability to interpret the written word, due to lesions in the posterior part of the left parieto-occipital region.

sentinel node biopsy (SNB)   procedure used in staging (mainly) breast cancer and melanoma where (blue) dye is injected at the primary tumour site and traced to the nearest nodal basin where the first node involved with tumour will accumulate the dye; resection of that node may improve the cure rate.

sepsis   infection of the body by pus-forming bacteria.

septal thickness   the thickness of the lead between the holes in a collimator of a gamma camera.

septic abortion   *see* **miscarriage**.

septicaemia   the multiplication of living bacteria in the bloodstream causing infection.

septic arthritis   arthritis caused by infection in the joint.

septic miscarriage   one associated with uterine infection.

septic shock   shock caused by infection.

septum   a partition between two cavities, e.g. between the nasal cavities.

sequestering agent   softens hard water, in developer EDTA sodium salt is used to prevent precipitation of calcium and magnesium salts onto the surface of the film.

sequestrum   a piece of dead bone which separates from the healthy bone but remains within the tissues.

serial port an external socket on older computers used to plug in a mouse or a modem.

serosa a serous membrane, e.g. the peritoneal covering of the abdominal viscera.

serotonin a monoamine formed from tryptophan (amino acid). Liberated by blood platelets after injury and found in high concentrations in the CNS and gastrointestinal tract. It is a vasoconstrictor, inhibits gastric secretion, stimulates smooth muscle and acts as a central neurotransmitter. It is also involved in pain transmission and perception, and sleep–wake cycles. Also called *5-hydroxytryptamine* (5-HT).

serous associated with serum.

serous membrane a lubricating membrane lining the closed cavities, and reflected over their enclosed organs.

server a central computer in a network that provides services and files to other computers, therefore enabling computers to communicate with each other.

service provider an organization that offers connections to the internet.

sesamoid bone a small area of bone formation in muscle tendons such as the patella.

set-up the accurate positioning of a patient in preparation for the delivery of radiotherapy treatment.

Sever's disease (calcaneal epiphysitis) occurs in children and is caused by damage to the bone–cartilage layer in the heel resulting in pain.

sexually acquired reactive arthritis (SARA, Reiter's disease) often caused by infection with *Chlamydia trachomatis*, but intestinal infections can also be the triggering event. Arthritis occurs together with conjunctivitis or uveitis, urethritis (or cervicitis in women), and sometimes psoriasis. *See also* **reactive arthritis**.

Sézary syndrome a leukaemic form of mycosis fungoides.

shaded surface display algorithms the generation of a three-dimensional outline of the surface of a patient or object from a set of stored images.

shadow mask a thin, perforated metal plate found in colour monitors to accurately focus the electron beam onto the phosphor and therefore improve image quality.

shadow tray a sheet of Perspex or perforated aluminium sheet in the form of a tray or table to hold shielding blocks during radiotherapy.

shared segment part of a computer network that is used by several nodes.

sharps a term used to define items that could cause harm to a person handling them, including needles, scalpels, broken ampoules, cannulae.

shelf operation an operation to deepen the acetabulum in developmental dysplasia of the hip, involving the use of a bone graft. Performed at 7–8 years, after failure of conservative treatment.

shell body temperature   that outside the body core. Varies between sites, for example, 35°C at the forehead and 20°C in the feet.

shells   *see* **beam direction shells, patient shell**.

Shenton's line   a line drawn along the medial border of the neck of femur and the superior border of the obturator foramen forming an even, continuous arc. If this arc is disrupted or displaced it indicates a fractured neck of femur or a hip dislocation.

shield   the shield forms the external casing of an X-ray tube.

shielding blocks   heavy metal blocks placed on a shadow tray to protect parts of the body that are in the beam of radiation but do not require treatment. They are a means of shaping the beam to individual volumes. *See also* **lead shielding, MCP blocks**.

shin bone   *see* **tibia**.

shock   a condition when the cardiovascular system is incapable of delivering oxygen and nutrients to the cells. Causes include haemorrhage and dehydration (*hypovolaemic shock*), heart failure (*cardiogenic shock*), infection (*septic shock*) and allergic reaction (*anaphylactic shock*). *See also* **anaphylactic shock, electric shock, cardiogenic shock, hypovolemic shock, vasovagal shock, medical shock, neurogenic shock, septic shock**.

short bone   bones that are cuboidal in shape and are formed by cancellous bone with a thin covering of compact bone, for example the carpal bones.

shoulder   a synovial ball and socket joint formed by the glenoid cavity of the scapula and the head of humerus. In photography the area of the characteristic curve where the film's reaction to exposure slows. *See also* **characteristic curve**.

shoulder girdle   formed by the clavicle and scapula on either side.

shrinking field technique   phased treatments, in radiotherapy, where a larger volume is treated first and then the volume is shrunk to allow higher doses to be delivered to the target volume while ensuring that tolerance doses to critical structures is not exceeded.

sialogram   radiographic image of the salivary glands and ducts, after injection of an opaque contrast agent.

sialography   the radiographic examination of the salivary glands following the direct injection of a contrast agent.

sialolith   a stone in a salivary gland or duct.

sickle cell disease   an inherited blood disorder.

side-effect   any physiological change other than the wanted one from a drug, e.g. oral iron causes the side-effect of black faeces. Also covers undesirable drug reactions. Some are predictable, being the result of a known metabolic action of the drug, e.g. hair loss with cytotoxic drugs.

Unpredictable reactions can be: (a) ***immediate***: anaphylaxis, angio-oedema, (b) ***erythematous***: all forms of erythema, including nodosum and multiforme and purpuric rashes, (c) ***cellular*** eczematous rashes and contact dermatitis, (d) ***specific***, e.g. light-sensitive eruptions with griseofulvin (antifungal).

siderosis   excess of iron in the blood or tissues. Inhalation of iron oxide into the lungs can cause one form of pneumoconiosis.

sievert (Sv)   the SI unit (International System of Units) for radiation dose equivalent. A measure of total biological effects of a beam of radiation. It has replaced the rem.

sighing   long, slow inspiration followed by rapid expiration.

sigmoid   shaped like the letter S.

sigmoid flexure   the S-shaped bend at the lower end of the descending colon. It is continuous with the rectum below.

sigmoidoscopy   the visual examination of the rectum and sigmoid colon using an instrument which contains a light.

sign test   a statistical test used to compare two sets of results using a normal distribution table and a sign test table; the results must be equal to or less than the results on the tables to be significant.

signal   in imaging it is the information required from the system, for example a radiograph, and the minimum-sized object that can be seen by a system.

signal gain   the electrical signal for a specific intensity of absorbed radiation.

signal-to-noise ratio   the ratio of the signal width to the unwanted energy (noise). In magnetic resonance imaging it can be improved by (a) increasing the number of signal excitations, (b) increasing the field of view, or (c) increasing the strength of the main magnetic field used.

significance   the numerical probability that the results of an experiment are meaningful.

silicone   a water-repellent compound. Used in dressings, as sheets, foams and gels, where it fits exactly the contours of the granulating wound to provide an ideal environment for wound healing. Also used as implants in breast reconstruction.

silicosis   a form of pneumoconiosis or industrial dust disease found in metal grinders, stone-workers, etc.

silver bromide   a chemical used as part of a film emulsion and has a peak sensitivity of 430 nm and is not sensitive to wavelengths above 480 nm.

silver collection   used fixing solution is stored and then collected in bulk along with unwanted radiographs to enable the silver to be commercially reclaimed.

silver estimating papers   special papers used to measure the quantity of silver remaining in a solution.

silver halides   silver compounds that have a natural spectral sensitivity in the blue part of the visible spectrum. *See also* **silver bromide**.

silver recovery   methods of recovering silver from either the fixer solution or unwanted radiographs. *See also* **silver collection, metal exchange, electrolytic silver recovery**.

simple fracture   a break in bone continuity where there is no break in the skin surface.

simulator   used in radiotherapy treatment localization and planning. This is a specialized unit housing a diagnostic X-ray tube to identify the treatment beam–patient geometry by using an image intensifier, an isocentric therapy unit and a collimation unit.

single photon emission computed tomography (SPECT)   a specialist gamma camera which rotates round the patient and a number of two-dimensional images are taken and stored on a computer. *See also* **positron-emission tomography**.

sinoatrial node   *see* **sinus node**.

sinus   a hollow or cavity within a bone, especially the nasal air sinuses. A channel containing blood, especially venous blood, e.g. the sinuses of the brain. Any abnormal blind tract or channel opening onto the skin or a mucous surface.

sinus arrhythmia   an increase of heart rate on inspiration, decrease on expiration.

sinusitis   inflammation of a sinus, used exclusively for the paranasal sinuses.

sinus node (sinoatrial)   the pacemaker of the heart. Part of the specialized tissue that forms the conducting system of the heart. It is situated at the junction of the superior vena cava and the right atrium. It initiates the wave of cardiac contraction. *See also* **pacemaker**.

sinusoid   a dilated channel into which arterioles or veins open in some organs, e.g. liver, and which act in place of the usual capillaries.

sinus rhythm   normal rhythm of the heart.

SIR (Serial Infra Red)   a wireless communication system for computers.

SI unit   abbreviation for the Système International d'Unités, the French name for the International System of Units. (See figures on p. 346).

skeleton   the bony framework of the body, supporting and protecting the soft tissues and organs and acting as attachments for muscles. *See also* **appendicular skeleton, axial skeleton**.

Skene's glands   two small glands at the entrance to the female urethra; the lesser vestibular or paraurethral glands.

skewed distribution   a statistical term that describes any distribution of scores where there are a greater number of values on one side of the mean than the other, i.e. not symmetrical. *See also* **normal distribution curve**.

SI base units[a]

Quantity	Unit of measurement	Symbol
Length	metre	m
Mass	kilogram	kg
Luminous intensity	candela	cd
Electric current	ampere	A
Amount of substance	mole	mol
Temperature	kelvin	K
Time	second	s

[a]From Principles of radiological physics, 3rd edn, 1996, D T Graham, Churchill Livingstone, Edinburgh, with permission.

Derived SI units and their definitions[a]

Quantity	Definition	SI unit	Scalar/vector
Speed	Distance travelled in unit time	metre per second $(m \cdot s^{-1})$	Scalar
Velocity	Distance travelled in unit time in a given direction	metre per second $(m \cdot s^{-1})$	Vector
Acceleration	Change of velocity in unit time	(metre per second)/per second $(m \cdot s^{-2})$	Vector
Force	The application of unit force to unit mass produces unit area	newton (N) $(kg \cdot m \cdot s^{-2})$	Vector
Pressure	Force applied per unit area	pascal (P)$(N \cdot m^{-2})$	Vector
Weight	Force acting on a body due to gravity	newton (N) $(kg \cdot m \cdot s^{-2})$	Vector
Work	Product of the force acting on a body times the distance the body moves	joule (J) $(N \cdot m)$	Scalar
Energy	Kinetic energy: work which can be done by a system because of its velocity	joule (J)	Scalar
	Potential energy: work which can be performed because of the position of state of a system	joule (J)	Scalar
Power	Rate of doing work	watt (W) $(J \cdot s^{-1})$	Scalar
Momentum	Product of the mass and the velocity of the body	$(kg \cdot m \cdot s^{-1})$	Vector

[a]From Principles of radiological physics, 3rd edn, 1996, D T Graham, Churchill Livingstone, Edinburgh, with permission.

skill mix the level, range and variety of skills of the staff in a department, unit or team which is needed to meet the organizational outcomes.

skin the tissue which forms the outer covering of the body; it consists of two layers, the outer epidermis (cuticle), dermis (true skin) and the appendages; nails, glands and hair.

skin fold thickness an anthropometric measurement used as part of nutritional assessment.

skin shedding skin is continually shedding its outer keratinized cells as scales. As the skin has a natural bacterial flora, the scales are a potential source of infection for susceptible patients. *See also* **psoriasis**.

skin-sparing effect seen in megavoltage radiotherapy treatment machines where the maximum radiation dose is delivered below the skin surface.

skull the bony framework of the head, the face and cranium.

slice a single, reconstructed CT image.

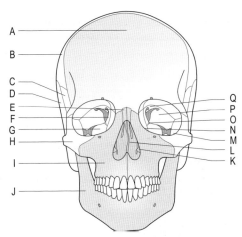

A – Frontal bone
B – Parietal bone
C – Greater wing of sphenoid bone
D – Temporal bone
E – Nasal bone
F – Ethmoid bone
G – Maxilla
H – Zygomatic bone
I – Maxilla

J – Mandible
K – Inferior nasal concha
L – Vomer
M – Zygomatic bone
N – Lacrimal bone
O – Palatine bone
P – Greater wing of sphenoid bone
Q – Lesser wing of sphenoid bone

Position of the bones of the skull (anterior aspect). From Bones and joints, 4th edn, Chris Gunn, 2002, Churchill Livingstone, Edinburgh, with permission.

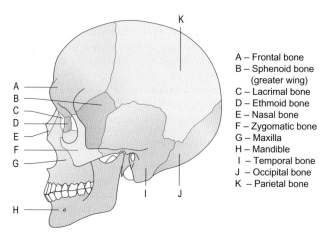

A – Frontal bone
B – Sphenoid bone
    (greater wing)
C – Lacrimal bone
D – Ethmoid bone
E – Nasal bone
F – Zygomatic bone
G – Maxilla
H – Mandible
I – Temporal bone
J – Occipital bone
K – Parietal bone

Position of the bones of the skull (lateral aspect). From Bones and joints, 4th edn, Chris Gunn, 2002, Churchill Livingstone, Edinburgh, with permission.

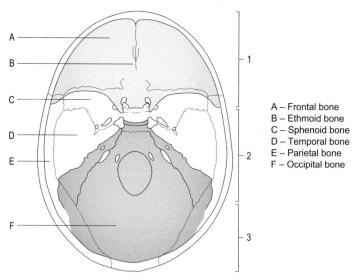

A – Frontal bone
B – Ethmoid bone
C – Sphenoid bone
D – Temporal bone
E – Parietal bone
F – Occipital bone

The floor of the cranial cavity is divided into three distinct sections:

1 – Anterior cranial fossa containing the frontal lobes of the brain.
2 – Middle cranial fossa containing the temporal lobes of the brain and the hypophysis cerebri (pituitary gland).
3 – Posterior cranial fossa containing cerebellum, pons and medulla oblongata.

Position of the bones of the skull (cranial cavity). From Bones and joints, 4th edn, Chris Gunn, 2002, Churchill Livingstone, Edinburgh, with permission.

slice interval in CT scanning, the distance between reconstructed slices.

slice thickness in modern CT scanners, reconstructed slice thickness can be selected to provide various slice thicknesses from a single data acquisition.

slip ring equipment to allow electrical power to be transferred from a stationary power source onto a continuously moving gantry to allow continuous motion; used in spiral or helical CT scanning.

slipped disc prolapsed intervertebral disc. *See also* **prolapse of an intervertebral disc**.

slipped epiphysis displacement of an epiphysis, especially the upper femoral one. *See also* **epiphysis**.

slough septic tissue which becomes necrosed and separates from the healthy tissue.

small bowel enema the examination of the small bowel by introducing barium sulphate via a nasogastric tube, directly into the duodenum or the first part of the jejunum.

small for dates small for gestational age.

small for gestational age (SGA) babies who weigh less than expected for a given gestational age. They are either constitutionally small or suffer from growth restriction. *See also* **low birthweight**.

Smith's fracture a fracture of the lower end of the radius and ulna with forward displacement of the radius. *See also* **Colles' fracture**.

Smith–Petersen nail a trifin, cannulated metal nail used to provide internal fixation for intracapsular fractures of the femoral neck.

'smudge' cells cells that have been ruptured when making a blood film.

snapping hip syndrome a snapping sensation either heard or felt in the hip during movement of the joint. The nature of the signs and symptoms will indicate whether the structure at fault is more likely to be the iliotibial band or the iliopsoas tendon.

sodium (Na) metallic element. A major extracellular cation concerned with the composition of fluid compartments and neuromuscular function.

sodium bicarbonate (sodium hydrogen carbonate) acts as a buffer in the blood. Administered intravenously to correct metabolic acidosis.

sodium chloride often used in intravenous fluids to replace fluids and correct electrolyte levels.

sodium citrate used as an in vitro anticoagulant, for example for stored blood.

sodium hydroxide a developer accelerator.

sodium hypochlorite a powerful disinfectant used, in suitable dilutions, in many situations, such as dealing with environmental contamination with blood and other body fluids.

sodium pump an active transport mechanism (needing ATP) that pumps sodium ions through semipermeable cell membranes.

sodium sulphite a fixer preservative.

soft palate situated at the posterior end of the palate and consisting of muscle covered by mucous membrane.

soft rollers part of the film transport system in an automatic film processor and are found where films crossover into another section and squeeze any excess liquid out of the film; they are made of a neoprene-type substance.

software the programs run by the computer.

solar keratosis a warty skin lesion due to sun exposure which may progress to cancer.

solar plexus a large network of sympathetic (autonomic) nerve ganglia and fibres in the upper abdomen. It supplies the abdominal organs.

solar plexus punch a blow to the abdomen that results in an immediate inability to breathe freely.

solarization when an increase in exposure results in a decrease in density on a film and therefore a reverse image can be obtained. *See also* **characteristic curve**.

solenoid consists of several coils of wire joined together to produce magnetic lines of force. If soft iron is placed inside the loops of wire it becomes magnetized.

solid state radiation detector a silicon diode used to measure the activity of electron beams or megavoltage photon beams.

solute substance dissolved in a solvent.

solution a fluid that contains a dissolved substance or substances. *saturated solution* one in which the maximum amount of a particular substance is dissolved.

solvent an agent that is capable of dissolving other substances (solutes). The component of a solution that is present in excess. In photography used to dilute chemicals for example when making up developer, developer replenisher and fixer; the solvent used is water.

solvent misuse the practice of inhaling volatile substances, such as those in some adhesives, solvents and fuels, to produce euphoria and intoxication. Characterized by odour on clothes and hair, redness and blistering around the nose and mouth, and behaviour changes. Dependence, local damage to the nasal mucosa and organ damage, e.g. the brain, may result. Death may be caused by asphyxia or toxicity. *See also* **drug misuse**.

somatic relating to the body such as somatic cells (body cells), as distinct from the gametes.

somatic nerves nerves controlling the function of voluntary, skeletal muscle.

somatostatin (growth hormone release-inhibiting hormone, GH-RIH) a peptide found in the brain where it is a nerotransmitter, the gastrointestinal tract and the pancreas.

somatostatin receptors are found in the pituitary, pancreas, upper gastrointestinal tract, small cell lung cancer, tumours of the ovary, cervix, endometrium, breast, kidney, larynx, paranasal sinus, salivary glands, some skin tumours and tumours in the salivary glands. They are useful in imaging a variety of tumours.

somatotrophin *see* **growth hormone**.

somnolence syndrome periods of drowsiness, lethargy, loss of appetite and irritability in children following radiotherapy treatment to the head.

sonograph graphic record of sound waves.

sonography the means by which a sonograph is recorded and interpreted.

sonolucent without echoes.

sound the result of mechanical energy travelling through matter as a wave, producing alternating compression and rarefaction resulting in vibration.

source isolation is used for patients who are sources of microorganisms that may be transmitted from them to infect others. *See also* **containment isolation, protective isolation**.

source organ an organ where radioactivity is accumulated and therefore irradiates associated organs.

source stick protocol the instructions to be followed if a machine housing a radioactive source remains in the 'beam on' position at the end of the planned exposure, i.e. the beam does not terminate.

Souttar tube an intubation tube which comprises flexible metal coils; the tube is pushed through an oesophageal tumour to enable the free passage of food and fluid.

spam unrequested email, usually advertising products or services.

spasticity marked rigidity of muscles.

spatial divided into partitions.

spatial detail *see* **spatial resolution**.

spatial distortion when a gamma camera does not accurately distinguish between an object and its surroundings.

spatial filtering a method of improving an electronic image by modifying the pixel values that surround the area.

spatial frequency the change in brightness value of a region of an electronic image per unit distance. If an area has low spatial frequency there is little change in brightness over distance but with high spatial values there can be a large change in brightness over a small distance.

spatial resolution the smallest distance between two objects that can be visually seen on an imaging system.

specific activity the ratio per unit mass of radioactive to non-radioactive atoms in an element.

specific dynamic action (SDA)   the increase in body temperature and metabolism that occurs when energy is used in the assimilation of ingested food. Protein foods in particular cause a sustained increase in basal metabolic rate that lasts for some hours.

specific gravity   the weight of a substance, as compared with that of an equal volume of pure water, the latter being represented by 1000.

specific heat   the energy in joules which is required to raise the temperature of 1 kilogram of the body by 1 kelvin unit.

specific ionization   the number of ion pairs produced per millimetre by a charged particle passing through a medium.

specificity   the ability of a detector to respond to a specific type and energy of radiation. The ability of a test to accurately identify non-affected individuals, such as a screening test.

specific resistance   of a substance is obtained when a current is measured after passing through opposing surfaces of a 1 metre cube of the material.

speckling   the graininess of an ultrasound image which is caused by scatter.

spectral Doppler trace   in ultrasound, a greyscale picture of a waveform showing all its components.

spectral emission   the colour of light emitted by an object. In intensifying screen, lanthanum oxybromide blue, gadolinium oxysulphide green, barium fluorochloride ultraviolet and calcium tungstate blue.

spectral sensitizing   increasing the spectral sensitivity of a film by adding impurities to the film emulsion, because it is done by adding coloured dyes and therefore can be called dye sensitizing, colour sensitizing or optical sensitizing.

spectral sensitivity   the range of wavelengths of electromagnetic radiation that a film emulsion or the human eye is sensitive to.

speculum   an instrument used to hold the walls of a cavity apart, so that the interior of the cavity can be examined or treated. *See also* **nasal speculum, vaginal speculum**.

speech recognition   software, which allows computers to be operated by human voice commands.

speech synthesis   software which allows computers to 'talk' to the user.

speed   distance travelled in unit time, unit metre per second. In photography, the *screen speed* is the ability of the phosphor to convert radiation to light, generally the faster the screen the less image detail when comparing the same phosphor, but this does not apply to comparisons between conventional and rare earth screens. The *film speed* is the ability of the film to respond to exposure, the faster the film, the less exposure will be required to produce a comparable image, on a characteristic curve; generally, the nearer the curve is to the vertical axis the faster the film. *See also* **characteristic curve**.

speed classification a means of comparing different film screen combinations, it is an arbitrary scale based on 100 and combinations range between 50 and 800.

sperm an abbreviated form of the word spermatozoon or spermatozoa.

sperm count an infertility test where semen is examined for volume, sperm numbers, morphology, motility and chemical composition.

spermatic associated with or conveying semen.

spermatic cord suspends the testis in the scrotum and contains the testicular artery and vein and the deferent duct (vas deferens).

spermatogenesis the process of development of spermatozoa, consisting of two stages, firstly spermatogonia become spermatocytes which develop into spermatids, secondly, spermiogenesis, the spermatids become spermatozoa.

spermatorrhoea involuntary discharge of semen without orgasm.

spermatozoon a mature, male gamete (germ cell).

sphenoid a wedge-shaped bone at the base of the skull containing the sphenoidal sinus.

spherical aberration the difference in focussing between the edge and the centre of a lens.

sphincter a circular muscle, contraction of which serves to close an orifice.

sphingolipid sphingosine combined with a lipid. A constituent of biological membranes, especially in the brain.

sphingomyelin a phospholipid formed from sphingosine found as part of biological membranes.

sphingomyelinase an enzyme concerned with the metabolism and storage of lipids.

sphingosine a constituent of sphingolipids and sphingomyelin.

sphygmomanometer an instrument used for non-invasive measurement of arterial blood pressure. Some utilize a column of mercury, but are generally being replaced with aneroid (not containing a liquid) devices.

spica a bandage applied in a figure-of-eight pattern.

spicule a small, spike-like fragment, especially of bone

spigot plastic peg used to close a tube.

spin echo the reappearance of a magnetic resonance signal after the initial signal has disappeared following a 90° radio-frequency pulse followed by the application of a 180° radiofrequency pulse.

spin-lattice relaxation time (T1, longitudinal relaxation time, T1 relaxation time) in magnetic resonance imaging, the time taken for the spins to give the energy obtained from the initial radio-frequency impulse, back to the surrounding environment and return to equilibrium. It represents the time required for the longitudinal magnetization (M_z) to go from 0 to 63% of its final maximum value.

spin-spin relaxation time (transverse or T$_2$ relaxation time) the time required for the transverse magnetization to decay to about 37% of its maximum value and is the characteristic time constant for loss of phase coherence among spins orientated at an angle to the static main magnetic field.

spina bifida a congenital defect in which there is incomplete closure of the neural canal, usually in the lumbosacral region.

spina bifida occulta a congenital defect that does not affect the spinal cord or meninges. It is often marked externally by pigmentation, a haemangioma, a tuft of hair or a lipoma which may extend into the spinal canal.

spina bifida cystica an externally protruding spinal lesion. It may vary in severity from meningocele to myelomeningocele. The condition can be detected during pregnancy by an increased concentration of alphafetoprotein in the amniotic fluid or by ultrasonography.

spinal associated with the spine.

spinal accessory nerve the eleventh pair of cranial nerves. They supply the muscles of the larynx and pharynx, and the muscles of the neck and shoulder to control movement of the head and shoulders.

spinal anaesthetic a local anaesthetic solution injected into the subarachnoid space, so that it renders the area supplied by the selected spinal nerves insensitive.

spinal column *see* **vertebral column**.

spinal cord a structure which lies in the spinal column, reaching from the foramen magnum to the first or second lumbar vertebra. It is a direct continuation of the nervous tissue of the medulla oblongata.

spinal cord compression (SCC) pressure on the spinal cord. Often caused by a tumour (which is commonly metastatic tumour from lung, breast or gastrointestinal cancers). Early diagnosis is vital to prevent permanent effects such as paralysis. Treatment usually involves corticosteroids and radiotherapy.

spinal nerves 31 pairs leave the spinal cord and pass out of the spinal canal to supply the periphery of the body.

spine a popular term for the bony spinal or vertebral column. A sharp process of bone.

spiral CT scan the patient table is moved at a constant speed through the CT gantry while the X-ray tube rotates around the patient; the technique improves the time taken to record the scan and improves contrast and opacification.

spiral fracture a break in a bone which twists round the bone, the most common site is the shaft of the tibia.

spiritual distress may occur when a person's spiritual beliefs are derived from a particular religion, which requires the person to observe certain practices in everyday living activities, e.g. the preparation of food, types of food eaten, fasting, attending public worship, prayer, personal hygiene and type of clothing. Distress is likely if they are unable to conform to the teachings of their religious faith such as might occur during illness and hospitalization.

spirometer   an instrument for measuring the air capacity of the lungs.

Spitz–Holter valve   a special valve used to drain hydrocephalus.

splanchnic   associated with or supplying the viscera.

spleen   a lymphoid, vascular organ immediately below the diaphragm, at the tail of the pancreas, behind the stomach. It is part of the monocyte-macrophage (reticuloendothelial) system. Functions include the destruction of worn out blood cells, filtering the blood of debris and providing a site for lymphocyte proliferation and antibody production.

splenocaval   associated with the spleen and inferior vena cava, usually referring to anastomosis of the splenic vein to the inferior vena cava.

splenomegaly   enlargement of the spleen.

splenoportal   associated with the spleen and hepatic portal vein.

splenoportogram   radiographic demonstration of the spleen and hepatic portal vein after injection of a radiopaque contrast agent. Superseded by ultrasound examination.

splenorenal   associated with the spleen and kidney, as anastomosis of the splenic vein to the renal vein; a procedure carried out in some cases of portal hypertension.

spindle cell sarcoma   malignant tumours of epithelial tissue.

splenomegaly   abnormal enlargement of the spleen.

splint   *see* **orthosis**.

split course therapy   radiotherapy where a gap is planned between the first and second halves of treatment to enable patients to recover from acute reactions to treatment.

split emulsion film   a film having two emulsions, one on top of each other on the same side of the base, one layer providing high contrast and the other high maximum density, used for mammography.

spondyl(e)   a vertebra.

spondylitis   inflammation of the spine. *See also* **ankylosing spondylitis**.

spondylography   a method of measuring and studying the degree of kyphosis by directly tracing the line of the back.

spondylolisthesis   forward displacement of lumbar vertebra(e).

spondylosis   degenerative disease of the whole spine, with osteophyte formation on either side of the intervertebral disc. Often associated with osteoarthritis of the apophyseal (facet) joints.

spontaneous abortion   *see* **spontaneous miscarriage**.

spontaneous emission   when an atom absorbs a photon and releases the absorbed energy as a photon of light.

spontaneous fracture one occurring without appreciable violence; may be synonymous with pathological fracture.

spontaneous miscarriage one which occurs naturally without intervention.

sprain injury to the soft tissues surrounding a joint, resulting in discoloration, swelling and pain. There is stretching or tearing of a ligament or capsular structure of a joint.

spreadsheet a program which allows forecasting and financial planning.

Sprengel's shoulder deformity congenital high scapula, a permanent elevation of the shoulder, often associated with other congenital deformities, for example the presence of a cervical rib or the absence of vertebrae.

squamous scaly.

squamous cell carcinoma carcinoma arising in squamous epithelium; epithelioma.

squamous epithelium the non-glandular epithelial covering of the external body surfaces.

SSL (Secure Socket Layer) a method of verifying the identity of system users and Web sites.

staging process of measuring how advanced a tumour is and to which sites it has spread; may be locally advanced or metastatic. In *stage 1* the tumour is confined to the organ of origin, *stage 2* local lymph nodes are invaded, *stage 3* distant lymph nodes are invaded or local spread beyond the original organ and *stage 4* blood-borne metastases are present. Usually involves imaging with computed tomography, bone scan and often surgery. It includes tumour (T) size, nodal (N) status and metastatic (M) sites present/absent.

standard a level or measure against which the performance of an activity can be monitored.

standard contrast emulsions once the most common film emulsion types with a low base fog, an average gradient of 2.6 and a maximum density of 3.5. *See also* **characteristic curve**.

standard deviation (SD) in statistics, a method of grouping data on either side of the mean of a graph, in a normal distribution curve 68% of the data will be covered in one standard deviation above and below the mean. A measure of dispersion of scores around the mean value. It is the square root of variance.

standard error (SE) in statistics, a measure of variability of many mean values of different samples from a population. Used to calculate the chance of a sample mean being smaller or bigger than that for the population.

standardized mortality rate the ratio of the observed numbers of deaths in a given region to the expected number of deaths in a given region multiplied by 100.

standardized mortality ratio (SMR) allows comparisons to be made between the death rates in populations with different demographic structures. It involves the application of national age-specific mortality rates to local populations so that a ratio of expected deaths to actual deaths can be calculated. The comparative national figure is, by convention, 100 and, for example, a local figure of 106 means that there is an increased risk of 6%, whereas a local figure of 94 indicates a risk 6% lower.

standby system a system which automatically shuts down sections of an automatic film processor when not in use to reduce running costs and conserve energy.

stapes the stirrup-shaped medial bone of the middle ear. *See also* **incus, malleus**.

staphylococci Gram-positive, non-mobile bacteria normally present on the skin and mucous membranes.

Starling's law of the heart states that the force of myocardial contraction is proportional to the length (stretching) of the ventricular muscle fibres. Increased stretching results in the next contraction being more powerful.

starter solution a solution containing a weak acid and bromide ions which is used with new developer in automatic processing machines to depress the activity of the developer until a number of films have been processed; the processed films produce bromide ions and therefore the solution will no longer need to be added.

start-up costs the costs, such as the purchase of equipment, that occur at the start of a project.

statement an instruction in a computer program.

Statistical Package for the Social Sciences (SPSS) software package often used in the analysis of quantitative data.

statistical significance in research, an expression of how likely it is that a set of results happened by chance, e.g. 0.05, 0.01 and 0.001 levels. *See also* **P value**.

statistics scientific study of numerical data collection and its analysis and evaluation.

status epilepticus a condition where there is a rapid succession of epileptic fits.

steatorrhoea the presence of excess fat in the faeces.

steering coils produce magnetic fields to ensure that an electron beam is positioned at the centre of a tube and that is then positioned on the correct aspect of the target in a linear accelerator.

Steinmann's pin an alternative to the use of a Kirschner wire for applying skeletal traction to a limb. It has its own introducer and stirrup.

stellate   star-shaped.

stellate ganglion   a large collection of nerve cells (ganglion) on the sympathetic chain in the root of the neck.

stellate ganglionectomy   surgical removal of the stellate ganglion.

stenosis   abnormal narrowing of a channel or opening.

stent   device used to provide a shunt or keep a tube or vessel open. For example stent insertion into the bile duct to relieve obstructive jaundice, stenting the ureters to overcome urinary obstruction, and stenting the oesophagus for palliation of dysphagia caused by oesophageal cancer. *See also* **transjugular intrahepatic portasystemic stent shunting**.

stepwedge   a piece of equipment which is made up of different thicknesses of aluminium with a layer of copper on the base; wedges are calibrated so that when radiographed each step produces an exact increase or decrease in density on the film. *See also* **characteristic curves**.

stercobilin   the brown pigment of faeces; it is formed from stercobilinogen which is derived from the bile pigments.

stereotactic radiotherapy   where multiple beams of radiation are given to a tumour over a number of days to destroy the tumour.

stereotactic surgery   where multiple beams of radiation are focused on a tumour and the total dose given destroys the tumour. *See also* **radiosurgery**.

sterile   free from microorganisms.

sterilization   activity that kills or removes all types of microorganisms including spores. It is accomplished by the use of heat, radiation, chemicals or filtration. Making incapable of reproduction.

sternoclavicular   associated with the sternum and the clavicle.

sternocleidomastoid muscle   a strap-like neck muscle arising from the sternum and clavicle, and inserting into the mastoid process of temporal bone.

sternocostal   associated with the sternum and ribs.

sternum   the breast bone.

steroids   a large group of organic compounds (lipids) that have a common basic chemical structure: three 6-carbon rings and a 5-carbon ring. They include: cholesterol, bile salts, vitamin D precursors, sex hormones and the corticosteroid hormones.

sterol   chemicals with the basic steroid structure combined with an alcohol group such as cholesterol.

stertorous   noisy breathing, cheeks puffed in and out with each breath.

stillbirth   birth of a baby, after 24 weeks' gestation, that shows no sign of life.

stillborn   born dead.

Still's disease   term seldom used, having been superseded by systemic onset juvenile idiopathic arthritis. *See also* **juvenile idiopathic arthritis**.

stimulant   an agent that causes functional activity of an organ.

stimulated emission   when an excited atom absorbs a photon and releases two light photons.

stochastic effect   one in which the probability of the effect occurring is governed by chance, therefore all doses of radiation carry some risk and the stochastic effects produced by radiation on an individual include radiation-induced cancer and genetic effects. *See also* **deterministic effects**.

stock control   the method of storing and recording purchased items for example film to ensure that the oldest is used first and all film is used before its expiry date.

stoma   the mouth; any opening. *See also* **colostomy, ileostomy, urostomy**.

stoma care nurse   specialist nurse who advises on the management of bowel and urinary stomas.

stomach   the most dilated part of the digestive tube, situated between the oesophagus and the duodenum; it lies in the epigastric, umbilical and left hypochondriac regions of the abdomen. The wall is composed of four coats: serous, muscular, submucous and mucous. It produces gastric juice containing digestive enzymes, hydrochloric acid and mucus.

stone   calculus; a hardened mass of mineral matter.

stool   faeces.

stove-in chest   there may be multiple anterior or posterior fractures of the ribs (causing paradoxical respiration) and fractures of sternum, or a mixture of such fractures.

straight line portion   the part of the characteristic curve which is used in radiography to determine the gamma, contrast, average gradient, useful exposure range, useful density range, film latitude and film speed. *See also* **sensitometry**.

strandquist isoeffect curves   a series of tolerance dose curves to relate total radiotherapy dose to overall treatment time.

strain   overuse or stretching of a part. A group of microorganisms within a species. To pass a liquid through a filter.

strangulated hernia   hernia in which the blood supply to the organ involved is impaired, usually due to constriction by surrounding structures.

Strategic Health Authority   a body responsible for strategic health planning for a geographical area with a population of many millions (for example, the English counties of Cambridgeshire, Norfolk and Suffolk). They are also responsible for the performance management of the Primary Care Trusts (PCTs) within that area.

strategic management   the management function concerned with longer-term future strategy. Financial and resource planning. *See also* **operational management**.

stratified arranged in layers.

stratum a layer or lamina, e.g. the various layers of the epithelium of the skin, i.e. stratum granulosum, stratum corneum.

streptococci Gram-positive spherical bacteria.

stress fracture (fatigue fracture) a bone fracture resulting from repeated loading with relatively low magnitude forces. Can be caused by a number of factors including overtraining, incorrect biomechanics, fatigue, hormonal imbalance, poor nutrition and osteoporosis.

stress incontinence occurs when the intra-abdominal pressure is raised as in coughing, giggling and sneezing; there is usually some weakness of the urethral sphincter muscle coupled with anatomical stretching and displacement of the bladder neck.

striae streaks; stripes; narrow bands. Occur when the abdomen enlarges such as with obesity, tumours and pregnancy, when the marks are called striae gravidarum they are red at first and then become silvery-white. Striae may also occur as a side-effect of corticosteroid therapy.

stricture a narrowing, especially of a tube or canal, due to scar tissue or tumour.

stridor a harsh breathing sound caused by partial obstruction of the larynx or trachea.

stroke (cerebrovascular accident) interference with the blood flow in the brain due to embolism, haemorrhage or thrombosis. Signs and symptoms range from weakness and tingling in a limb through to paralysis of limbs, incontinence of faeces and urine and loss of speech.

stroke volume (SV) the volume of blood pumped out of the heart by each ventricular contraction.

stroma the blood supply and supporting structures of a tumour above the size of about 2 mm.

strontium (Sr) a metallic element present in bone. Isotopes of strontium are used in radionuclide scanning of bone.

strontium-90 (^{90}Sr) a radioisotope with a half-life of 28 years produced during atomic explosions. It is dangerous when it becomes integrated within bone tissue where turnover is slow. Used to treat the cornea by being incorporated in a rolled silver foil and bonded into a silver applicator.

structure localization a method of accurately locating small, impalpable lesions using ultrasound, CT scanning or using a localizing grid and conventional radiography.

structure mottle an uneven radiographic image due to the fact that it is not possible to evenly disperse the phosphor crystals throughout the binder when manufacturing intensifying screens and therefore light from the intensifying screens is not uniformly produced.

Stryker bed   a proprietary bed. Designed to allow rotation of patients to the prone or supine position. Main uses include spinal injuries and burns.

Student's paired test   a parametric test for statistical significance. Used to test differences in mean values for two related measurements such as those obtained from the same subject. *See also* **Wilcoxon test**.

Student's t test for independent groups   a parametric test for statistical significance. Used to test differences in mean values of two groups. *See also* **Mann–Whitney test**.

stupor   a state of semi-unconsciousness, occurs in some mental illnesses when the patient does not move or speak and makes no response to stimuli.

styloid   long and pointed; resembling a pen or stylus.

subarachnoid haemorrhage (SAH)   the loss of blood from a vessel in the brain which leaks into the subarachnoid space. This is typically due to an intracerebral aneurysm or arteriovenous malformation and can be fatal. Blood is present in the cerebrospinal fluid (CSF).

subarachnoid space   the space beneath the arachnoid membrane, between it and the pia mater. It contains cerebrospinal fluid.

subcarinal   below a carina, usually referring to the carina tracheae.

subclavian   beneath the clavicle.

subcostal   beneath the rib.

subcutaneous   beneath the skin.

subdural   beneath the dura mater; between the dura and arachnoid membranes.

subdural haematoma (SDH)   the accumulation of blood beneath the dura lining the skull that can occur after head trauma. It develops slowly and may present as a space-occupying lesion with vomiting, papilloedema, fluctuating level of consciousness, weakness, usually hemiplegia on the opposite side to the clot. Finally there is a rise in blood pressure and a fall in pulse rate.

subendocardial   immediately beneath the endocardium.

subhepatic   beneath the liver.

subject contrast   the contrast seen on a radiograph varies with the body part being imaged and will change with the size of the area, the density and atomic number of the tissue, the quality of radiation and the use of contrast agents.

subjective contrast   the observer's opinion of the contrast seen on an image; it depends on the viewing conditions, and the observer's ability to see differences on the film.

sublethal damage   damage caused by radiation that is insufficient to cause death of the cell.

subliminal   inadequate for perceptible response. Below the level of consciousness.

sublingual   beneath the tongue.

subluxation   incomplete dislocation of a joint.

submandibular   below the mandible.

submaxillary   below the maxilla.

submucosa   the layer of connective tissue beneath a mucous membrane.

submucous   beneath a mucous membrane.

submucous resection (SMR)   surgical correction of a deviated nasal septum.

suboccipital   beneath the occiput; in the nape of the neck.

subperiosteal   beneath the periosteum of bone.

subphrenic   beneath the diaphragm.

subroutine   a self-contained part of a computer program which can be returned to time and time again.

substrate   a chemical acted upon and changed by an enzyme in a chemical reaction.

substratum   an adhesive layer that attaches the emulsion to the film base, or the phosphor layer to the reflective layer of an intensifying screen.

succenturiate lobe   an accessory lobe of the placenta.

sucrase   intestinal enzyme that converts sucrose to glucose and fructose.

sucrose   a disaccharide that is hydrolysed into glucose and fructose during digestion. It occurs naturally in sugar and is added to many manufactured foods. Frequent consumption of sucrose causes dental disease.

suction   the process of sucking. The removal of gas or fluid from a cavity by means of reduced pressure.

sudden infant death syndrome (SIDS, cot death)   the unexpected sudden death of an infant, usually occurring overnight while sleeping in a cot, but may occur under other situations. The commonest mode of death in infants between the ages of 1 month and 1 year, neither clinical nor postmortem findings being adequate to account for death. Overheating, sleeping in the prone position, respiratory illness and infection, and being in an environment where people smoke, have all been implicated as risk factors. Parents/carers are now recommended to put babies to sleep on their backs, at the foot of the cot to prevent them wriggling under bedclothes, not to overheat the room, not to smoke in the same room and to seek advice from a health professional if the baby seems unwell.

sulcus   a furrow or groove, particularly those separating the gyri (convolutions) of the cerebral cortex.

sulphuric acid   chemical used as the acid in a fixer solution with aluminium sulphate hardener.

superadditivity   the combined activities of two chemicals is greater than the sum of their separate activities, for example phenidone and hydroquinone used in developer.

supercilium   the eyebrow.

supercoat   a thin layer of gelatine that is coated on the outer surface of a film or the thin layer of cellulose acetobiturate on an intensifying screen, to protect from mechanical damage.

superficial   near the surface such as the superficial veins of the leg.

superior   in anatomy, the upper of two parts.

supernumerary   in excess of the normal number; additional. ***supernumerary bones*** include os trigonum, os tibial externum and os vesalii. Such abnormalities of sesamoid bones and supernumerary bones rarely directly cause problems in the paediatric foot but may result in soft-tissue lesions. Their presence is confirmed radiographically.

supernumerary digits   *see* **polydactyly**.

superparamagnetic   a substance which is 100–1000 times more susceptible to magnetism than a paramagnet. *See also* **diamagnetic, paramagnetic, superparamagnetic, ferromagnetic**.

supervised area   a type of designated area where a person is likely to receive a dosage of radiation in excess of one third the dose in a controlled area; access to the area is limited to those people whose presence is necessary.

supinate   turn or lay face or palm upward. *See also* **pronate**.

supinato   that which supinates, usually applied to a muscle. *See also* **pronator**.

supine   lying on the back with face upwards, of the hand with palm upwards. *See also* **prone**.

suppository   medicine, contained in a base that melts at body temperature, placed inside the rectum.

supraclavicular   above the clavicle.

supracondylar   above a condyle.

supracondylar fracture   a fracture affecting the lower end of the humerus or femur. The former may interfere with the blood supply to the forearm.

supraorbital   above the orbits.

supraorbital ridge   the ridge covered by the eyebrows.

suprapubic   above the pubis.

suprarenal   above the kidney. *See also* **adrenal**.

suprasternal above the sternum.

surface applicator used in brachytherapy where the external surface of the patient is treated by locally applied sources held in shaped applicators.

surfactant a mixture of phospholipids secreted by type II pneumocytes. It reduces surface tension in the alveoli, allows lung inflation and prevents alveolar collapse between breaths. *See also* **pneumocytes**.

surgical mask a mask to cover the nose and mouth to prevent contamination of a sterile area by droplet infection. Worn to protect the wearer from airborne infection.

survey a data collection method. Includes: interview, postal, telephone, or via the internet.

survival rate the proportion of patients who survive for a certain number of years, usually five, used for measuring the success of treatment for cancer.

suspensory ligaments supporting or suspending such as those supporting the lens of the eye.

suture the junction of cranial bones. In surgery, a stitch or series of stitches used to appose the edges of a surgical or traumatic wound. Also describes the placement of such stitches. *See also* **ligature**.

swab a small piece of cotton wool gauze. *See also* **filamented swab**.

swallowing (deglutition) part voluntary and part involuntary activity with three stages: oral (buccal), pharyngeal and oesophageal. *See also* **dysphagia**.

sweat the secretion from the sweat (sudoriferous) glands. Contains water, electrolytes (mainly sodium and chloride) and waste. Sweat production is primarily concerned with temperature regulation but has a small excretory role.

sweat gland *see* **apocrine glands, eccrine**.

swept gain used in ultrasound scanners to give an image of even brightness when scanning homogeneous tissue.

sympathetic nervous system part of the peripheral nervous system (PNS), it describes a division of the autonomic nervous system (ANS). It is composed of a chain of ganglia on either side of the vertebral column and nerve fibres having thoracolumbar outflow. It opposes the parasympathetic nervous system and is usually involved with body stimulation. Its action is augmented by adrenaline (epinephrine) and noradrenaline (norepinephrine).

symphalangism the fusion of phalanges in one digit.

symphysis a fibrocartilaginous union of bones such as the symphysis pubis.

symptoms any indication of disease perceived by a patient.

synapse   the gap between the axon of one neuron and the dendrites of another, or the gap between the axon and a gland or muscle. Most operate chemically but a few are electrical. The synapse permits the passage of an impulse across the gap. This is achieved chemically by the release of calcium ions and a neurotransmitter such as acetylcholine.

synarthroses   fibrous joints with virtually no movement.

synchondrosis   a type of cartilaginous joint with minimal movement, for example, the sternocostal joints.

synchronous   at the same time.

syncope   a simple faint or loss of consciousness due to cerebral ischaemia.

syncytium   a mass of tissue with several nuclei. Boundaries between individual cells are absent or poorly defined.

syndactyly (syndactylism, syndactylia, zygodactyly, webbed toes)   a term applied to a total or partial fusion of adjacent digits. It is very common, usually bilateral and often familial. Multiple syndactyly occurs in hands and feet associated with other anomalies, as in Apert's syndrome, an autosomal dominant disorder – acrocephalosyndactyly. Treatment is not required for webbing of the toes.

syndesmoses   joints held together by a ligament or membrane, for example inferior tibiofibular joint.

syndrome   a group of signs and symptoms typical of a distinctive disease, which often occur together and form a distinctive clinical picture.

synergism (synergy)   the harmonious working together of two agents, such as drugs, microorganisms, muscles, etc.

synergistic action   that brought about by the cooperation of two or more muscles, neither of which could bring about the action alone.

synovial cavity   the potential space in a synovial joint.

synovial fluid   the fluid secreted by the membrane lining a freely movable joint cavity.

synovial joint (diarthroses)   the main group of joints found in the body; the ends of the bone are covered with articular hyaline cartilage and there is synovial fluid within the joint cavity which is secreted by the synovial membrane which lines the fibrous capsule that surrounds the joint.

synovial membrane   the membrane lining the intra-articular parts of bones and ligaments. It does not cover the articular surfaces.

synovioma   a tumour of synovial membrane; it can be benign or malignant.

synovitis   inflammation of a synovial membrane.

syntax error   two words which are shown on the computer display when an incorrect input or statement has been made.

syphilis   a sexually transmitted disease.

syringe   an instrument for holding fluid or air for injection, for aspirating fluid or irrigating body cavities. It is a hollow tube with a tight-fitting piston; a hollow needle or a thin tube can be fitted to the end.

syringe shield   a device made of either metal with a high atomic number or thick Perspex which is designed to protect the hands of staff when handling syringes containing radioactive material.

syringomyelia   a disease of the spinal cord with associated muscular wasting of the upper limbs.

syringomyelocele   the most severe form of meningeal hernia (spina bifida). The central canal is dilated and the thinned-out posterior part of the spinal cord is in the hernia.

syrinx   a cyst-like cavity in the spinal cord.

systematic review   a systematic approach to literature reviews of both published and unpublished material that lessens bias and random errors.

Système International d'Unités (SI, International System of Units)   system of measurement used for scientific, technical and medical purposes. There are seven base units: ampere, candela, kelvin, kilogram, metre, mole and second, and various derived units, e.g. pascal, becquerel, etc. (See figures on p. 346)

systemic circulation   oxygenated blood leaves the left ventricle and, after flowing through the aorta throughout the body tissues, returns deoxygenated to the right atrium of the heart.

systole   the contraction phase of the cardiac cycle, as opposed to diastole.

systolic function   the measurement of the ventricular contraction of the heart.

systolic murmur   a cardiac murmur occurring between the first and second heart sounds due to valvular disease, e.g. mitral systolic murmur.

T

· ·

T_1 relaxation time (T_1, spin-lattice relaxation time, longitudinal relaxation time) in magnetic resonance imaging, the time taken for the spins to give the energy obtained from the initial radio frequency impulse, back to the surrounding environment and return to equilibrium. It represents the time required for the longitudinal magnetization (M_z) to go from 0 to 63% of its final maximum value.

T_2 relaxation time (transverse or spin-spin relaxation time) the time required for the transverse magnetization to decay to about 37% of its maximum value and is the characteristic time constant for loss of phase coherence among spins orientated at an angle to the static main magnetic field.

table incrementation time the time taken for the patient's couch to move from one slice location to the next in sequential (non-spiral) CT scanning.

tabular grains are 'flattened' grains that are used only in sensitized film emulsions in screen film technology; they have a large surface area and small volume. The added dye can increase the amount of absorption resulting in a high-speed, high-resolution film with relatively low silver coating weights.

tachycardia excessively heart beat (in excess of 100 beats per minute in adults). Can occur following shock, haemorrhage, heart condition, hyperthermia or the action of certain drugs.

tachypnoea rapid, shallow respiration.

tactile relating to the sense of touch. *See also* **taenia**.

taenia a flat band.

taenia coli three flat bands running the length of the large intestine and consisting of the longitudinal muscle fibres.

talipes any of a number of deformities of the foot and ankle.

talipes calcaneovalgus a condition usually caused by intrauterine posture. The foot has been fixed in an upturned position with the sole against the uterine wall. Improvement and usually complete recovery occurs with active movement after birth.

talipes equinovarus (club foot) the heel is drawn up, the foot inverted and the hindfoot adducted.

talus situated between the tibia proximally and the calcaneus distally, thus directly bearing the weight of the body. It is the second largest bone of the ankle.

tangential   when a beam enters the body at an angle to avoid critical structures, for example, in the treatment technique for carcinoma of the breast.

target   thin tungsten plate on the anode of an X-ray tube which, when bombarded with electrons, produces X-rays.

target angle   the angle between the X-ray beam and the face of the target, the target of an X-ray tube is set at an angle to maximize the target area and minimize the geometric unsharpness.

target organ   the organ that a dose of radiation is calculated for.

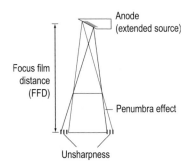

Target angle and geometric unsharpness. From Radiographic imaging, 3rd edn, Chris Gunn, 2002, Churchill Livingstone, Edinburgh, with permission.

tarsal bones   short bones, the seven bones which lie between the metatarsal bones and the ankle joint in the foot.

tarsal coalition (peroneal spastic flat foot)   an anomaly in which adjacent tarsal bones are fused together. Fusion may be bony or cartilaginous. The most common occurs between the calcaneus and the navicular with union across the mid-tarsal joint. Talocalcaneal coalition also occurs.

tarsalgia   pain in the foot.

tarsometatarsal   relating to the tarsal and metatarsal region.

tarsus   the seven small bones of the foot. The dense connective tissue found in each eyelid, contributing to its form and support.

tartar   *see* **calculus**.

taste (gustation)   a chemical sense closely linked with smell.

taste buds   sensory receptors found on the tongue, epiglottis and pharynx.

tattoos   permanent skin markings to facilitate accurate daily set up of patients during a course of radiotherapy.

T cell   *see* **lymphocyte**.

TE (echo time)   the time between the centre of the excitation pulse and the peak of the echo.

tears   the secretion produced by the lacrimal gland. Tears contain the bactericidal enzyme lysozyme.

technetium (Tc)   a radioactive element which is produced by irradiation of molybdenum, an isotope of technetium ($^{99}Tc^{m}$) is used in radionuclide imaging for brain scanning.

technetium generator   used to produce radionuclides artificially by bombarding the nuclei of elements with particles. Molybdenum-98 is placed in a

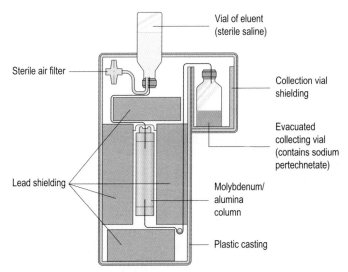

Vial of eluent
(sterile saline)

Sterile air filter

Collection vial
shielding

Evacuated
collecting vial
(contains sodium
pertechnetate)

Lead shielding

Molybdenum/
alumina
column

Plastic casting

Principal features of a technetium-99 m generator. From Principles of radiological physics, 3rd edn, D T Graham, 1996, Churchill Livingstone, Edinburgh, with permission.

neutron stream and neutrons are absorbed to produce molybdenum-99 which results in the emission of gamma rays; the molybdenum decays to form technetium-99 m and this is removed from the generator as sodium pertechnetate which is used for radionuclide imaging.

teeth   the 32 adult (see figure on p. 370) or 20 childhood teeth lie in the alveolar ridge of the mandible and the maxilla.

teething   lay term for the discomfort during the eruption of the primary dentition in babies.

tegument   the skin or covering of the body.

telangiectasia   the dilatation of thin-walled, superficial blood vessels.

teleisotope unit   equipment containing a radioactive source producing X or γ rays for teletherapy.

telemetry   the electronic transmission of data including clinical measurement between distant sites. May be used for cardiac monitoring.

teleradiology   the electronic transfer of images and reports to remote centres, for example, general practitioner practices.

Teletex   the sending of documents at high speed electronically.

Teletext   the non-interactive public information service on television; BBC transmits Ceefax, the ITA transmits Oracle.

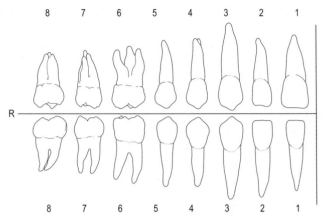

1 2 – Incisors; 3 – Canine; 4 5 – Premolars; 6 7 8 – Molars

Permanent teeth right upper and lower quadrants. From Bones and joints, 4th edn, Chris Gunn, 2002, Churchill Livingstone, Edinburgh, with permission.

teletherapy   when an external source of radiation (X-rays or γ-rays) is directed to a tumour to give the maximum radiation dose to the tumour and the minimum dose to the surrounding healthy tissue.

temple   that part of the head situated between the outer angle of the eye and the top of the pinna.

temporal   relating to the temple.

temporal bones   one on each side of the skull below the parietal bone, containing the middle ear.

temporomandibular   relating to the temporal region or bone, and the lower jaw, such as the joint between the temporal bone and mandible.

temporomandibular joint (TMJ) syndrome   pain in the region of the temporomandibular joint frequently caused by malocclusion of the teeth, resulting in malposition of the condylar heads in the joint and abnormal muscle activity, and by bruxism.

tendinitis   inflammation of a tendon.

tendon   a band of white, fibrous connective tissue that joins muscle to bone.

tenesmus   a feeling of incomplete emptying of the bowel.

tennis elbow   a painful condition affecting the extensor muscle of the forearm at the attachment of the lateral epicondyle of the humerus.

tension pneumothorax   a valve-like wound or tear in the lung allows air to enter the pleural cavity with each inspiration, but not to escape on expiration, thus progressively increasing intrathoracic pressure and constituting an acute medical emergency. Signs are of hyperinflation, midline shift and increasing respiratory distress.

tenosynovitis inflammation of the thin synovial lining of a tendon sheath, as distinct from its outer fibrous sheath. It may be caused by mechanical irritation or by bacterial infection.

tenth-value thickness the thickness of a substance that will transmit exactly one-tenth of the intensity of radiation falling on it.

tentorium cerebelli a fold of dura mater between the cerebellum and cerebrum. Damage during birth may result in intracranial bleeding.

teratoma commonly a tumour of the testis or ovary. It is of embryonic origin and usually malignant. Some testicular tumours have both seminoma and teratoma components. The cure rate for germ cell tumours has increased 10-fold with use of platinum-based chemotherapy.

termination of pregnancy (TOP) *see* **abortion.**

tesla a unit for measuring the strength of a magnetic field. A magnetic flux density of 1 tesla exists if the force on a 1 metre long straight wire, carrying a current of 1 ampere, is 1 Newton and the wire is placed at right angles to the direction of magnetic flux.

testicle *see* **testis.**

testis a male gonad. One of the two glandular structures contained in the scrotum of the male; they produce spermatozoa and the male sex hormones. ***undescended testis*** the testis remains within the bony pelvis or inguinal canal. *See also* **cryptorchism.**

testosterone the major androgen, a steroid hormone produced by the testes. It is responsible for the development of the male secondary sexual characteristics and reproductive functioning.

tetradactylous having four digits on each limb.

tetraplegia (quadriplegia) paralysis of all four limbs.

TFT (Thin Film Transistor) the technology used in laptop screens.

thalamus a collection of grey matter at the base of the cerebrum. Sensory impulses from the whole body pass through the thalamus en route to the cerebral cortex.

thalassaemia an inherited disease due to abnormal haemoglobin causing haemolytic anaemias.

thallium activator luminescent centres where about 10–15% of the energy deposited is converted to light energy. Used with sodium iodide as a scintillator crystal.

theca an enveloping sheath, especially of a tendon, or the dura mater.

thenar relating to the palm (hand) and the sole (foot). ***thenar eminence*** the palmar eminence below the thumb.

therapeutic ablation   a dose of radiation given to destroy harmful tissue.

therapeutic abortion   *see* **abortion**.

therapy verification film   an X-ray film shielded by a lead sheet, which is placed behind the patient during one treatment to verify the area being treated. *See also* **portal imaging**.

thermal capacity   the heat energy in joules which is required to raise the temperature of the body by 1 kelvin unit.

thermal effect of ultrasound   the heating of tissue by breaking down the air bubbles and cavities in the tissues.

thermionic emission   the process of releasing electrons from an emitter.

thermionic emitter   a substance that releases electrons when heated.

thermographic printing   utilizes a film containing silver behenate that when exposed to light the resultant heat activates the silver and produces the image. *See also* **photo-thermographic printing**.

thermography   an investigation that detects minute temperature differences over different body areas by use of an infrared thermograph that is sensitive to radiant heat. The uses include the study of blood flow and detection of cancers, such as breast cancer.

thermoluminescence   a substance that when irradiated stores energy, when heated photons of light are produced in proportion to the energy stored.

thermoluminescent dosimetry   small disks containing lithium fluoride can be attached to a patient's body, the disks are then heated and the amount of light produced is compared to a standard to ascertain the amount of radiation received by the patient. A badge containing two lithium fluoride disks worn by radiation workers to estimate the radiation dose they have received to the skin and the whole body dose.

thermometer   equipment for measuring temperature.

thermostat   equipment for controlling temperature.

thoracic   associated with the thorax.

thoracic cage   framework of bones that protects the thoracic structures and provides muscle attachments.

thoracic duct   a channel conveying lymph (chyle) from the cisterna chyli in the abdomen to the left subclavian vein. ***thoracic inlet syndrome*** (cervical rib) a supernumerary rib in the cervical region, which may present no symptoms or it may press on nerves of the brachial plexus.

throracic vertebrae   the 12 bones of the spine that articulate with the ribs.

Thoraeus filter *see* **compound filters**.

thorax the chest cavity.

threatened miscarriage loss of pregnancy characterized by slight vaginal bleeding while the cervix remains closed.

three-dimensional reconstruction a digitally produced image that shows the depth, height and width of an object or objects.

three-dimensional ultrasound the creation of a computerized, reconstructed ultrasound image which represents the anatomical structure being investigated, for example, used to visualize the fetal face and the adult heart valves.

three phase a form of alternating current formed by three phases of current and voltage to enable more power to be supplied for static X-ray equipment. The line voltage is 398 volts in a three-phase supply.

threshold the point at which a film first shows a reaction to exposure. *See also* **sensitometry**.

thrombin the active enzyme formed from prothrombin. Thrombin is formed during both the extrinsic and intrinsic coagulation pathways; it converts fibrinogen to fibrin. *See also* **coagulation, prothrombin, thromboplastin**.

thrombocyte (platelet) plays a part in the clotting of blood. *See also* **blood**.

thrombocytopenia a reduction in the number of platelets in the blood.

thrombosis the unwanted, intravascular formation of a blood clot. *See also* **coronary thrombosis, deep-vein thrombosis**.

thromboxanes regulatory lipids derived from arachidonic acid (fatty acid). They are released from platelets and cause vasospasm and platelet aggregation during platelet plug formation. *See also* **haemostasis**.

thymocytes cells found in the dense lymphoid tissue of the thymus gland.

thymoma a tumour arising in the thymus.

thymopoietin peptide hormone secreted by the thymus gland.

thymosin peptide hormone secreted by the thymus gland.

thymus a lymphoid gland lying behind the sternum and extending upward as far as the thyroid gland. It is well developed in infancy and attains maximum size during puberty; and then the lymphatic tissue is replaced by fatty tissue. It produces thymic hormones (thymosins and thymopoietin) that ensure the proper development of T lymphocytes. The autoimmune condition myasthenia gravis results from pathology of the thymus gland.

thyratron a gas-filled device allowing current to flow in one direction only, containing an anode, a cathode and a grid. A negative potential on the grid can stop the electron flow and therefore can act as an on–off switch.

thyristor   a solid-state replacement for a thyraton which can act as an electric switch.

thyroglobulin   a colloid stored in the thyroid follicles used for the production of thyroxine.

thyroglossal   associated with the thyroid gland and the tongue.

thyroglossal cyst   a retention cyst caused by blockage of the thyroglossal duct: it appears on one or other side of the neck.

thyroglossal duct   the embryonic passage from the thyroid gland to the back of the tongue. In this area thyroglossal cyst or fistula can occur.

thyroid   associated with the thyroid gland.

thyroid antibody test   the presence and severity of autoimmune thyroid disease is diagnosed by the levels of thyroid-stimulating immunoglobulins in the blood.

thyroid gland   a two-lobed endocrine gland, either side of the trachea. It secretes three hormones: triiodothyronine (T_3) and thyroxine (T4) under pituitary control, which stimulate metabolism, and calcitonin from the follicular cells, which helps to regulate calcium and phosphate homeostasis. *See also* **hyperthyroidism, hypothyroidism**.

thyroid-stimulating hormone (TSH)   pituitary hormone that stimulates the secretion of the thyroid hormones thyroxine and triiodothyronine. ***thyroid-stimulating hormone assay*** radioimmunoassay of the level of thyroid stimulating hormone in the serum. Used in the diagnosis of hypothyroidism.

thyrotoxicosis   a disease of the thyroid gland resulting in the overproduction of thyroid hormones.

thyrotrophic   describes any substance that stimulates the thyroid gland, for example, thyrotrophin (thyroid-stimulating hormone, TSH) secreted by the anterior pituitary gland.

thyroxine (T_4)   the principal hormone of the thyroid gland, it contains four atoms of iodine. It is essential for metabolism and development. Used in the treatment of hypothyroidism. *See also* **triiodothyronine**.

TI (inversion time)   the time after the middle of a 180° radio frequency inverting pulse and the inversion recovery sequence to the middle of the 90° read pulse which monitors the amount of longitudinal magnetization.

tibia   the shin bone; the larger of the two bones in the lower part of the leg; it articulates with the femur, fibula and talus.

tibial   relating to the tibia, as in the artery and vein.

tibiofibular   associated with the tibia and the fibula.

tidal air/volume (TV)   the volume of air that passes in and out of the lungs in normal breathing.

tied numbers   results of the same value.

TIFF (Tif, Tagged Information File Format) a graphics or picture computer file used for photographs. The file is not compressed and therefore the picture quality is good but the file size is very large.

time bomb a device used by some software suppliers to prevent piracy of programmes.

time gain control (TGC) a method of compensating for the attenuation of ultrasound as it passes through the tissues so that the deep echoes appear equally as reflective as superficial echoes.

time-of-flight angiography a technique in magnetic resonance imaging to enhance the blood flowing into a slice by ensuring that the blood does not become saturated by previous radio-frequency pulses.

time scale sensitometry a method of producing a characteristic curve by keeping all exposure factors constant, covering the film with a piece of lead rubber and exposing the film a number of times, moving the rubber to reveal more film for each exposure or producing darkened strips on the film by doubling the exposure time for each subsequent step.

tinnitus ringing or buzzing sound in the ears.

tissue a collection of cells or fibres of similar function, forming a structure, often in a background connective tissue.

tissue–air ratio the ratio of the dose rate at a point in the patient to that at the same point in air without the patient being present.

tissue compensator an attenuator placed in the primary beam during radiotherapy of irregular parts of the body, to maintain the dose distribution and the skin sparing effect.

tissue Doppler imaging the analysis of the Doppler signals from a moving structure, for example, the myocardium of the heart, exhibiting a large amplitude but low frequency.

tissue equivalent material a substance that interacts with ionizing radiation in the same way that a patient would interact with the radiation, it therefore has the same scattering and absorption properties of human tissue.

tissue harmonic imaging in ultrasound, using the secondary frequencies sent back to the probe by tissue or contrast media such as air bubbles to improve contrast and spatial resolution in larger subjects as the far field is improved. *See also* **contrast, spatial resolution**.

tissue phantom ratio the ratio of the axis dose rate at a depth d in a phantom to the axis dose rate at a reference depth in the same phantom.

TNM classification a description of the primary tumour, the nodal spread and the distant metastases which summarizes the extent of the malignancy in a patient (see box on p. 376).

token part of a computer network that indicates if a node can write to the network.

TNM classification

T1–3	Generally based on the size and/or extent of the primary
T4	The most advanced local disease, often with invasion of adjacent structures
N0	No nodes palpable
N1	Mobile nodes on the same side as the primary
N1a	Nodes not considered to contain tumour
N1b	Nodes considered to contain tumour
N2	Mobile nodes on the opposite side (N2a and N2b as above)
N3	Fixed, involved nodes
M0	No evidence of distant metastasis
M1	Distant metastasis present

From Walter and Miller's textbook of radiotherapy, 6th edn, 2003, C K Bomford and I H Kunkler (eds), Churchill Livingstone, Edinburgh, with permission.

---

token ring the circular computer network which carries the tokens enabling them to signal to the nodes.

tomography a radiographic technique to produce a sharp plane within the body by blurring the structures above and below the image by moving the X-ray tube and film around a fulcrum.

tone a quality of sound, or the normal, healthy state of tension.

tongue the mobile muscular organ situated in the mouth; it is concerned with mastication, swallowing, taste and speech.

tonsillopharyngeal relating to the tonsils and pharynx.

tonsils small aggregations of lymphoid tissue located around the pharynx. Forming part of body defences they contain macrophages and are a site for lymphocyte proliferation. There are lingual tonsils under the tongue, nasopharyngeal tonsils located on the posterior wall of the nasopharynx (called adenoids when enlarged) and the palatine tonsils found in the oropharynx, one on each side in the fauces between the palatine arch. *See also* **Waldeyer's ring**.

tooth hard calcified structures in the mouth used for masticating food. Composed largely of dentine with enamel covering the crown and cementum covering the root surface. The pulp occupies the cavity at the core of the crown (pulp chamber) and the channel running along the length of the root (root canal). The primary (deciduous, milk) and secondary (permanent, adult) dentitions consist of 20 and 32 teeth, respectively.

tophus a small, hard concretion forming on the ear lobe, on the joints of the phalanges, etc. in gout.

topography a description of the regions of the body.

torsion   the process of twisting.

total body imaging   the radionuclide imaging of the whole of the body to detect metastatic spread from carcinomas.

total body irradiation (TBI)   the aim of the treatment is to deliver a uniform dose to the whole body, using megavoltage photons and tissue compensation. Used prior to bone marrow transplants.

total efficiency   the ability of a phosphor to produce light; it is dependent of its ability to absorb energy and convert it to light.

total linear attenuation coefficient (μ)   the fraction of the X-rays removed from a beam per unit thickness of the attenuating material.

total mass attenuation coefficient graphs   the sum of the individual mass attenuation processes, that is: energy spectrum of the X-ray beam, density and atomic number of the tissue passed through and the separation of the patient, plotted as a graph of energy against incidence.

total quality management (TQM)   a whole organization approach to quality where all employees are expected to take responsibility for quality. It aims to ensure quality at every interface and improve effectiveness and flexibility throughout the organization.

total scanning time   with multi-slice CT this is commonly reduced to the time of data acquisition as large volumes can be scanned in a single breath hold.

tourniquet   equipment for compressing the blood vessels in a limb for the control of bleeding or the removal of blood from a vein.

trabeculae   the septa or fibrous bands projecting into the interior of an organ, for example, the spleen.

tracer   a substance or instrument used to gain information. Radioactive tracers are used in the diagnosis of some cancers, for example, brain, and thyroid disease.

trachea (windpipe)   the fibrocartilaginous tube lined with ciliated mucosa passing from the larynx to the bronchi. It is about 115 mm long and about 25 mm wide.

tracheobronchial   associated with the trachea and the bronchi.

tracheo-oesophageal   associated with the trachea and the oesophagus.

tracheo-oesophageal fistula   usually occurs in conjunction with esophageal atresia. The fistula usually connects the distal oesophagus to the trachea.

tracheostomy   surgical opening between the front of the neck and the trachea to create an artificial airway. It is kept open with a tracheostomy tube.

tracheotomy   a vertical slit in the anterior wall of the trachea at the level of the third and fourth cartilaginous rings.

traction   a drawing or pulling on the patient's body to overcome muscle spasm and to reduce or prevent deformity. A steady pulling exerted on some part (limb or head) by means of weights, pulleys and cords in conjunction with a variety of splints or frames. *skeletal traction* applied on a bone by means of a wire or pin passed through the lower fragment. *skin traction* or extension involves the application of weights to foam or extension plaster attached to the skin. *See also* **beam, Braun's frame, hoop traction, halopelvic traction**.

tragus   the projection in front of the external auditory meatus.

transabdominal   through the abdomen.

transamniotic   through the amniotic membrane and fluid, as a transamniotic transfusion of the fetus for haemolytic disease.

transcription   first stage in protein synthesis where genetic information is transferred from DNA to mRNA. *See also* **translation**.

transducer (probe)   device that converts one form of energy into another to facilitate its electrical transmission. A hand-held instrument composed of multiple elements of piezo-electric material each with its own electrodes, used in ultrasound imaging.

transferrin   a protein that binds iron for safe transport in the blood.

transfer tubes   tubes used to connect catheters to an afterloading machine.

transformer   is a piece of equipment that either raises or lowers electric current in a circuit, a *step-up transformer* raises current, a *step-down transformer* reduces current.

transformer efficiency   is the ratio of output power to input power of the transformer.

transfusion   the introduction of fluid into the tissue or into a blood vessel. *See also* **blood transfusion, intrauterine transfusion**.

transhiatal   across the opening.

transistor   a solid-state replacement of a diode which consists of an emitter, a base and a collector; it allows current to flow in one direction only.

transjugular intrahepatic portasystemic stent shunting (TIPSS)   a stent placed between the hepatic portal vein and the hepatic vein in the liver to reduce hepatic portal pressure by providing a shunt between the hepatic portal and systemic circulations. Performed to prevent further bleeding from oesophageal varices.

translation   the second stage of protein synthesis in which tRNA and rRNA translate the base sequence required to make a new protein. The movement of a body or system in such a way that all points are moved in a parallel direction through equal distances. *See also* **transcription**.

translation table   a method of modifying digital pixel values to adjust the contrast of a CT image; the table is loaded into the video interface of the display system.

translational   movement along a path.

translumbar through the lumbar region. Route used for injecting aorta prior to aortography.

translumbar aortography the radiographic investigation of the aorta and its major branches by the direct injection of a contrast agent into the abdominal aorta.

transluminal angioplasty a method of dilating arterial narrowing by passing a guide wire through the lesion and then a catheter over the guidewire to dilate the artery.

transmethylation a process in which methyl groups are donated by amino acids and transferred to other compounds.

transmitted when photons pass through an object without interacting with it. *See also **transmitted light, transmitted beam**.*

transmitted beam the radiation leaving an object.

transmitted light the light seen by the viewer after it has passed through an X-ray film, used to calculate the opacity of the film. *See also **opacity**.*

transmitter bandwidth the range of frequencies within a radiofrequency pulse delivered by the transmitter in magnetic resonance imaging.

transnasal through the nose.

transoesophageal echo a tiny ultrasound probe on the end of an endoscope, used in cardiac work to examine the heart valves.

transonic a material that allows the passage of a beam of ultrasound without any reflection back to the transducer.

transport system the part of an automatic film processor that moves the film through the system and comprises a number of various diameter. *See also **hard roller, soft rollers**.*

transrectal through the rectum.

transrectal ultrasonography (TRUS) method used to perform an ultrasound examination of the prostate.

transthoracic across or through the chest, as in transthoracic needle biopsy of a lung mass.

transthoracic echo the examination of the heart through the thorax with the probe in the parasternal and apical positions.

transvaginal probe an ultrasound probe that is inserted into the vagina to allow imaging of the cervix, fallopian tubes, uterus, ovaries and related structures.

transverse fracture a horizontal break in a bone.

transverse plane a horizontal plane that divides the body into superior and inferior parts, it lies at right angles to the median sagittal plane. Also called the horizontal plane.

transverse relaxation time (T$_2$ or spin-spin relaxation time) the time required for the transverse magnetization to decay to about 37% of its maximum value and is the characteristic time constant for loss of phase coherence among spins orientated at an angle to the static main magnetic field.

trapezium   one of the eight carpal bones of the wrist; it lies under the base of the thumb.

trapezius   large muscle of the neck and thorax.

trapezoid   one of the eight carpal bones of the wrist.

traumatic occlusion   any malocclusion resulting in damage to the teeth or periodontal tissues.

treated volume   the volume of tissue inside an isodose surface that is appropriate to receive a radiation dose during radiotherapy treatment.

Trendelenburg's position   lying on an operating or examination table, where the patient is tilted so that the feet are higher than the head.

triceps   the three-headed muscle on the back of the upper arm.

tricuspid   having three cusps. *tricuspid valve* the right atrioventricular valve of the heart.

trigeminal   triple; separating into three sections, for example, the trigeminal nerve, the fifth cranial nerve, which has three branches, ophthalmic, maxillary and mandibular.

triglyceride (triacylglycerol)   a lipid with three fatty acids and a glycerol molecule. The major source of stored energy in the body.

trigone   a triangular area, especially applied to the bladder base, bounded by the ureteral openings at the back and the urethral opening at the front.

triiodothyronine (T_3)   a thyroid hormone that plays a part in maintaining the body's metabolic processes. It contains three iodine atoms and is formed from thyroxine.

trimester   a period of 3 months. Applied especially to pregnancy.

triode   a device allowing current to flow in one direction only, containing an anode, a cathode and a grid in a vacuum, a negative potential on the grid can stop the electron flow and therefore can act as an on−off switch.

triploidy   a fetus with three sets of chromosomes instead of two, usually abort spontaneously in the first trimester.

triquetral   one of the eight carpal bones of the wrist.

tritiated water   when one hydrogen atom is replaced with tritium, an isotope of hydrogen-3. It is used to study electrolyte and water absorption problems.

Triton tumour   a rare, benign tumour of the trigeminal nerve.

trocar   a pointed rod which fits inside a cannula used for the introduction of a guide wire/catheter into a vessel. *See also* **guidewire**.

trochanters   two processes, the larger one (greater trochanter) on the outer, the other (lesser trochanter) on the inner side of the femur between the neck and shaft; they provide attachment for muscles.

trochlea any part which is like a pulley in structure or function.

trochlear nerves the fourth pair of cranial nerves. They innervate the muscle that moves the eyeball in an outwards and downward direction.

trophic associated with nutrition.

tropomyosin one of the proteins located in the thin filaments of a muscle myofibril.

troponin one of the proteins present in a muscle myofibril.

true pelvis that part of the pelvis below the brim.

trypsin active proteolytic enzyme. *See also* **trypsinogen**.

trypsinogen inactive form of trypsin secreted by the pancreas. Activated by enterokinase (enteropeptidase).

t-test a statistical test used to compare two sets of results using a t-test table. If the results are equal to or greater than the value on the tables the results are significant.

tubal associated with a tube.

tubal abortion *see* **tubal miscarriage**.

tubal ligation tying of both uterine (fallopian) tubes as a means of sterilization. **tubal pregnancy**. *See also* **ectopic pregnancy**.

tubal miscarriage an ectopic pregnancy that dies and is expelled from the fimbriated end of the uterine (fallopian) tube.

tube insert an evacuated tube which contains a negative cathode, which when heated produces a stream of electrons, and a positive anode or target that when bombarded by electrons produces a beam of radiation.

tubercle a small rounded prominence, usually on bone. The specific lesion produced by *Mycobacterium tuberculosis*.

tuberculide, tuberculid a small lump. Metastatic manifestation of tuberculosis, producing a skin lesion, for example, papulonecrotic tuberculide, rosacea-like tuberculide.

tuberculoma a caseous tubercle, usually large, its size suggesting a tumour.

tuberculosis (TB) chronic granulomatous infection caused by *Mycobacterium tuberculosis* (human type). Incidence, especially of multidrug resistant tuberculosis (MDR-TB), is increasing, in Asia and Africa, in association with poverty and homelessness, and in those who are immunocompromised. *See also* **bovine tuberculosis**.

tuberosity a bony prominence.

tubo-ovarian associated with or involving both tube and ovary, for example, tubo-ovarian abscess.

tubule a small tube.

tumor swelling: one of the five classic local signs and symptoms of inflammation, the others are calor, dolor, loss of function and rubor.

tumour a swelling. A mass of abnormal tissue which resembles the normal tissues in structure, but which fulfils no useful function and which grows at the expense of the body. Benign, simple or innocent tumours are encapsulated, do not infiltrate adjacent tissue or cause metastases and are unlikely to recur if removed. ***malignant tumour*** not encapsulated, infiltrates adjacent tissue and causes metastases. *See also* **cancer**.

tumour lysis syndrome (TLS) may occur following intensive chemotherapy treatment for some haematological malignancies. As cancer cells are destroyed there is release of cellular breakdown products. This results in metabolic problems (for example, hyperkalaemia, hypocalcaemia, hyperuricaemia, hyperphosphataemia) that may cause renal failure and possibly circulatory and respiratory failure.

tumour marker chemical detected in the serum that may be associated with a specific cancer or sometimes non-malignant diseases. They include: alphafetoprotein, CA-125, carcinoembryonic antigen and prostate specific antigen. They may be used for monitoring disease progress and efficacy of treatment, but are of limited use for population screening.

tumour necrosis factor (TNF) a cytokine that is toxic to cancer cells and activates other leucocytes. It causes profound metabolic effects that include inflammatory responses, pyrexia and weight loss.

tumourocidal dose a dose of radiation capable of destroying a tumour.

tumour suppressor gene a gene that, when it is absent or non-functioning in a cell, permits the abnormal development of the cell.

tunica a lining membrane; a coat.

tunica adventitia the outer coat of an artery or vein.

tunica intima the lining of an artery or vein.

tunica media the middle muscular coat of an artery or vein.

turbinate shaped like an inverted cone.

turbinate bones three on either side forming the lateral nasal walls. Also called ***nasal conchae***.

Turner's syndrome the absence of one X chromosome in women, resulting in ovarian failure, webbing of the neck, short metacarpals.

turnkey a term used to denote a company which will provide all the necessary software and hardware and back-up support to enable the user to '*turn a key*' and use the equipment.

turtle a wheeled mechanical device, used for graphics, attached to a computer via cables.

two-tailed hypothesis a theory which predicts an outcome but does not state the direction it will take.

tylosis palmaris a scaling condition of the palms of the hands.

tylosis plantaris a scaling condition of the soles of the feet.

tympanic associated with the tympanum.

tympanic membrane (eardrum)   separates the outer from the middle ear.

tympanic thermometer   accurate body temperature recorded by means of an electronic probe introduced into the external auditory canal.

tympanum   the cavity of the middle ear.

type I error (α error)   in research, rejecting a null hypothesis that is true.

type II error (β error)   in research, not rejecting a null hypothesis that is false.

tyrosine   an amino acid.

ulcer an erosion or loss of continuity of the skin or mucous membrane.

ulcerative associated with or of the nature of an ulcer.

ulcerative colitis superficial inflammatory condition affecting the colon. It always involves the rectum and spreads continuously for a variable distance. Long-standing disease predisposes to colorectal cancer.

ulna the inner bone of the forearm.

ulnar associated with the ulna as in artery, vein and nerve.

ultrasonic relating to mechanical vibrations of very high frequency.

ultrasonography formation of a visible image from the use of ultrasound. A controlled beam of sound is directed into the relevant part of the body. The reflected ultrasound is used to build up an electronic image of the various structures of the body. Routinely offered during pregnancy to monitor progress and detect fetal and placental abnormalities. *See also* **ultrasound, diagnostic ultrasonography, real-time ultrasonography**.

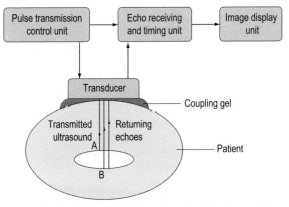

Block diagram showing the basic functions of a pulse-echo ultrasound imager. For clarity the return echoes have been displaced to the right. From Principles of radiological physics, 3rd edn, D T Graham, 1996, Churchill Livingstone, Edinburgh, with permission.

ultrasound   sound waves with a frequency of over 20 000 Hertz, not audible to the human ear.

ultraviolet rays (UV)   short wavelength electromagnetic rays outside the visible spectrum.

umbilical cord   the cord connecting the fetus to the placenta. It contains a vein and two arteries.

umbilical hernia (omphalocele)   protrusion of a portion of intestine through the area of the umbilical scar.

umbilicus (navel)   the abdominal scar left by the separation of the umbilical cord after birth.

unconscious   incapable of responding to sensory stimuli. That part of mental activity concealed from the consciousness by the psychological sensor.

undescended testis   the testis remains within the bony pelvis or inguinal canal. *See also* **cryptorchism**.

uniaxial joint   a joint with movement round one axis only, for example, flexion and extension.

unicellular   consisting of only one cell.

uniformity   the variations in count rate detected by a gamma camera when it is exposed to a regular source of gamma rays emitted from a radionuclide.

unilateral   relating to or on one side only.

unit cost   an average cost for a specific activity, for example, a surgical procedure, or a home visit. It is calculated by dividing the total cost of the service by the number of outputs.

univariate statistics   descriptive statistics that analyse one variable, such as frequency distributions.

unrelated   the whole groups of data are roughly matched but the individual samples are not.

unsharpness   blurring on a radiograph (photographic unsharpness) which can be caused by movement unsharpness, screen unsharpness and/or geometric unsharpness.

upgrade   an improvement to a computer system which allows the most recent information to be added to a programme.

upper motor neuron   the cell is in the motor cortex and the axon terminates in the anterior horn of the spinal cord.

upper respiratory tract infection (URTI)   the upper respiratory tract is the commonest site of infection in all age groups. The infections include rhinitis – usually viral – sinusitis, tonsillitis, adenoiditis, pharyngitis, otitis media and croup (laryngitis), often involving the tonsils and cervical lymph nodes. Such infections seldom require hospital treatment, but epiglottitis can be rapidly fatal.

uptake count   for a particular organ, is expressed as a percentage of the total radiation administered to the patient for radionuclide imaging purposes.

urachus   the stem-like structure connecting the bladder with the umbilicus in the fetus; after birth it becomes a fibrous cord situated between the apex of the bladder and the umbilicus, known as the median umbilical ligament.

uraemia   an excess of urea, creatinine and nitrogenous end products of protein and amino acid metabolism in the blood. The entire complex of signs and symptoms of chronic renal failure.

urate   any salt of uric acid.

urea   the main nitrogenous end product of protein metabolism; produced in the liver it is excreted in the urine.

urease   bacterial enzyme that splits urea.

ureter   the tube passing from each kidney to the bladder for the conveyance of urine; its average length is 25–30 cm.

ureterolith   a calculus in the ureter.

ureterovaginal   associated with the ureter and vagina.

ureterovesical   associated with the ureter and urinary bladder.

urethra   the passage from the bladder through which urine is excreted.

urethrography   radiological examination of the urethra. Can be an inclusion with cystography either retrograde (ascending) or during micturition.

uric acid   substance formed during purine metabolism which is present in nucleic acids and some foods and beverages. Uric acid is excreted in the urine and may give rise to kidney stones. High levels of uric acid in the blood may be due to faulty excretion of uric acid, excessive cell breakdown, or associated with high purine intake. *See also* **gout**.

urinal   a vessel used for urination if a patient is unable to walk, a static unit for urination.

urinary   associated with urine.

urinary bladder   a muscular distensible bag situated in the pelvis. It receives urine from the kidneys via two ureters and stores it until micturition occurs.

urinary catheter   a catheter inserted into the urinary bladder to drain urine.

urinary system   comprises two kidneys, two ureters, one urinary bladder and one urethra. The kidneys produce urine of variable content; the ureters convey the urine to the bladder, which stores it until there is sufficient volume to elicit reflex emptying or the desire to pass urine and it is then conveyed to the exterior by the urethra.

urinary tract infection (UTI)   the second most prevalent infection in hospital, but the most common hospital-acquired infection. It occurs most frequently in the presence of an indwelling catheter. It is most commonly caused by the bacterium *Escherichia coli*, suggesting that self-infection via the peri-urethral route is a common pathway.

urine the clear straw-coloured fluid excreted by the kidneys. Urine contains water, nitrogenous waste and electrolytes. Normally adults produce about 1500 mL every 24 h, but this depends on fluid intake, activity and age. Usually slightly acidic (pH 6.0), but varies between 4.5 and 8.0. The specific gravity is usually within the range 1005–1030.

URL (Uniform Resource Locator) the address of internet files.

urobilin a brownish pigment excreted in the faeces. Formed by the oxidation of urobilinogen.

urobilinogen (stercobilinogen) a pigment formed from bilirubin in the intestine by bacterial action. It may be reabsorbed into the circulation and converted back to bilirubin in the liver and re-excreted in the bile or urine.

urodynamics the method used to study bladder function. *See also* **cystometry**.

urogenital (urinogenital) associated with the urinary and the genital organs.

urography radiographic visualization of the renal pelvis and ureter by injection of a contrast agent. The medium may be injected into the bloodstream whence it is excreted by the kidney (***intravenous urography***) or it may be injected directly into the renal pelvis or ureter by way of a fine catheter introduced through a cystoscope (***retrograde*** or ***ascending urography***). *See also* **intravenous urography**.

urokinase an enzyme which dissolves fibrin clot. It is used therapeutically in vitreous haemorrhage (eye), thrombosed arteriovenous shunts and other thromboembolic conditions.

urticaria (nettlerash, hives) skin eruption characterized by multiple, circumscribed, smooth, raised, pinkish, itchy weals, developing very suddenly, usually lasting a few days and leaving no visible trace. The cause is unknown in most cases. *See also* **angio-oedema**.

USB (Universal Serial Bus) a serial port on a computer used to attach hardware such as the mouse, keyboard or a scanner.

useful density range the range of densities, between 1.36 and 2.16 that make up a radiographic image; above and below this range it is not possible to determine differences visually between adjacent densities. *See also* **useful exposure range**.

useful exposure range the range of exposures that make up a radiographic image; above and below this range it is not possible to determine differences visually between adjacent densities. To calculate the range the characteristic curve of the film is used at a particular kV, a vertical line is drawn from density 1.36 and 2.16, the antilogs of the range of values on the horizontal, log It, axis gives the useful exposure range in mAs. *See also* **characteristic curve**.

uterine   associated with the uterus. ***uterine supports*** muscles of the pelvic floor, the peritoneum and various ligaments; pubocervical, round, transverse cervical (Mackenrodt's or cardinal) and the uterosacral ligaments that hold the uterus in the correct anteverted and anteflexed position.

uterine cavity   that of the uterus, the base extending between the orifices of the uterine tubes.

uterine tubes (fallopian tubes, oviducts)   two tubes opening out of the upper part of the uterus. Each measures 10 cm and the distal end is fimbriated and lies near the ovary. They are the site of fertilization and they convey the ovum to the uterus.

uteroplacental   associated with the uterus and placenta.

uterorectal   associated with the uterus and the rectum.

uterosacral   associated with the uterus and sacrum.

uterosalpingography (hysterosalpingography)   radiological examination of the uterus and uterine tubes involving retrograde introduction of an opaque contrast agent during fluoroscopy. Used to investigate patency of uterine (fallopian) tubes. Is being superseded by ultrasound examination.

uterovaginal   associated with the uterus and the vagina.

uterovesical   associated with the uterus and the urinary bladder.

uterus   the womb, a hollow muscular organ into which the ovum is received through the uterine (fallopian) tubes and where it is retained during development, and from which the fetus is expelled through the vagina. *See also* **bicornuate**.

utricle   a little sac or pocket. A fluid-filled sac in the internal ear. Part of the vestibular apparatus. *See also* **saccule**.

uvea   the pigmented middle coat of the eye, includes the iris, ciliary body and choroid.

uvula   the central tag hanging down from the free edge of the soft palate.

V

vacuum space entirely without matter.

vacuum bag a sealed plastic bag containing small expanded polystyrene spheres, the patient is positioned on the bag which has the air pressure reduced until it is hardened. This mould can be used during radiotherapy to accurately immobilize the patient and enable daily reproducibility of positioning. *See also* **patient immobilization**.

vagal associated with the vagus nerve.

vagina literally, a sheath; the musculomembranous passage extending from the cervix uteri to the vulva.

vaginal speculum used to examine the vagina and cervix, for taking high vaginal swabs and cervical smears and for some treatments. Types include Cuscoe's bivalve and Sim's speculum.

vagus nerve the tenth cranial nerve, composed of both motor and sensory fibres, with a wide distribution in the neck, thorax and abdomen, sending important parasympathetic branches to the heart, lungs, stomach, etc.

valence band a band which contains the outer electrons of an atom and may be partially or completely full.

valency the ability of one atom to join another.

valency bond the electron linkage between two atoms.

valgus (valga, valgum) exhibiting angulation away from the midline of the body, e.g. hallux valgus.

validity (external) a term that indicates the degree to which research findings can be generalized to other populations and in other settings.

validity (internal) in research, a term that indicates the extent to which a method or test measures what it intends to measure.

Valsalva manoeuvre the maximum intrathoracic pressure achieved by forced expiration against a closed glottis; occurs in activities such as lifting heavy objects, changing position and during defecation: the glottis narrows simultaneously with contraction of the abdominal muscles.

value for money (VFM) a means of obtaining the best quality of service within the resource allocation. It involves economy, efficiency and effectiveness.

valve a fold of membrane in a passage or tube permitting the flow of contents in one direction only.

variable   a research term that describes any factor or circumstance that is part of the study. ***confounding variable*** one that affects the conditions of the independent variables unequally. ***dependent variable*** one that depends on the experimental conditions. ***independent variable*** the variable conditions of an experimental situation, e.g. control or experimental. ***random variable*** background factors such as environmental conditions that may affect any conditions of the independent variables equally.

variance   a mathematical term used in statistics. The distribution range of a set of results around the mean. *See also* **standard deviation**.

varicocele   a swelling of the pampiniform venous complex of the spermatic cord.

varices   dilated, tortuous vein.

varus (vara, varum)   displaying displacement or angulation towards the midline of the body, for example coxa vara.

vas   a vessel.

vas deferens (deferent duct)   the excretory duct of the testis.

vasa vasorum   the minute nutrient vessels of the artery and vein walls.

vascular   supplied with vessels, especially referring to blood vessels.

vascularization   the acquisition of a blood supply; the process of becoming vascular.

vasoconstriction   narrowing of the lumen of a blood vessel.

vasodilation   widening of the lumen of a blood vessel.

vasography   the investigation of male infertility by injecting radiographic contrast agent into the vas deferens.

vasomotor   relating to nerves and muscles that control vessel lumen size.

vasomotor centre (VMC)   a centre, located in the medulla oblongata, concerned with controlling lumen size of peripheral arterioles, it operates through sympathetic activity in response to baroreceptor signals.

vasopressin   formed in the hypothalamus and stored in the posterior lobe of the pituitary gland. It is the antidiuretic hormone (ADH).

vasospasm   constricting spasm of vessel walls.

vasovagal shock   shock caused by the loss of vascular tone and therefore dilatation of the blood vessels as a result of severe pain or fright. Used to be called ***neurogenic shock***.

vein   a vessel conveying blood from the capillaries back to the heart. It has the same three coats as an artery, the inner one modified to form valves.

velocity   distance travelled in unit time in a given direction, unit metre per second.

vena cava   one of two large veins emptying into the right atrium of the heart.

venepuncture   insertion of a needle into a vein.

venesection   surgical blood letting by opening a vein or introducing a wide-bore needle, performed on blood donors and to reduce the risk of thrombosis.

venography (phlebography)   radiological examination of the venous system involving injection of an opaque medium. Mostly replaced by ultrasound.

venous   associated with the veins.

venous haemorrhage   the loss of blood from a vein.

ventilation   the mechanical process of breathing, the supply of fresh air. *See also* **pulmonary ventilation**.

ventilation perfusion ratio (V/Q)   the ratio between gases in the alveoli (alveolar ventilation) and blood flow in the pulmonary capillaries (pulmonary perfusion).

ventilator (life support machine)   specialized equipment for mechanically inflating a patient's lungs. Used to support or replace a patient's own breathing.

ventral   associated with the abdomen or the anterior surface of the body.

ventral decubitus radiograph   the patient lies prone and the central ray passes through the body from side to side.

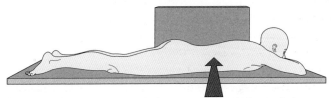

Ventral decubitus. From Pocketbook of radiographic positioning, 2nd edn, Ruth Sutherland, 2003, Churchill Livingstone, Edinburgh, with permission.

ventricle   a small belly-like cavity.

ventricles of the brain   four cavities filled with cerebrospinal fluid within the brain.

ventricles of the heart   the two lower muscular chambers of the heart.

ventricular fibrillation   fine, rapid twitching of the ventricles of the heart, if uncontrolled leads to circulatory arrest.

ventriculoatrial shunt   creating a pathway between the atria of the heart and the cerebral ventricles to drain cerebrospinal fluid.

ventriculoperitoneal shunt   creating a pathway between the peritoneum and the cerebral ventricles to drain cerebrospinal fluid.

ventriculostomy   an artificial opening into a ventricle. Usually refers to a drainage operation for hydrocephalus.

venule   a small vein.

verification   the process of confirming the accuracy of radiotherapy planning prior to treatment taking place.

vermiform   wormlike.

vermiform appendix   the vestigial, hollow, wormlike structure attached to the caecum.

vernix caseosa   the fatty substance which covers and protects the skin of the fetus.

vertebra   one of the irregular bones making up the spinal column.

vertebra prominens   the seventh cervical vertebra.

vertebral column (spinal column)   made up of 33/34 vertebrae, articulating with the skull above and the pelvic girdle below. The vertebrae are so shaped that they enclose a cavity (spinal canal, neural canal) which houses the spinal cord.

vertex   the top of the head.

vertigo   feeling of loss of balance. *See also* **Menière's syndrome**.

vesical   associated with the urinary bladder.

vesicle   a small bladder, cell or hollow structure. A skin blister.

vesico-ureteric reflux   the passing of urine backwards up the ureter during micturition.

vessel   a tube, duct or canal, holding or conveying fluid, especially blood and lymph.

vestibule   the middle part of the internal ear, lying between the semicircular canals and the cochlea. The triangular area between the labia minora. The area of the mouth between the lips and the gums/teeth.

vestibulocochlear   relating to the vestibule and the cochlear.

vestibulocochlear nerve auditory nerve   the eighth pair of cranial nerves. There are two branches: the vestibular, which transmits impulses from the vestibular apparatus of the ear to the cerebellum, and the cochlear, which transmits impulses from the cochlea in the ear to the auditory cortex situated in the temporal lobe of the cerebrum.

vestibulo-ocular reflex   compensatory eye movement stimulated by head movement to stabilize gaze in space.

vibration syndrome   cysts in the wrist or sometimes the hand, caused by using vibrating machinery.

videotext   the interactive public information service broadcast on television, known as Prestel.

vignetting   shading round an image.

villonodular synovitis a joint problem, usually affecting the hips or knees where the lining of the joint becomes swollen and extra synovial fluid is secreted causing swelling and pain.

villus a microscopic fingerlike projection; found in the mucosa of the small intestine or on the outside of the chorion of the embryonic sac.

virement financial term meaning to move money from one expenditure category to another.

virus a unique class of infectious agents, consisting of genetic material surrounded by protein and in some cases, with an outer membranous envelope. They cause many diseases including measles, AIDS, hepatitis and evidence suggests that some may be capable of causing cancer. A computer program designed to cause malfunction in a computer which often arrives as an attachment to an email and opening the attachment will release the virus to corrupt the main program.

viscera the internal organs.

visible spectrum the small part of the electromagnetic spectrum containing the range of wavelengths that can be seen by the human eye (see figure on p. 396).

visual acuity the ability of a person to see small objects.

visually handicapped a loss or reduction of sight.

vital capacity (VC) the amount of air expelled from the lungs after a deep inspiration.

vitallium an alloy used in the manufacture of nails, plates, etc., used in orthopaedic and other surgical procedures.

vitamins organic substance or group of substances that have specific biochemical functions in the body. They are either fat-soluble, vitamins A, D, E and K, or water-soluble, vitamin B complex and vitamin C. They are essential for normal metabolism and are provided by the diet. Some vitamins can also be synthesized in the body, e.g. vitamin D. Their absence causes deficiency diseases.

vitreous resembling glass.

vitreous chamber the cavity inside the eyeball and behind the lens.

vitreous humour (body) the jelly-like substance contained in the vitreous chamber.

vocal cords membranous folds stretched anteroposteriorly across the larynx. They vibrate as air from the lungs passes between them to produce the voice.

Volkmann's canals canals joining the haversian systems in compact bone.

volt (V) the derived SI unit (International System of Units) for electromotive force (also known as *potential difference* or *electrical potential*). It is the potential that exists at a point when 1 joule of work is done in moving coulomb of positive charge from infinity to that point; volt of potential difference exists between two points if 1 joule of work is done moving coulomb of positive charge from one point to the other.

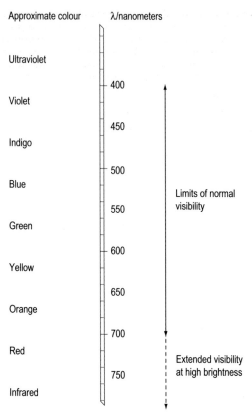

The visible spectrum. From Radiographic imaging, 3rd edn, Chris Gunn, 2002, Churchill Livingstone, with permission.

voltage   the number of volts in a circuit; in Britain the mains voltage is 240 volts for the domestic supply and 398 volts for a three-phase supply.

volumetric reconstruction   the production of a three-dimensional image in CT scanning.

volvulus   a loop of bowel causing an obstruction.

vomer   a flat bone forming the postero-inferior aspect of the bony nasal septum.

vomiting centre   a centre in the medulla oblongata that has overall control of vomiting. It responds to various stimuli such as those from the gastrointestinal organs.

Von Recklinghausen's disease (Recklinghausen's disease)   describes two conditions: (a) ***osteitis fibrosa cystica*** – the result of hyperparathyroidism leading to decalcification of bones and formation of cysts; (b) ***multiple neurofibromatosis*** – the tumours can be felt beneath the skin along the course of nerves. There may be pigmented spots (café au lait) on the skin and neurofibroma in the endocrine glands and the gastrointestinal tract.

voxel   a three-dimensional pixel.

vulva   the external genitalia of the female.

vulvovaginal   associated with the vulva and the vagina.

Waldeyer's ring   a lymphoid tissue circle surrounding the pharynx. *See also* **tonsils**.

WAN (Wide Area Network)   the connection of a group of computer networks.

WAP (Wireless Application Protocol)   a standard to allow text messages from the web to be available to mobile phones.

washing   in film processing is to remove fixer solution and the remaining soluble silver complex salts from the film surface.

water phantom   a water tank containing a small ionization chamber; the radiation beam can enter the tank either horizontally or vertically. The signal is displayed on a television monitor and the image is analysed for radiotherapy treatment planning.

watt (W)   derived SI unit (International System of Units) for electrical power, watts equal volts times amps (W=VI).

waveguide   a series of chambers with small iris diaphragms between them and varying distance apart. The function is to control the velocity of the electron beam that passes through it. *See also* **magnetron, klystron**.

wavelength (λ)   the distance travelled in one complete cycle, usually expressed in millimetres; it is dependent on the frequency and propagation of speed. The term can refer to electricity or ultrasound. *See also* **propagation speed**.

wave theory   the theory of electromagnetic radiation which considers that the radiation is produced as a sinusoidal wave consisting of an electrical field with a magnetic field at right angles to it.

web server   a computer which fetches or stores images or web pages and makes them available over the internet or intranet on request.

wedge   a wedge-shape piece of metal used to attenuate the beam over part of the field during radiotherapy treatment.

wedge angle   for a particular wedge is the angle that the 50% isodose line makes with the central axis of the X-ray beam. The angle defined at a specific depth of tissue in a patient, usually 10 cm.

wedged pair dose distribution   when two beams of the same wedge angle are used to produce an ideal dose distribution when used with a hinge angle of (180–200) degrees.

wedge factor the increase in set monitor units required to the same dose at D_{max} with a wedge as without the wedge present for the same field size.

weight force acting on a body due to gravity, unit newton.

weighted capitation the allocation of resource based on the number of people in an area but adjusted for the age profile or the relative economic and social conditions, e.g. areas with a high level of social deprivation would be allocated extra resource.

well counter a scintillation counter containing a sodium iodide crystal with a depression cut out of it, a bottle containing the sample is placed in the depression and the gamma emission from the sample is measured.

wetting agent an addition to the film emulsion to reduce the surface tension and allow the easy penetration of chemicals, an addition to developer to reduce the surface tension of the film.

Wharton's jelly embryonic connective tissue contained in the umbilical cord.

wheezing a whistling or rasping breathing sound, occurs when air is forced through fluid. Associated with the bronchospasm of asthma and other conditions.

white matter white nerve tissue of the CNS, the myelinated fibres. *See also* **grey matter**.

white muscle a term used to describe muscle consisting mainly of fast-twitch fibres. It is white because there is very little myoglobin and a less abundant blood supply than in red muscle.

Wilcoxon test a statistical test used to compare two sets of results using a Wilcoxon test table and a normal distribution table. The results must be equal to or less than the reading on the tables to be significant. A non-parametric alternative to Student's paired test.

Wilms' tumour the commonest abdominal tumour of childhood, and one which usually affects the kidneys. Usually diagnosed during the pre-school period. Prognosis is uncertain and depends on the stage of the tumour and child's age at onset of diagnosis and treatment. *See also* **nephroblastoma**.

winchester disk a large-capacity *hard* disk, is housed in a hermetically sealed container, as any ingress of dust or dirt, no matter how microscopic, could possibly destroy very large amounts of data.

window the range of grey scale (or colour scale) values displayed in a digital image.

window centre the central point in a range of grey scale (or colour scale) values.

window level the centre of the window width, another term for window centre.

window mean the average range of pixel values in an image.

window width the range of displayed pixel values in a digital image.

windowing   *see* **window**.

windpipe   *see* **trachea**.

WinZip   a computer program that is used to compress computer files prior to storage or sending to another computer thus saving on storage space or transmission time.

wire diaphragms   an additional set of wires attached to a simulator to accurately display the edges of the treatment area.

wisdom tooth   lay term for the molar tooth placed eighth from the midline in the secondary dentition. The last teeth to erupt.

Wiskott–Aldrich syndrome   an immunodeficiency disorder resulting in increased susceptibility to viral, bacterial and fungal infections.

womb   the uterus.

work   the product of the force acting on a body times the distance the body moves, unit joule.

WORM (Write Once Read Many)   optical disks which are used once to receive data for archiving and can subsequently be read as often as is required.

wound healing   there are four stages/phases in normal wound healing: haemostasis, inflammation, proliferation and maturation, which may take many months. Wound healing may be delayed by local factors, e.g. mechanical stress, inadequate blood supply, or by general factors that include: malnutrition, ageing, drugs such as corticosteroids, etc. Wound healing may be by first/primary intention in a clean wound with the edges in apposition. There is minimal scarring and deformity; second intention when the wound edges are not in apposition, the gap must be filled by granulation tissue before epithelialization can take place; or by third intention when a wound is left open until local factors such as infection have been treated before the wound edges are brought together.

wrap around (aliasing, fold-over)   an artefact that occurs in magnetic resonance imaging due to the image-encoding process. It occurs when the field of view is smaller than the area being imaged.

wrist   the carpal bones.

wrist drop   paralysis of the muscles which raise the wrist, caused by damage to the radial nerve.

write protect   a method of protecting a computer file or disk to prevent the contents being altered or deleted.

WWW (World Wide Web)   an information and resource centre for the internet.

xanthine an intermediate product formed during the breakdown of nucleic acids to uric acid. It is excreted in the urine.

xanthogranuloma a tumour of granulation tissue.

xanthoma a benign, fatty, fibrous tumour that develops in the subcutaneous layers of skin, usually round a tendon.

xerophthalmia dry eye.

xeroradiography a method of image recording using a re-usable, electrically charged selenium plate which is sprayed with blue powder and the image is transferred to paper; was used for soft tissue imaging, including mammography. Now obsolete.

xerostomia dryness of the mouth caused by the inhibition of normal salivary secretions.

X-rays short wavelength, penetrating rays of electromagnetic spectrum, produced by electrical equipment. The word is popularly used to mean radiographs.

X-ray tube equipment formed by either a stationary or rotating anode and a cathode assembly in an evacuated glass envelope which is contained in an oil-filled, lead-lined housing.

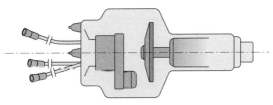

A rotating anode tube insert and shielding (housing). From Principles of radiological physics, 3rd edn, D T Graham, 1996, Churchill Livingstone, Edinburgh, with permission.

Y

yolk sac a circular structure seen on ultrasound scans at 6 weeks which supplies the fetal pole with nutrients; it is used to confirm an intrauterine pregnancy.

yttrium-90 (^{90}Y) a substance emitting beta particles with a half-life of 64 hours. Implantations of this in bone wax are left in the pituitary fossa after hypophysectomy for breast cancer. Also used in a number of interstitial cancer treatments.

Z

zap a small alteration to a computer program.

zona a zone; a girdle; herpes zoster.

zona pellucida membrane around the oocyte.

zonule small zone, belt or girdle. Suspensory ligament attaching the periphery of the lens of the eye to ciliary body.

zoster an inflammatory skin reaction to the herpes virus characterized by a vesicular rash in the area of the distribution of a sensory nerve. Also called shingles.

zygoma a long slender process of the temporal bone. The zygomatic bone that forms the cheek.

zygomatic arch the cheekbone.

zygomatic bone a bone forming the bony cheek and the lateral walls and the floor of the orbit.

zygote the fertilized ovum. The diploid cell derived from the fusion after fertilization of the female and male nuclei, each of which has one set of chromosomes (the haploid).

References

Ball John, Price Tony 1995 Chesneys' radiographic maging, 6th edn. Blackwell Science, Oxford

Ballinger Philip W, Frank Eugene D 2003 Pocket guide to radiography, 5th edn. Mosby, St Louis

Bomford C K, Kunkler I H 2003 Walter and Miller's textbook of radiotherapy radiation physics, therapy and oncology, 6th edn. Churchill Livingstone, Edinburgh

Brooker Chris Ed 2003 Pocket medical dictionary. Churchill Livingstone, Edinburgh

Bryan Glenda J 1996 Skeletal Anatomy 3rd edn. Churchill Livingstone, Edinburgh

Bushlong Stewart C 2004 Radiologic science for technologists, 8th edn. Mosby, St Louis

Fauber Terri L 2000 Radiographic imaging and exposure. Mosby, St Louis

Graham Donald T 1996 Principles of radiological physics, 3rd edn. Churchill Livingstone, Edinburgh

Gunn Chris 2001 Using maths in health sciences. Churchill Livingstone, Edinburgh

Gunn Chris 2002 Bones and joints, a guide for students. Churchill Livingstone, Edinburgh

Gunn Chris 2002 Radiographic imaging, a practical approach, 3rd edn. Churchill Livingstone, Edinburgh

Gunn C, Jackson C S 1991 Guidelines on patient care in radiography, 2nd edn. Churchill Livingstone, Edinburgh

Hutton Andrew 2004 Pocket medical terminology. Churchill Livingstone, Edinburgh

Kenyon Jonathan, Kenyon Karen 2004 The physiotherapist's pocket book. Churchill Livingstone, Edinburgh

Morris Caroline 2000 Getting on board the net. The NHS Confederation, London

Morris Samantha 2001 Radiotherapy physics and equipment. Churchill Livingstone, Edinburgh

Mosby 2002 Mosby's pocket dictionary of medicine, nursing, and allied health, 4th edn. Mosby, St Louis

Oakley Jason 2003 Digital imaging a primer for radiographers, radiologists and health care professionals. Cambridge University Press, Cambridge

O'Halloran David, Guyers Kathryn, Henderson Jill 2004 Notes on anatomy and oncology. Churchill Livingstone, Edinburgh

Resnick D, Kransdorf M J 2005 Bone and joint imaging, 3rd edn. Elsevier Saunders, Philadelphia

Saunders Roger C 1984 Clinical sonography, a practical guide, 2nd edn. Little Brown, Boston

Sutherland Ruth 2003 Pocketbook of radiographic positioning, 2nd edn. Churchill Livingstone, Edinburgh

Sutton David 1987 A textbook of radiology and imaging, vol 1, 4th edn. Churchill Livingstone, Edinburgh

Sutton David 1988 Radiology and imaging for medical students, 5th edn. Churchill Livingstone, Edinburgh

Sutton David 2002 Textbook of radiology and imaging, vol 2, 7th edn. Churchill Livingstone, Edinburgh

Waugh Anne, Grant Allison 2001 Ross and Wilson's anatomy and physiology in health and illness. Churchill Livingstone, Edinburgh

Webb Richard W, Brant William E, Helms Clyde A 1991 Fundamentals of body CT, 2nd edn. Saunders, Philadelphia

Weller Barbara F Ed 2000 Bailliere's nurses' dictionary, 23rd edn. Bailliere Tindall, Edinburgh

Appendix 1: **Radionuclide applications**

Radionuclide	Chemical form	Application
Chromium-51	Sodium chromate solution	Red blood cells Spleen Glomerular filtration rate
Cobalt-57	Cyanocobalamin	Pernicious anaemia Vitamin B_{12}
Cobalt-58	Cyanocobalamin	Gastrointestinal malabsorption
Gallium-67	Gallium citrate	Infections Tumour seeking
Indium-111	Indium oxine labelled white cells	Infections Abscesses
Iodine-123	Sodium iodide capsules and solutions	Renography Thyroid
Iodine-125	o-Iodohippurate Human serum albumin	Plasma volume
Iodine-131	Sodium iodide	Thyroid diagnosis and treatment
Iodine-131 hippuran	o-Iodohippurate	Renography
Iodine-123 MIBG	Meta-iodo-benzylguanidine	Adrenals
Krypton-81 m	Gas	Pulmonary ventilation
Phosphorus-32	Sodium phosphate	Treatment of polycythaemia vera
Selenium-75	Seleno-norcholesterol	Adrenals
Selenium-75 (seHCAT)	23-seleno-25-homo-taurocholate Selenium-tagged bile salt	Diarrhoea Bile salt absorption
Technetium-99 m	Sodium pertechnetate	Brain Thyroid

(Continued)

Radionuclide	Chemical form	Application
Technetium-99 m	Exametazine HMPAO	Cerebral blood flow Leucocyte labelling
Technetium-99 m colloid	Tin colloid	Liver Sites of gasterointestinal bleeds
Technetium-99 m	Succimer (DMSA)	Static renal imaging
Technetium-99 m	Pentetate (DTPA)	Renal imaging, lung ventilation
Technetium-99 m	Etefenin (EHIDA) injection	Biliary function
Technetium-99 m	Albumin aggregated (MAA) Albumin microspheres (HAM)	Perfusion lung scanning
Phosphates labelled with technetium-99 m	HDP hydroxydisophosphate	Bone scanning
Technetium-99 m pertechnetate	Sodium pertechnetate	Testicular torsion Thyroid Salivary glands Meckel's diverticulum (pockets of acid-secreting cells in the stomach lining and the small bowel)
Technetium-99 m Pyrophosphates	Phosphonates and phosphates	Acute myocardial infarct Myocardial imaging
Technetium-99 m	Glucoheptonate	Brain Kidneys
Technetium-99 m	Stannous fluoride	Heart blood pool
Technetium cardiolite	Thallous chloride	Myocardial ischaemia
Xenon-133	Gas	Pulmonary ventilation Cerebral blood flow

Appendix 2: **Abbreviations**

A	ampere
AAA	abdominal aortic aneurysm
Ab	abortion
AC	alternating current, abdominal circumference
ACL	anterior cruciate ligament
ACTH	adrenocorticotrophic hormone
ADE	acute demyelinating encephalitis
ADH	antidiuretic hormone
ADI	acceptable daily intake
ADPKD	adult dominant polycystic kidney disease
ADR	adverse drug reaction
AE title	application entry title
AFB	acid-fast bacillus
AfC	Agenda for Change
AFI	amniotic fluid index
AFP	alphafetoprotein
AFW	alternative folder wrapped (film)
Ag^+	silver ion
AgBr	silver bromide
AgCl	silver chloride
AgI	silver iodide
AGM	annual general meeting
$AgNO_3$	silver nitrate
Ag_2S	silver sulphide
AHF	antihaemophilic factor
AHP	allied health profession
AIDS	acquired immune deficiency syndrome
ALARA	as low as reasonably achievable
$AlCl_3$	aluminium chloride
ALL	acute lymphoblastic leukaemia
ALLO	atypical legionella-like organisms
$Al_2(SO_4)_3$	aluminium sulphate
ALU	arithmetic logic unit
AMI	acute myocardial infarction
AML	acute myeloid leukaemia
ANA	antinuclear antibody
ANLL	acute non-lymphoblastic leukaemia
ANSI	American National Standards Institute
APD	automated peritoneal dialysis
APH	ante partum haemorrhage
APKD	adult polycystic kidney disease
ARDS	acute respiratory distress syndrome

ARF	acute renal failure, acute respiratory failure
ARM	artificial rupture of the membranes
ARSAC	Administration of Radioactive Substances Advisory Committee
ASCII	American standard code for information interchange
ASD	atrial septal defect
ASHD	arteriosclerotic heart disease
ASRT	American Society of Radiologic Technologists
ATM	asynchronous transfer mode
ATN	acute tubular necrosis
ATP	adenosine triphosphate
AVB	atrioventral block
AVH	acute viral hepatitis
AVM	arteriovenous malformation
AVR	aortic valve replacement
BASIC	**B**eginners **A**ll-purpose **S**ymbolic **I**nstruction **C**ode
BaFCl	barium fluorochloride
BaFCl.Eu	barium fluorochloride with europium activator
BAMRR	British Association of Magnetic Resonance Radiographers
BBA	born before arrival (at hospital)
BBB	bundle branch block
BBV	blood-borne virus
BED	biological effective dose
BEL	breech, legs extended
BFL	breech, legs flexed
BI	bone injury
BID	brought in (to hospital) dead
BIPAP	biphasic positive airways pressure
BLS	basic life support
BMD	bone mineral density
BME	benign myalgic encephalomyelitis
BMI	body mass index
BMR	basal metabolic rate
BMT	bone marrow transplant
BMUS	British Medical Ultrasound Society
BNF	British National Formulary
BO	bowels open
BOD	biochemical oxygen demand
BPD	biparietal diameter
BPI	blood pressure index
bpm	beats per minute
Br^-	bromide ion
BS	British Standard

BSE	bovine spongiform encephalopathy, breast self-examination
BSR	blood sedimentation rate
Bq	becquerel
c	velocity
Ca	calcium, carcinoma
CAD	coronary artery disease, computer aided drawing, computer aided detection
CAPD	continuous ambulatory peritoneal dialysis
CAT	computer assisted tomography
$CaWO_4$	calcium tungstate
CBA	cost–benefit analysis
CBF	cerebral blood flow
CBP	chronic back pain
CCF	congestive cardiac failure
CCU	coronary care unit
CD	controlled drugs
cd	candela
CDH	coronary heart disease, congenital dislocation of hip
CD-R	compact disk recordable
CD-ROM	compact disk read only memory
CD-RW	compact disk re-writable
CEA	carcinoembryonic antigen
CEO	chief executive officer
CF	cystic fibrosis
CFC	chlorofluorohydrocarbons
CFM	cerebral function monitor
CHAI	commission for healthcare audit and inspection – now known as the healthcare commission
CHD	coronary heart disease
CHF	congestive heart failure
$C_6H_6O_2$	hydroquinone
Ci	curie
CIBD	chronic inflammatory bowel disease
CIN	cervical intraepithelial neoplasm
CJD	Creutzfeldt-Jakob disease
CLL	chronic lymphocytic leukaemia
CML	chronic myeloid (granulocytic) leukaemia
CNS	central nervous system
CO (CI)	cardiac output (cardiac index)
COAD	chronic obstructive airways disease
COPD	chronic obstructive pulmonary disease
COSHH	control of substances hazardous to health
CPAP	continuous positive airways pressure
CPB	cardiopulmonary bypass
CPC	choroid plexus cyst
CPD	continuing professional development

CPR	cardiopulmonary resuscitation
CPU	central processing unit
CR	computed radiology/radiography
CRE	cumulative radiation effect
CRF	chronic renal failure
CRL	crown–rump length
CRS	care records service
CRT	cathode ray tube
CSF	cerebrospinal fluid
CSM	Committee on Safety of Medicines
CSRT	craniospinal radiotherapy
CSSD	central sterile supplies department
CSSU	central sterile supply unit
CT	computed tomography
CTG	cardiotocography
CTV	clinical target volume
Cv	critical value
CVA	cerebrovascular accident
CVP	central venous pressure
CVS	chorionic villus sampling
CVVH	continuous veno-venous haemofiltration
CVVHD	continuous veno-venous haemodiafiltration (haemodialysis)
CXR	chest X-ray
D	density
d	distance
D and C	dilatation and curettage
DC	direct current
DCIS	ductal carcinoma in situ
DCR	digitally composite radiographs
D and E	dilatation and evacuation
DDH	developmental dysplasia of the hip
DEL	dose-equivalent limit
Dev	developer
DIC	disseminated intravascular coagulation
DICOM	digital imaging and communications in medicine
DIN	Deutsche Industrie Normen
DM	diabetes mellitus
Dmax	maximum density
DMWL	DICOM modality worklist
DNA	deoxyribonucleic acid
DOA	dead on arrival
DoH	Department of Health
dors	dorsal
DQE	detected quantum efficiency
DRR	digitally reconstructed radiographs
DSH	deliberate self-harm
DVD	digital versatile disk

DVT	deep vein thrombosis
DXRT	deep X-ray therapy
e^-	electron
E	energy or exposure
EBM	evidence-based medicine, expressed breast milk
EBV	Epstein–Barr virus
ECG	electrocardiogram
ECT	electroconvulsive therapy
EDD	expected date of delivery
EDTA	ethylene diamine tetra-acetic acid
EEG	electroencephalogram
EFAs	essential fatty acids
EGF	epidermal growth factor
ELISA	enzyme-linked immunosorbant assay
EMF	electromotive force
EMI	elderly mentally ill
EMRSA	epidemic methicillin-resistant *Staphylococcus aureus*
ENT	ear, nose and throat
EORTC	European Organization for Research on Treatment of Cancer
EOS	ecologically optimized system
EPA	environmental protection act
EPR	electronic patient record
ER	oestrogen receptor
ERCP	endoscopic retrograde cholangio-pancreatography
ERPC	evacuation of retained products of conception
ESCC	epidural spinal cord compression
ESR	erythrocyte sedimentation rate
ETL	echo train length
Eu	europium
EUA	examination under anaesthetic
EV	exposure value
F	farad or field size
f	frequency of radiation
FAP	familial adenomatous polyposis
FAQ	frequently asked question
FAS	fetal alcohol syndrome
FB	foreign body
FDD	focus to diaphragm distance, floppy disk drive
FDDI	fibre distribution data interface
Fe	iron
FEV	forced expiratory volume
FFD	focus–film distance
FHR	fetal heart rate
FL	femur length
FLAIR	fluid attenuation inversion recovery
FMNF	fetal movements not felt

FN	false negative
FNA	fine needle aspiration
FNAC	fine needle aspiration cytology
FOD	focus–object distance
FOI	freedom of information
FOV	field of view
FP	false positive
FID	free induction decay
FSD	focus skin distance
FSH	follicle-stimulating hormone
FVC	forced vital capacity
FW	folder wrapped (film)

$\bar{G}$	average gradient
GBM	glomerular basement membrane
GBS	Guillain–Barré syndrome
Gbytes	gigabytes
Gd	gadolinium
Gd_2O_2S	gadolinium oxysulphide
$Gd_2O_2S.Tb$	gadolinium oxysulphide with terbium activator
GE	gradient echo
GFR	glomerular filtration rate
GH	growth hormone
GHRF	growth hormone releasing factor
GHIF	growth hormone inhibiting factor
GIRSIG	gastrointestinal radiographers special interest group
GIT	gastrointestinal tract
GnRH	gonadotrophin-releasing hormone
GOO	gastric outlet obstruction
GRE	gradient echo
GSL	general sale list medicine
GTT	gestational trophoblastic tumour
GTV	gross tumour volume
GU	gastric ulcer
GUM	genitourinary medicine
Gy	gray

H^+	hydrogen ion
h	Planck's constant
HADS	hospital anxiety and depression scale
HAI	hospital-acquired infection
HBr	hydrogen bromide
HBO	hyperbaric oxygen
HC	head circumference
HCAIs	healthcare-associated infections
HCG	human chorionic gonadotrophin
H & D	Hurter and Driffield (curve in sensitometry)
HDD	hard disk drive
HDR	high dose rate

HDU	high dependency unit
HGH	human growth hormone
HIS	hospital information system
HL	health level
HNPCC	hereditary non-polyposis colorectal cancer
HOCM	hypertrophic obstructive cardiomyopathy
HPC	history of present complaint, Health Professions Council
HPV	human papilloma virus
HR	human resources
HRCT	high-resolution computerized tomography
HRmax	maximum heart rate
HRT	hormone replacement therapy
HSDU	hospital sterilization and disinfection unit
HSE	Health and Safety Executive
HSSU	hospital sterile supply unit
HSV	herpes simplex virus
HU	heat unit
HVT	half-value thickness
Hz	Hertz
I	intensity
IAM	internal auditory meatus
IBD	inflammatory bowel disease
IBS	irritable bowel syndrome
ICP	intracranial pressure
ICSH	interstitial cell stimulating hormone
ICU	intensive care unit
IDDM	insulin dependent diabetes mellitus
Ig	immunoglobulin
IEP	isoelectric point
IF	intensifying factor
IHD	ischaemic heart disease
IHE	integrated health enterprise
IMRT	intensity modulated radiotherapy
in	inch
Io	incident light
IOFB	intraocular foreign body
IOP	intraocular pressure
IORT	intraoperative radiotherapy
IPH	intrapartum haemorrhage
IPPV	intermittent positive pressure ventilation
IR	inversion recovery
IRR	ionizing radiation regulations
ISD	interventricular septal defect
ISO	International Standards Organization
ITU	intensive therapy unit
IUCD	intrauterine contraceptive device
IUD	intrauterine device, intrauterine death

IUGR	intrauterine growth restriction/retardation
IVC	inferior vena cava
IVD	intervertebral disc
IVF	in vitro fertilization
IVU	intravenous urogram

J	joules
JCA	juvenile chronic arthritis
JPEG	joint photographic expert group

K	degrees Kelvin (degrees centigrade + 273)
KBr	potassium bromide
KeV	kiloelectron volt
Kerma	kinetic energy released per unit mass
kg	kilogram
KNO_3	potassium nitrate
K_2SO_3	potassium sulphite
kV	kilovolt
kVp	kilovoltage peak
Kw	equilibrium constant of water

l	litre
λ	decay constant or wavelength
La	lanthanum
LABC	locally advanced breast cancer
LAC	linear attenuation coefficient
LAN	local area network
LAO	left anterior oblique
LaOBr	lanthanum oxybromide
LaOBr.Tb	lanthanum oxybromide with terbium activator
LASER	light amplification by stimulation emission of radiation
LBD	light beam diaphragm
LBP	low back pain
LCD	liquid crystal display
LCIS	lobular carcinoma in situ
LD	lymphocyte depleted
LDH	lactate dehydrogenase
LDR	low dose rate
LED	light-emitting diodes
LET	linear energy transfer
LFT	liver function test
LH	luteinizing hormone
LLL	left lower lobe
LLO	legionella-like organisms
LMP	last menstrual period
LOA	left occipitoanterior
logIt	logarithm of light intensity (intensity $\times$ time)
LP	lymphocyte predominant, lumbar puncture
lp mm^1	line pairs per millimetre

LRTI	lower respiratory tract infection
LUL	left upper lobe
lux	1 lumen per square metre
μ	micron, total linear attenuation coefficient
m	metre
M	mega
mA	milliamps
MABP	mean arterial blood pressure
MAC	mass attenuation coefficient
MALT	mucosa-associated lymphoid tissue
mAs	milliamps per seconds
Mbytes	megabytes
MC	mixed cellularity
MDR1	multiple drug resistance gene
MDR-TB	multidrug-resistant tuberculosis
MENSoR	minority ethnic network of the Society of Radiographers
MFH	malignant fibrous histiocytoma
MHz	megahertz
MI	myocardial infarction, mitral incompetence, mitral insufficiency
MIPS	maximum intensity projections
mol	mole (molecular weight in grams)
MPAP	mean pulmonary artery pressure
MPD	maximum permissible dose
MPNST	malignant peripheral nerve sheath tumour
MPR	multi-planar reconstruction
MR	mitral regurgitation
MRA	magnetic resonance angiography
MRI	magnetic resonance imaging
MRSA	methicillin-resistant *Staphylococcus aureus*
MS	multiple sclerosis
MSI	musculoskeletal injury
MSP	Munchausen syndrome by proxy
MSU	mid-stream urine
MTC	magnetization transfer contrast
MTF	modulation transfer function
MTI	malignant teratoma intermediate
MTT	malignant teratoma trophoblastic
MTU	malignant teratoma undifferentiated
MUGA scan	multigated acquisition scan
MVD	mitral valve disease
Mx	mastectomy
M_z	longitudinal magnetization
n	nano
N	Newton
N_a	absorption efficiency (QDE)

NAD	nothing abnormal detected
NAI	non-accidental injury
NAR	nasal airway resistance
$Na_2S_2O_3$	sodium thiosulphate
Na_2SO_3	sodium sulphite
N_c	conversion efficiency
NCAM	neural cell adhesion molecule
ND	net density
N_e	emission efficiency
NEB	noise equivalent bandwidth
NEQ	noise equivalent quanta
NFS	no fracture seen
NG	new growth
NGU	non-gonococcal urethritis
$(NH_2CH_2COOH)_n$	gelatine
NHL	non-Hodgkin's lymphoma
$(NH_4)_2S_2O_3$	ammonium thiosulphate
NICE	National Institute for Clinical Excellence
NICU	neonatal intensive care unit
NIF	non-interleaved film
NIPPV	non-invasive intermittent positive pressure ventilation
nm	nanometres
NMR	nuclear magnetic resonance
NNU	neonatal unit
NPfIT	national programme for information technology
NPL	National Physical Laboratory
NRDS	neonatal respiratory distress syndrome
NREM	non-rapid eye movement
NRPB	National Radiological Protection Board
NS	nodular sclerosing
NSAIDs	non-steroidal anti-inflammatory drugs
NSCLC	non-small cell lung cancer
NSD	nominal standard dose
NSU	non-specific urethritis
N_t	total efficiency
NVQ	national vocational qualifications
NWB	non-weight-bearing
OA	osteoarthritis
OC	oral contraceptive
OE	on examination
OER	oxygen enhancement ratio
OES	occupational exposure standard
OFD	object to film distance
OH^-	hydroxyl ion
ORIF	open reduction internal fixation
Ortho	orthochromatic
OSI	operating systems interconnect

P	phenidone or phosphor or pascal or pharmacy medicines
^{32}p	radioactive phosphorus
PACS	picture archiving and communication system
PAFC	pulmonary artery flotation catheter
PALS	paediatric advanced life support, patient advice and liaison service
PAS	periodic acid–Schiff
Pb	lead
PBD	peak bone density
PC	personal computer, phase contrast, politically correct
PCI	peripheral component interconnect
PCL	posterior cruciate ligament
PCT	Primary Care Trust
PDA	patent ductus arteriosus
PDD	percentage depth dose
PDGF	platelet derived growth factor
PDR	pulsed dose-rate technique, personal development review
PDT	photodynamic therapy
PE	pulmonary embolism
PET	positron emission tomography, pre eclampsic toxaemia
PFI	private finance initiative
PFO	patent foramen ovale
PgR	progesterone receptor
pH	measure of acidity/alkalinity of a solution
PHT	pulmonary hypertension
PI	pulsativity index
PID	pelvic inflammatory disease, prolapse of an intervertebral disc
PIH	pregnancy-induced hypertension
PLAP	placental alkaline phosphate
PLDR	potentially lethal damage recovery
PMS	patient management system
PNET	primitive neuroectodermal tumour
PNS	post-nasal space
POM	prescription-only medicine
PPH	post-partum haemorrhage
PPNET	peripheral primitive neuroectodermal tumour
PQ	phenidone hydroquinone
PR	per rectum
PRB	pay review body
PRF	pulse repetition frequency
PROM	premature rupture of membranes
P s/n	probability of positive response to noise
P s/s	probability of positive response to signal
PSA	prostate-specific antigen
PTB	pulmonary tuberculosis

PTE	pulmonary thromboembolism
PTRF	post-transplant renal failure
PTV	planning target volume
PUO	pyrexia of unknown origin
PV	per vaginam
PWB	partial weight bearing
Q	hydroquinone or total charge of one sign
QA	quality assurance
QALYs	quality-adjusted life years
QARC	Quality Assurance Review Centre
QCA	Qualifications Curriculum Authority
QCE	quantum conversion efficiency
QDE	quantum detection efficiency
QoL	quality of life
Q/R	query retrive density of a medium
RAS	renal artery stenosis
RAW	Radiography Awareness Week
RB	recurrent bleed
RBBB	right bundle branch block
RBC	red blood cell
RCT	randomized controlled trial
RDS	respiratory distress syndrome
RF	radio frequency
RGB	Red, green, blue (output)
RI	resistivity index
RIDDOR	reporting of injuries, disease and dangerous occurrences regulations
RIP	raised intracranial pressure
RIS	radiology information system
RLL	right lower lobe
ROC	receiver operating characteristics
RPA	radiation protection advisor
RPN	renal papillary necrosis
RPOC	retained products of conception
RPS	radiation protection supervisor
RS	Reed–Sternberg (cells)
RSI	repetitive strain injury
RTA	road traffic accident
RTP	radiation treatment planning
RUL	right upper lobe
S	speed
s	seconds
SAH	subarachnoid haemorrhage
SAM	systolic anterior motion of anterior mitral valve leaflet
SARA	sexually acquired reactive arthritis
SCBU	special care baby unit
SCC	spinal cord compression, squamous cell carcinoma

ScE	scintillation efficiency
SCLC	small-cell lung cancer
SCP	service class provider
SCU	service class user
SD	standard deviation
SDH	subdural haemorrhage/haematoma
SDT	signal detection theory
SE	spin echo, standard error
SI	Système International d'Unités
SIDS	sudden infant death syndrome
SIOP	International Society of Paediatric Oncology
SLD	sublethal damage
SLDR	sublethal damage recovery
SMART	stereotactic multiple arc radiotherapy
SMR	standardized mortality ratio, submucous resection
SNR	signal-to-noise ratio
SOL	space-occupying lesion
SOP	service object pair
SoR	Society of Radiographers
SPECT	single-photon-emission computed tomography
Sr	strontium
SSD	source–skin distance
Sv	sievert
SV	stroke volume
θ	variable field compensation factor
T_3	triiodothyronine
T_4	thyroxine
t	time
T	transmitted (light), tesla
TAR	tissue–air ratio
Tb	terbium
TB	tuberculosis
TBG	thyroid-binding globulin
TBI	total body irradiation
TD	teratoma differentiated
TDF	time, dose and fractionation
TDS	total dissolved solids
TE	echo time
TGF	transforming growth factor
THI	tissue harmonic imaging
TI	inversion time
TIA	transient ischaemic attack
TiO_2	titanium dioxide
TKR	total knee replacement
TLD	thermoluminescent dosimetry
TLS	tumour lysis syndrome
TMJ	temporomandibular joint
TN	true negative

TNF	tumour necrosis factor
TNM	tumour, node (lymph) and metastasis
TOE	transoesophageal echo
TOF	tracheo-oesophageal fistula, time of flight, tetralogy of Fallot
TOP	termination of pregnancy
TP	true positive
TR	repetition time
TRH	thyroid releasing hormone
TRIR	total radiation intensity range
TSH	thyroid-stimulating hormone
TSS	toxic shock syndrome
TUC	trades union council
TURP	transurethral resection of prostate
TVT	tenth-value thickness
TVL	tenth-value layer
Tx	transplant

σ	scattering cross-section
UICC	International Union Against Cancer
Ug	geometric unsharpness
Um	movement unsharpness
Up	photographic unsharpness
URTI	upper respiratory tract infection
Us	screen unsharpness
USB	universal serial bus
Ut	total unsharpness
UTI	urinary tract infection
UV	ultraviolet

v	object speed (velocity)
VDU	visual display unit
VEB	ventricular ectopic beats
VEGF	vascular endothelial growth factor
vent	ventral, above
VIN	vulval intraepithelial neoplasm
VLBW	very low birth weight
VSD	ventricular septal defect

ω	frequency of oscillation
W	watt
WAN	wide area network
WB	weight bearing
WBC	white blood count, white blood cell
WG	Wegener's granuloma
WHA	World Health Assembly
WHO	World Health Organization

| Y | yttrium |
| YST | tissue resembling yolk sac |

| Z | atomic number, acoustic impedance |